Books are to be returned on or before
the last date below.

Vascular Disease

METHODS IN MOLECULAR MEDICINE™

John M. Walker, SERIES EDITOR

METHODS IN MOLECULAR MEDICINE™

Vascular Disease

Molecular Biology and Gene Therapy Protocols

Edited by

Andrew H. Baker

Bristol Heart Institute
University of Bristol, Bristol, UK

Humana Press ※ **Totowa, New Jersey**

© 1999 Humana Press Inc.
999 Riverview Drive, Suite 208
Totowa, New Jersey 07512

This publication is printed on acid-free paper. ∞
ANSI Z39.48-1984 (American Standards Institute) Permanence of Paper for Printed Library Materials.

Cover illustration: Fig. 1 from "In Vitro Detection of Apoptosis in Isolated Vascular Cells," by Shiu-Wan Chan and Martin R. Bennett.

Cover design by Patricia F. Cleary.

For additional copies, pricing for bulk purchases, and/or information about other Humana titles, contact Humana at the above address or at any of the following numbers: Tel: 973-256-1699; Fax: 973-256-8341; E-mail: humana@humanapr.com, or visit our Website at www.humanapress.com

Photocopy Authorization Policy:

Printed in the United States of America. 10 9 8 7 6 5 4 3 2 1

Library of Congress Cataloging in Publication Data

Main entry under title:

Methods in molecular medicine™.
Vascular disease: molecular biology and gene therapy protocols / edited by Andrew H. Baker.
        p.   cm.—(Methods in molecular medicine ; 30)
    Includes bibliographical references and index.
    ISBN 0-89603-731-2 (alk. paper)
    1. Blood-vessels—Diseases—Molecular aspects—Laboratory manuals. 2. Blood-vessels—Diseases—Gene therapy—Laboratory manuals. 3. Blood-vessels—Diseases—Genetic aspects—Laboratory manuals. I. Baker, Andrew H. II. Series.
    [DNLM: 1. Vascular Diseases—genetics. 2. Molecular Biology—methods. WG 500 V33128 1999]
    RC691.4.V36   1999
    616.1'3042—dc21
    DNLM/DLC
    for Library of Congress   98-55168
                                           CIP

Preface

Molecular biology has revolutionized research into vascular disease. Over the past 20 years molecular techniques have enabled us to both elucidate molecular mechanisms in vascular disease and identify appropriate therapies. The vast explosion in technical knowledge and the array of protocols that become more advanced and intricate by the day lead us into new and exciting areas of research that were previously unobtainable.

Vascular Disease: Molecular Biology and Gene Therapy Protocols describes today's most powerful molecular methods for the investigation of the pathogenesis of vascular disease. The protocols are highly detailed, allowing beginners who have little experience in either vascular biology or molecular biology to embark on new molecular projects. This book is also suited to more experienced molecular biologists who wish to grasp new methods for studying the involvement of genes in normal vascular physiology and in diseased states.

It is well established that cardiovascular disease progression has a substantial genetic influence. Part I describes three methods that have been used successfully to identify specific mutations in candidate genes involved in cardiovascular disorders. These mutations include both single-stranded conformational polymorphism analysis and heteroduplex detection methods. In addition, technology to map new genes to specific regions of chromosomes by high-resolution mapping is described.

Identification of new genes and their corresponding full length cDNA species is an absolute requirement to further the understanding of cardiovascular disease progression and, hence, to identify potential new therapies. Part II describes methods to identify novel genes and to generate full-length cDNAs as tools for further experimentation. Such recent techniques as differential display and representative cDNA analysis are detailed. These techniques allow rapid identification of genes expressed differentially by directly comparing two or more mRNAs. Similarly, techniques to subsequently isolate full-length clones of the corresponding genes for functional studies are described.

One of the most important initial experiments to be performed on novel genes is to determine how the gene is expressed in individual vascular cells. Cloning of the promoters of individual genes is critical to this understanding, and Part III details such techniques as gel shift and nuclear run-on analyses to study gene transcription and promoter activity easily and effectively.

In any one cell, there are up to 15,000 genes (of a potential 100,000) that may be expressed. It is therefore critical to determine, first, whether a "gene" is expressed in different cell types important in the vasculature. Second, owing to such local influences as flow, occlusion, lipid deposition, or mechanical injury, it is critical to ascertain accurately the level of expression of the gene within individual cell types in different pathophysiological conditions. Part IV describes detailed protocols for accurate quantification and localization of this expression within vascular cells and tissue, including Northern blotting, RT-PCR, and *in situ* hybridization.

One of the most important observations in cardiovascular disease is the potential role of programmed cell death or apoptosis. Although apoptosis was first described over 20 years ago, it has only been recently, with advances in molecular tools and methods, that the quantification and analysis of apoptosis in cardiovascular disease have been made possible. Methods for the assessment of apoptosis have been used extensively with differing results. Chapters in Part V highlight technical difficulties and describe accurate methods to quantify apoptosis in both cultured cells and pathological specimens.

Parts I–V provide the basis for extensive studies into the identification and molecular characterization of genes involved in cardiovascular disease. Parts VI and VII are dedicated to gene transfer in cardiovascular disease. Gene transfer enables investigators to gage many important features and potential therapeutic applications of key genes. For example, gene transfer leads into the exciting area of gene therapy for cardiovascular disease. Modern advances described here may ultimately lead to clinical gene therapy. In particular, nonviral delivery methods have become substantially more efficient, although, currently, high-level in vivo gene transfer is still provided by viral vectors. The protocols described in Parts VI and VII provide details for transferring genes into different vascular cell types in culture and in vivo. Future studies based on these protocols will provide vital information on the potential of individual genes to reverse or prevent vascular disease progression, with a final aim of providing realistic clinical treatments.

Finally, I would like to acknowledge John M. Walker and Humana Press for this opportunity and my family for their patience during the editorial processing of this book.

Andrew H. Baker

Contents

Contributors

PAUL J. ADAM • *Department of Molecular Physiology and Biological Physics, University of Virginia, Charlottesville, VA*

ANDREW H. BAKER • *Bristol Heart Institute, University of Bristol, Bristol, UK*

MARTIN R. BENNETT • *Department of Medicine, Addenbrooke's Hospital, University of Cambridge, Cambridge, UK*

TODD BOURCIER • *Vascular Medicine and Atherosclerosis Unit, Boston, MA*

LEE D. K. BUTTERY • *Department of Histochemistry, RPMS, London, UK*

MAURIZIO C. CAPOGROSSI • *Laboratory of Vascular Pathology, Rome, Italy*

ANA CENARRO • *Department of Biochemistry and Cellular Molecular Biology, University of Zaragoza, Zaragoza, Spain*

SHIU-WAN CHAN • *Department of Medicine, Addenbrooke's Hospital, University of Cambridge, Cambridge, UK*

DAXIN CHEN • *Department of Immunology, Imperial College School of Medicine, London, UK*

FERNANDO CIVEIRA • *Department of Internal Medicine, Hospital Miguel Servet, Zaragoza, Spain*

DAVID CROSSMAN • *Section of Cardiology, Department of Medicine, Clinical Sciences Centre, Northern General Hospital, Sheffield, UK*

CSILLA CSORTOS • *Department of Medicine, Indiana Univeristy School of Medicine, Indianapolis, IN*

DAVID C. CUMBERLAND • *Cardiovascular Medicine, Clinical Sciences Centre, Northern General Hospital, Sheffield, UK*

THOMAS O. DANIEL • *Department of Cell Biology, Vanderbilt University, Nashville, TN*

CLARE DOLLERY • *The Hatter Institute, Department of Academic and Clinical Cardiology, University College Hospital, London, UK*

ROSALIND P. FABUNMI • *Department of Physiology, University of Texas Southwestern Medical Center, Dallas, TX*

JAMES E. FABER • *Department of Physiology, University of Carolina, Chapel Hill, NC*

SHEILA E. FRANCIS • *Division of Cardiology, Department of Medicine, Clinical Sciences Centre, Northern General Hospital, Sheffield, UK*

MASON W. FREEMAN • *Lipid Metabolism Unit, Massachusetts General Hospital, Boston, MA*

JOACHIM FRUEBIS • *Genset, La Jolla, CA*

GUILIO GABBIANI • *Department of Pathology, University of Geneva, Geneva, Swizterland*

EMILIO GARCIA • *Lawrence Livermore Laboratories, Livermore, CA*

JOE G. N. GARCIA • *Department of Medicine, Indiana Univeristy School of Medicine, Indianapolis, IN*

SARAH J. GEORGE • *Bristol Heart Institute, University of Bristol, Bristol, UK*

JULIAN GUNN • *Section of Cardiology, Department of Medicine, Clinical Sciences Centre, Northern General Hospital, Sheffield, UK*

ADRIANO HENNEY • *Cardiovascular, Musculoskeletal and Metabolism Research Department, Zeneca Pharmaceuticals, Cheshire, UK*

BARBARA HERREN • *The Wolfson Institute for Biomedical Research, University College London, London, UK*

MIKKO O. HILTUNEN • *AI Virtanen Institute, University of Kuopio, Kuopoi, Finland*

KUNIO HIWADA • *Department of Internal Medicine 2, Ehime University School of Medicine, Ehime, Japan*

CATHERINE HOLT • *Section of Cardiology, Department of Medicine, Clinical Sciences Centre, Northern General Hospital, Sheffield, UK*

RACHEL JOHNATTY • *Department of Surgical Sciences, University of Sheffield Medical School, Northern General Hospital, Sheffield, UK*

YASUFUMI KANEDA • *Institute of Molecular and Cellular Biology, Osaka University, Suita, Japan*

MICHEAL-CHRISTOPHER KEOGH • *Department of Biological Chemistry and Molecular Pharmacology, Harvard Medical School, Boston, MA*

YUKATA KITAMI • *Department of Internal Medicine 2, Ehime University School of Medicine, Ehime, Japan*

MARK KOCKX • *Department of Pathology, A Z Middelheim, Antwerp, Belgium*

MICHIEL KNAAPEN • *Department of Pathology, A Z Middelheim, Antwerp, Belgium*

RALF KRAHE • *Deparment of Medical Microbiology and Immunology, Division of Human Cancer Genetics, Ohio State University, Columbus, OH*

DARREN LAMBERT • *Cardiovascular Medicine, Clinical Sciences Centre, Northern General Hospital, Sheffield, UK*

ULLRICH LAUFS • *Klinik III für Innere Medizin, Universität zu Köln, Köln, Germany*

VIRGINIE LAZAR • *Department of Medicine, Indiana University School of Medicine, Indianapolis, IN*

JAMES K. LIAO • *Cardiovascular Division, Brigham and Women's Hospital, Harvard Medical School, Boston, MA*

MARK E. LIEB • *Cardiovascular Institute, Mount Sinai School of Medicine, New York, NY*

TREVOR LITTLEWOOD • *Imperial Cancer Research Fund, London, UK*

CARMEL M. LYNCH • *Targeted Genetics Corporation, Seattle, WA*

JEAN R. MCEWAN • *The Hatter Institute, Department of Academic and Clinical Cardiology, University College Hospital, London, UK*

JAMES MIANO • *Department of Physiology, Cardiovascular Research Centre, Medical College of Wisconsin, Milwaukee, WI*

CHEN MINGYI • *Department of Biosciences, National Cardiovascular Centre Research Institute, Osaka, Japan*

KATHRYN J. MOORE • *Lipid Metabolism Unit, Massachusetts General Hospital, Boston, MA*

JOHANNES MUHRING • *Department of Pathology, A Z Middelheim, Antwerp, Belgium*

PASCAL NEUVILLE • *Department of Pathology, University of Geneva, Geneva, Swizterland*

CHRISTOPHER M. H. NEWMAN • *Division of Cardiology, Department of Medicine, Clinical Sciences Centre, Northern General Hospital, Sheffield UK*

STUART A. NICKLIN • *Bristol Heart Institute, University of Bristol, Bristol, UK*

ANTONINO PASSANITI • *National Institute of Aging (NIH), Gerontology Research Centre, Laboratory of Biological Chemistry,Baltimore, MD*

STELLA PELENGARIS • *Imperial Cancer Research Fund, London, UK*

MIGUEL POCOVI • *Department of Biochemistry and Cellular Molecular Biology, University of Zaragoza, Zaragoza, Spain*

JANET M. POLAK • *Department of Histochemistry, RPMS, London, UK*

JACQUES POUYSSÉGUR • *Centre Biochimie, Université de Nice, Nice, France*

DANIÈLE ROUX • *Centre Biochimie, Université de Nice, Nice, France*

TATSUYA SAWAMURA • *Department of Biosciences, National Cardiovascular Centre Research Institute, Osaka, Japan*

SPIROS SERVOS • *The Wolfson Institute for Biomedical Research, University College London, London, UK*

CATHERINE SHANAHAN • *Department of Medicine, Addenbrooke's Hospital, University of Cambridge, Cambridge, UK*

RONG-FONG SHEN • *Program in Human Genetics and Department of Pediatrics, University of Maryland, Baltimore MD*

KEIKO TAKAHASHI • *Department of Cell Biology, Vanderbilt University, Nashville, TN*

TAKAMUNE TAKAHASHI • *Department of Cell Biology, Vanderbilt University, Nashville, TN*

MARK B. TAUBMAN • *Cardiovascular Institute, Mount Sinai School of Medicine, New York, NY*

CATHERINE F. TOWNSEND • *Division of Cardiology, Department of Medicine, Clinical Sciences Centre, Northern General Hospital, Sheffield, UK*

MIKKO P. TURUNEN • *AI Virtanen Institute, University of Kuopio, Kuopio, Finland*

KERRY TYSON • *Department of Medicine, Addenbrooke's Hospital, University of Cambridge, Cambridge, UK*

SHULI WANG • *Department of Physiology, University of Carolina, Chapel Hill, NC*

NENGYU YANG • *Department of Physiology, University of Carolina, Chapel Hill, NC*

SHU YE • *Wessex Human Genetics Institute, Southampton University School of Medicine, Southampton General Hospital, Southampton, UK*

SEPPO YLÄ-HERTUALLA • *AI Virtanen Institute, University of Kuopio, Kuopoi, Finland*

YOSHIKAZU YONEMITSU • *Ion Transport Unit, National Heart and Lung Institute, Imperial College School of Medicine, London, UK*

IAN ZACHARY • *The Wolfson Institute for Biomedical Research, University College London, London, UK*

I

GENETICS IN VASCULAR DISEASE

1

Detection of Mutations and DNA Polymorphisms in Genes Involved in Cardiovascular Diseases by Polymerase Chain Reaction–Single-Strand Conformation Polymorphism Analysis

Shu Ye and Adriano M. Henney

1. Introduction

Over the last 15 years, there has been remarkably rapid progress in defining the molecular basis of inherited disorders. Many disease genes (the majority of which are genes responsible for monogenic Mendelian diseases) have now been identified, predominately through linkage analysis and positional cloning approaches. With the continuing expansion in this research area, the number of genes to be screened for disease-causing mutations will continue to increase, especially as there are now worldwide efforts aiming to identify the gene lesions that contribute to complex diseases, such as hypertension, diabetes mellitus, and coronary artery diseases, each of which involves many susceptibility genes.

Disease-causing mutations can be broadly classified into two groups: those causing a significant change in chromosome or gene structures (e.g., large deletions, insertions, and rearrangements) and those involving only one or a few nucleotides (e.g., point mutations, and small deletions and insertions) *(1)*. The former group of mutations can be detected using, for example, cytogenetic techniques, pulsed field gel electrophoresis, and Southern blotting. Detection of the latter group of mutations, however, require different methodologies. DNA sequencing will be the ultimate technique for identifying such mutations. However, despite automation, sequencing remains a relatively slow procedure and is not cost-effective. Therefore, a number of different mutation detection techniques have been developed, such as ribonuclease A cleavage analysis and

From: *Methods in Molecular Medicine, vol. 30: Vascular Disease: Molecular Biology and Gene Therapy Protocols*
Edited by: A. H. Baker © Humana Press Inc., Totowa, NJ

chemical cleavage analysis, both of which involve cleavage of heteroduplex molecules at the site of mismatched base pairs resulting from a point mutation; denaturing gradient gel electrophoresis and temperature gradient gel electrophoresis, which assess the differences in the melting point of heteroduplex molecules; and single-strand conformation polymorphism analysis and heteroduplex analysis (*see* Chapter 2), which rely on the differences in gel electrophoretic mobility between wild-type and mutant DNA molecules *(1,2)*.

Of these different techniques, single-strand conformation polymorphism (SSCP) analysis, originally developed by Orita et al. *(3,4)*, is currently the most widely used method for mutation detection. It relies on the fact that, under nondenaturing conditions, single-stranded DNA adopts a folded conformation that is stabilised by intrastrand interactions. Because DNAs with different nucleotide compositions may adopt different conformations, the electrophoretic mobility of a single-stranded DNA fragment in a non-denaturing polyacrylamide gel will depend not only on its size but also on its nucleotide composition. To search for mutations in a given DNA sequence, polymerase chain reaction (PCR) is first carried out using DNA templates from different individuals under study (*see* **Subheading 3.1.**). The PCR products are then denatured to separate the two single strands, and fractionated by nondenaturing polyacrylamide gel electrophoresis (*see* **Subheadings 3.2.** and **3.3.**). Where mutations exist, the PCR products are expected to migrate at different speeds. The different mobility patterns are detected by autoradiography (**Fig. 1**).

2. Materials
2.1. Amplification of Target Sequences by PCR

1. 25–250 ng/mL of genomic DNA.
2. Forward and reverse PCR primers: 20mer oligonucleotides, dissolved in distilled water or TE at a concentration of 1 µg/µL, store at –20°C.
3. 2 mM dNTP mix, store at –20°C.
4. 10 mCi/mL [α-^{32}P] dCTP or [α-^{33}P] dCTP. Caution: follow local rules for handling, storage, and disposal of radioactivity.
5. 10× PCR buffer: 500 mM potassium chloride, 100 mM Tris-HCl, pH 8.3, 0.01% w/v gelatin.
6. 25 mM magnesium chloride.
7. *Taq* DNA polymerase, store at –20°C.
8. Mineral oil.
9. Agarose.
10. 10× TAE buffer: 400 mM Tris-HCl, 10 mM EDTA, adjust to pH 8.0 with glacial acetic acid.
11. 6× sample loading buffer: 15% (w/v) Ficoll-400, 0.05% (w/v) bromophenol blue, 0.05% (w/v) xylene cyanol.

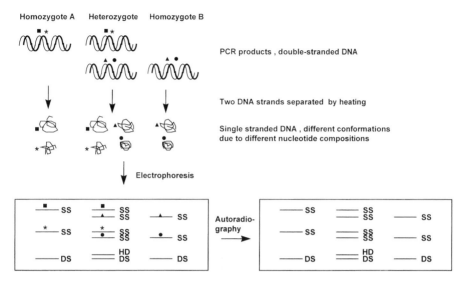

Fig. 1. Single-strand conformation polymorphism (SSCP) analysis. The sequence to be screened for mutations is amplified by PCR using DNA templates from different individuals. The two DNA strands of the PCR products are then separated by heating. Single-stranded DNA molecules with a point mutation (marked ● on the sense strand and ▲ on the antisense strand) have different conformations as compared with single stranded DNA molecules of the wild-type (marked ★ on the sense strand and ■ on the antisense strand). Denatured PCR products are subjected to native polyacrylamide gel electrophoresis. Because of the different conformations, single stranded DNA molecules deriving from the mutant and wild-type have different mobility. The different mobility patterns are detected by autoradiography. SS, single-strand; DS, double-strand; HD, heteroduplex (reannealed double-stranded DNA: one strand from the wild-type and the other from the mutant).

12. Ethidium bromide: dissolved in distilled water to 10 mg/mL. **Caution:** Ethidium bromide is a suspected carcinogen.
13. DNA size marker: e.g., 1 kb ladder (Gibco BRL, Grand Island, NY), store at –20°C.
14. Thermal cycler.
15. Horizontal gel electrophoresis apparatus.
16. UV transilluminator.

2.2. Nondenaturing Polyacrylamide Gel Electrophoresis

1. 49% (w/v) acrylamide stock solution: 49% (w/v) acrylamide and 1% (w/v) bisacrylamide, store at 4°C. **Caution:** unpolymerized acrylamide is a neurotoxin; wear gloves.
2. 10× TBE buffer: 89 mM Tris-borate, 2 mM EDTA, pH 8.3.
3. 20% (w/v) ammonium persulphate: freshly prepared with distilled water.
4. NNN'N'-tetramethylethylenediamine (TEMED).

5. Glycerol.
6. 2% dimethyldichlororosilane. **Caution:** used in fume hood cabinet.
7. 0.1% (w/v) SDS in 10 mM EDTA.
8. 2× formamide loading buffer: 95% formamide, 20 mM EDTA, 0.05% (w/v) bromophenol blue and 0.05% (w/v) xylene cyanol, store at –20°C.
9. Detergent (e.g., Alconox, Alconox plc, New York, NY).
10. Whatman 3MM filter paper.
11. Plastic wrap, e.g., Saran Wrap.
12. X-ray films, e.g., Hyperfilm MP (Amersham, UK).
13. Vertical polyacrylamide gel electrophoresis apparatus with approx 30 cm (width) by 40 cm (length) glass plates, and 0.4 mm (thick) spacers and shark's-tooth comb.
14. Gel dryer.

3. Methods

Preparation of the PCR reactions takes 1–2 h; PCR amplification 2–3 h; preparation of agarose checking gel, sample preparation, loading and running another 2–3 h. All these can be carried out on d 1. In addition, the nondenaturing polyacrylamide gel(s) can be prepared (it takes approx 1 h) during PCR amplification, and run at room temperature overnight. On d 2, more nondenaturing polyacrylamide gel(s) can be prepared, and run at 4°C for several hours.

3.1. Amplification of Target Sequence by PCR (see Notes 1 and 2)

When setting up multiple PCR reactions, prepare a premix containing all reagents listed below (scaled up correspondingly) except template DNA, and dispense 23 μL aliquots into microcentrifuge tubes each containing 2 μL of DNA sample. In parallel with PCR reactions of tested samples, set up the following controls:

    a. PCR negative control: a PCR reaction without template DNA.
    b. SSCP positive control: a PCR reaction with DNA from an individual known to carry a mutation in the target sequence, if available.

1. For each PCR, set up the following 25 μL reaction in a microcentrifuge tube (or a microtiter plate): 2.0 μL template DNA (0.025–0.25 μg/μL), 0.2 μL forward primer (1 μg/μL), 0.2 μL reverse primer (1 μg/μL), 2.5 μL 2 m M dNTP, 0.3 μL [α-^{32}P] dCTP (10 μCi/μL), 2.5 μL 10 × PCR buffer, 1.5 μL 25 mM magnesium chloride (*see* **Note 3**), 0.2 μmL Taq DNA polymerase (5 U/μL) (to be added last), 15.6 μL sterile distilled water.
2. Mix well, and overlay each solution with 30 μL of mineral oil.
3. Place the tubes in a thermal cycler, and program it to perform the following cycling (*see* **Note 1**): Initial step: 94°C for 3 min; 30 cycles of: 94°C for 30 s (denaturation), 55°C for 1 min (annealing), 72°C for 1 min (extension); final step: 72°C for 10 min.
4. Prepare a 1.5% (v/w) agarose gel with 1× TAE buffer and 0.5 μg/mL ethidium bromide.

5. Take a 5-µL aliquot from each PCR reaction, and mix it with 1 µL of 6× sample loading buffer.
6. Load the mixtures, as well as a DNA size marker, onto separate wells in the agarose gel.
7. Run the gel in 1× TAE buffer until the bromophenol blue tracking dye is approx 5 cm away from the wells.
8. Observe the gel on a UV transilluminator.
9. Proceed to nondenaturing polyacrylamide gel electrophoresis (**Subheading 3.3.**) or store PCR products at –20°C.

3.2. Preparation of Nondenaturing Polyacrylamide Gel (see Note 4)

1. Clean two glass plates (first wash thoroughly with detergent and tap water, rinse with distilled water, and dry, then wipe with absolute ethanol).
2. Treat one side of one of the plates with dimethyldichlorosilane (in a fume hood cabinet, pipet approx 5 mL of 2% dimethyldichlorosilane onto the plate surface and spread evenly over the entire surface with a Kimwipe tissue). Leave the plate in the fume hood cabinet until dry.
3. Place the two plates together with the dimethyldichlorsilane-treated surface facing inward. Insert two 0.4-mm-thick spacers, one on each side. Seal the sides and bottom with tape.
4. Prepare a 4.5% nondenaturing acrylamide gel mix (*see* **Note 5**): 9 mL 49% acrylamide stock solution, 10 mL 10× TBE buffer, 91 mL distilled water. Mix well. Add 100 µL of 20% ammonium persulfate and 100 µL TEMED; 5% or 10% glycerol may be added in the gel mix (*see* **Note 6**).
5. With the plate tilted from the horizontal, slowly inject the acrylamide mix into the space between the plates using a 50-mL syringe without forming air bubbles. Insert Shark's-tooth comb with the flat side facing downward, and clipped in place to form a flat surface at the top of the gel.
6. Let the gel set.
7. Between 2 and 24 h after the gel is poured, remove the clips, tape, and comb.
8. Fix the plates in a vertical electrophoresis apparatus.
9. Add 1× TBE buffer to the top and bottom tanks.
10. Using a pipet, flush the flat gel surface with TBE buffer.
11. Reinsert the comb with teeth downward and just in contact with the gel surface.

3.3. Sample Preparation and Electrophoresis

1. Dilute PCR products 5–20 folds (depending on the efficiency of PCR reaction) with 0.1% SDS/10 mM EDTA (omit this step if using ^{33}P instead of ^{32}P in PCR reaction) (*see* **Note 7**).
2. Transfer a 5-µL aliquot of the diluted sample (or undiluted PCR products if using ^{33}P) into a fresh tube containing 5 µL of 2× formamide loading buffer, and mix gently.
3. Heat at 95°C (e.g., on a heating block or a thermal cycler) for 3 min.
4. Snap chill on a ice/water mixture.

5. Load 3 µL of each sample onto the nondenaturing polyacrylamide gel. Also load 3 µL of an undenatured (unheated) sample.
6. Connect the electrophoresis apparatus to a power supply, and carry out electrophoresis at a constant current of 30 mA at 4°C for 3–6 h (for gels without glycerol) or 15 mA at room temperature for 12–16 h (for gels containing glycerol) (*see* **Note 8**).
7. Disconnect power and detach plates from the electrophoresis apparatus.
8. Place the plates on a flat surface and insert a spatula into the space between the two plates and carefully pry them apart.
9. Lay a sheet of Whatman 3MM paper on the gel, press gently, and carefully lift up the 3MM paper to which the gel has adhered.
10. Turn the 3MM paper over and cover the gel with plastic wrap.
11. Dry the gel at 80°C in a gel dryer for 1–2 h.
12. Expose an X-ray film to the gel for several hours to days at room temperature without intensifying screens.

3.4. Data Interpretation

Typically, each DNA fragment deriving from a wild-type or mutant homozygous sample produces three bands, two corresponding to the two different single-stranded DNA molecules and the remainder corresponding to the double-stranded. Usually the fastest migrating band represents the double-stranded DNA, but there are exceptions. Corunning an undenatured sample helps to identify the position of the double-stranded DNA. In some cases, there are more than three bands for each fragment, presumably because a same single-stranded DNA can adopt more than one conformation. Although DNA fragments from wild-type and mutant homozygous samples have the same number of bands, the positions of the bands corresponding to one or both single-stranded molecules differ. A heterozygous sample, in contrast, will have all bands of a wild-type and all bands of a mutant homozygote. In addition, the double-stranded DNA from a heterozygous sample sometimes produces two or three bands, respectively, representing the fast migrating homoduplex band and one or two slowly migrating heteroduplex bands. **Figure 2** shows a typical SSCP autoradiograph.

SSCP analysis can only indicate that there are sequence variations within the DNA fragment being studied. It does not reveal the position and nature of the mutations. To obtain such information, DNA sequencing is required. PCR products used for SSCP analysis can be used as templates in DNA sequencing (*5*). Alternatively, DNA in mutant bands on SSCP gels can be recovered, reamplified by PCR, and used as templates in sequencing analysis (*6,7*).

Fig. 2. Autoradiograph of SSCP analysis. A 433 bp sequence in the stromelysin gene promoter was PCR amplified. The amplicon was cleaved into two fragments, sized 181 bp and 258 bp. respectively, with restriction endonuclease *Eco*RI. The

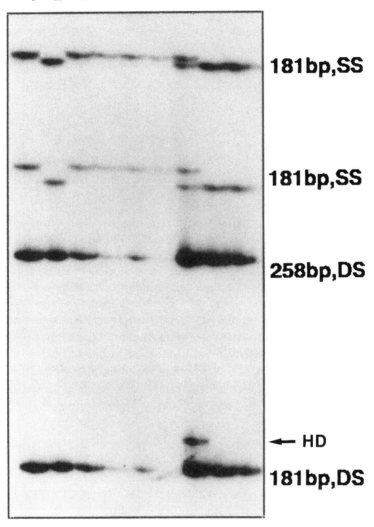

digests were denatured and then subjected to nondenaturing polyacrylamide gel electrophoresis. Shown in the figure are the two single-strands (SS) and double-strand (DS) of the 181 bp fragment, and the DS of the 258 bp fragment. Both SSs of the 181 bp fragment in lanes 1, 3, 4, 5, and 6 migrate more slowly than those in lanes 2, 8, and 9. Both fast and slowly migrating bands of the two SSs of the 181 bp are present in lane 7. Also seen in lane 7 is an extra band immediately above the DS of the 181 bp fragment, which represents the formation of heteroduplex (HD). DNA sequencing has revealed that the variation in mobility of single-stranded DNA is due to a single nucleotide difference. Samples 1, 3, 4, 5, and 6 are wild-type homozygotes, samples 2, 8, and 9 are mutant homozygotes, and sample 7 is a heterozygote.

4. Notes

1. The fidelity and efficiency of PCR reactions are affected by a number of factors, such as the amount of template DNA, the amount and melting temperature (*Tm*) of the primers, Mg^{2+} concentration, annealing temperature, and cycling number. *(8)*. PCR conditions should therefore be optimised individually for each set of primers, and the conditions described in **Subheading 3.1.** can be used as a starting point for optimization. Because nonspecific bands complicate the interpretation of SSCP results, it is worth making the efforts to optimize the PCR conditions so that there are only minimal spurious products (ideally there should be only a single major band on an agarose checking gel).
2. The ability to detect mutations decreases with increasing fragment length. Estimated sensitivity approx 90% for 100–300 bp fragments, but drops significantly for fragments over 300 bases (67% for 300–450 bp fragments) *(9–12)*. Therefore, DNA fragments between 100 and 300 bases are used. If the PCR amplicon is too long, it can be cleaved into smaller fragments with suitable restriction endonucleases prior to denaturation and polyacrylamide gel electrophoresis *(13)*.
3. If there are significant nonspecific bands, reduce the Mg^{2+} concentration and/or the number of amplification cycles, and/or increase the annealing temperature. If, on the other hand, the expected PCR product cannot be seen, increase the Mg^{2+} concentration and/or number of amplification cycles, and/or reduce the annealing temperature. In some difficult situations, "hot start" or "touch down" PCR might be preferable.
4. SSCP analysis can also be carried out using smaller polyacrylamide gels, although the sensitivity is likely to decrease. It has been reported that mutations can be detected using 9% mini-gels (0.75 mm × 6 cm × 8 cm) *(14,15)*. In addition to autoradiography, other methods, such as silver staining *(6,15)*, ethidium bromide staining *(16)*, and fluorescence labeling *(17–19)*, have been applied successfully to detect DNA bands in SSCP analysis.
5. The ratio of acrylamide to bisacrylamide determines the percentage of crosslinking. A ratio of 49:1 is commonly used for SSCP.
6. In some cases, the addition of 5% or 10% glycerol in the gel increases mobility shift *(3)*. Gels containing glycerol tend to produce somewhat diffused bands.
7. A total of 40 samples (including tested samples, and positive and negative controls) can be loaded onto a 30-cm-wide gel, and two or even more gels can be run at once. Therefore, 70 samples can be analyzed within two days, although autoradiographs may not be ready for another day or two, depending on the strength of signals.
8. Some mutations are detected more readily at room temperature, others at 4°C *(20)*. Therefore, usually each DNA fragment is analyzed on at least two different conditions. A useful combination is a glycerol containing gel run at room temperature and a gel without glycerol run at 4°C *(3,4)*.

References

1. Spanakis, E., and Day, I. N. M. (1997) The molecular basis of genetic variation: mutation detection methodologies and limitations, in *Genetics of Common Diseases* (Day, I. N. M. and Humphries, S. E., eds.), BIOS Scientific Publishers, Oxford, pp. 33–74.
2. Cooper, D. N. and Krawczak, M. (1993) *Human Gene Mutation*, BIOS ScientificPublishers, Oxford.
3. Orita, M., Iwahana, H., Kanazawa, H., Hayashi, K., and Sekiya, T. (1989) Detection of polymorphisms of human DNA by gel electrophoresis as single-strand conformation polymorphisms. *Proc. Natl. Acad. Sci. USA* **86,** 2766–2770.
4. Orita, M., Suzuki, Y., Sekiya, T., and Hayashi, K. (1989) Rapid and sensitive detection of point mutations and DNA polymorphisms using the polymerase chain reaction. *Genomics* **5,** 874–879.
5. Demers, D. B., Odelberg, S. J., and Fisher, L. M. (1991) Identificatiion of a factor IX point mutation using SSCP analysis and direct sequencing. *Nucleic Acids Res.* **18,** 5575.
6. Calvert, R. J. (1995) PCR amplification of silver-stained SSCP bands from cold SSCP gels. *Biotechniques* **18,** 782–784.
7. Suzuki, Y., Sekiya, T., and Hayashi, K. (1991). Allele-specific PCR: A method for amplification and sequence determination of a single component among a mixture of sequence variants. *Anal. Biochem.* **192,** 82–85.
8. Erlich, H. A. (1989) *PCR Technology. Principles and Applications for DNA Amplification,* Stockton Press, New York.
9. Hayashi, K. (1991) PCR-SSCP: a simple and sensitive method for detection of mutations in the genomic DNA. *PCR Methods Appl.* **1,** 34–38.
10. Hayashi, K. and Yandell, D. W. (1993) How sensitive is PCR-SSCP? *Hum. Mutat.* **2,** 338–346.
11. Sheffield, V. C., Beck, J. S., Kwitek, A. E., Sandstrom, D. W., and Stone, E. M. (1993) The sensitivity of single-strand conformation polymorphism analysis for the detection of single base substitutions. *Genomics* **16,** 325–332.
12. Liu, Q., Feng, J., and Sommer, S. S. (1996) Bi-directional dideoxy fingerprinting (Bi-ddF): a rapid method for quantitative detection of mutations in genomic regions of 300–600bp. *Hum. Mol. Genet.* **5,** 107–114.
13. Liu, Q. and Sommer, S. S. (1995) Restriction endonuclease fingerprinting (REF): a sensitive method for screening mutations in long, contiguous segment of DNA. *Biotechniques* **18,** 470–477.
14. Ainsworth, P. J., Surh, L. C., and Coulter-Mackie, M. B. (1991) Diagnostic single strand conformational polymorphism (SSCP): a simplified non-radioisotopic method as applied to a Tay-Sachs B1 variant. *Nucleic Acids Res.* **19,** 405.
15. Oto, M., Miyake, S., and Yuasa, Y. (1993) Optimization of nonradioisotopic single strand conformation polymorphism analysis with a conventional minislab gel electrophoresis apparatus. *Anal. Biochem.* **213,** 19–22.

16. Hongyo, T., Buzard, G. S., Calvert, R. J., and Weghorst, C. M. (1993) 'Cold SSCP': a simple, rapid and non-radioactive method for optimized single-strand conformation polymorphism analyses. *Nucleic Acids Res.* **21**, 3637–3642.
17. Makino, R., Yazyu, H, Kishimoto, Y., Sekiya, T., and Hayashi, K. (1992) F-SSCP: A fluorescent polymerase chain reaction-single strand conformation polymorphism (PCR-SSCP) analysis. *PCR Methods Appl.* **2**, 10–13.
18. Takahashi-Fujii, A., Ishino, Y., Shimada, A., and Kato, I. (1993) Practical application of fluorescence-based image analyzer for PCR single-stranded conformation polymorphism analysis used in detection of multiple point mutations. *PCR Methods Appl.* **2**, 323–327.
19. Iwahana, H., Yoshimoto, K., Mizusawa, N., Kudo, E., ans Itakura, M. (1994) Multiple fluorescence-based PCR-SSCP analysis. *Biotechniques* **16**, 296–305.
20. Glavac, D. and Dean, M. (1993) Optimization of the single-strand conformation polymorphism (SSCP) technique for detection of point mutations. *Hum. Mutat.* **2**, 404–414.

2

Analysis of Genetic Variants in Cardiovascular Risk Genes by Heteroduplex Analysis

Ana Cenarro, Fernando Civeira, and Miguel Pocovi

1. Introduction

As an increasing number of human diseases are linked to the effects of altered genes, new methods are being sought for detection of mutations and their relationship to the presence of disease. Since total genomic DNA usually cannot be analyzed directly, target sequences are amplified by the polymerase chain reaction (PCR). Several methods have been reported that allow detection of small changes in DNA sequence *(1)*. Among them, one of the most commonly used is the heteroduplex analysis method (HA) *(2–5)*.

HA is a screening method based on the different conformation of DNA molecules containing a mismatch in their double strands. This different DNA conformation of homoduplexes and heteroduplexes can be detected by electrophoresis on a nondenaturing polyacrylamide gel. To create heteroduplexes, the genomic DNA from a heterozygous subject is amplified by PCR, heated to denature, and allowed to reanneal at a lower temperature. This reannealing permits the formation of four different products: two homoduplexes (normal double strand, mutant double strand) and two heteroduplexes (normal sense/mutant antisense, and normal antisense/mutant sense). When separated on a nondenaturing polyacrylamide gel electrophoresis, heteroduplexes migrate through the gel at a different rate than homoduplexes, because the region of mismatch forms a "bubble" in the DNA. Therefore, heteroduplex strands frequently appear on the gel as a distinct band, separated from the corresponding homoduplexes, as their mobility is different. There are several detection methods for heteroduplex strands after electrophoresis, but ethidium bromide staining or fluorescence, combined with an automated DNA sequencer, are, in our experience, the best choices.

From: *Methods in Molecular Medicine, vol. 30: Vascular Disease: Molecular Biology and Gene Therapy Protocols*
Edited by: A. H. Baker © Humana Press Inc., Totowa, NJ

In order to decide which method of mutation detection is better to use, it can help to know the different advantages and disadvantages of each method *(6)*. The main advantages of the HA method are:

1. Simplicity. HA and single-strand conformation polymorphism (SSCP, *see* Chapter 1) are the simplest methods currently used for mutation detection.
2. Few requirements. No special equipment is required, only the usual for conventional electrophoresis. For this reason HA is not expensive.
3. HA does not require radioactive material.
4. Assay conditions do not have to be determined for each PCR fragment.
5. HA can be performed in combination with SSCP, because the same PCR fragments can be studied for SSCP or doubled-stranded (HA) on the same gel *(7,8)*.
6. HA allows separation of the mutant DNA from the wild-type, and therefore it permits isolation for further studies.

The disadvantages of this method are the following:

1. HA does not localize the exact position of the mutation in the DNA fragment nor the type of the mutation.
2. Although HA sensitivity for mutation detection has not been clearly established, it is probably about 80%. For this reason it has been suggested to be used in combination with another technique such as SSCP to improve the mutation detection.
3. The HA method can only be applied to fragments that are relatively short, less than 500 bp. The optimal size range for detecting mutations is between 200 and 450 bp (*see* **Note 1**).
4. Homozygosity cannot be detected by HA, but, when suspected, wild-type DNA can be added to the DNA analyzed, to generate "artificial" heteroduplexes by a denaturation–renaturation step.

The HA protocol can be modified to give a more sensitive method known as conformation sensitive gel electrophoresis (CSGE), which uses partially denaturing polyacrylamide gels *(9)*. The differences in mobility of homoduplexes and heteroduplexes are increased and therefore, the sensitivity of mutation detection is improved with respect to HA.

CSGE is based in the concept that mildly denaturing solvents can produce DNA conformational changes at different concentrations, when their concentration is not enough to promote complete DNA denaturation *(10)*. CSGE takes advantage of the fact that mildly denaturing gels promote rotation of one mismatched base out of the double helix to produce a "bend" in the helix and a greater difference in the electrophoretic mobility than the "bubble" obtained by the nondenaturing gel used in HA. CSGE has proved to be highly sensitive (approx 90%) in the detection of mutation in DNA fragments below 800 bp *(9,11)*. Some recent modifications in CSGE technique seem to improve sensitivity to 100% *(12,13)*.

In this chapter, we describe how the combination of PCR and HA can be used as a rapid and simple detection of point mutations in genomic DNA, by means of manual or automated DNA sequencer. Main modifications to the HA protocol to carry out CSGE are also described.

2. Materials

All solutions should be made to the standard required for molecular biology. Use molecular biology grade reagents and sterile distilled water.

2.1. PCR Reaction for Heteroduplex Analysis

1. Oligonucleotide primers (with fluorescent label attached in 5' position if automated sequencer is used): Appropriate primers for PCR were synthesized on a DNA synthesizer (Pharmacia Biotech, Uppsala, Sweden). For PCR, 10 μM stock solutions are used. The design of these primers is critical to the success of the PCR reaction (*see* **Note 2**).
2. Genomic DNA: The concentration of DNA is determined spectrophotometrically. Store as a 0.1 μg/μL stock at –20°C.
3. Standard PCR 50 μL reaction mixture: This contains 200 μM of each dNTP, 10 pmol of each primer, 20 mM Tris-HCl, pH 8.4, 1.5 mM $MgCl_2$, 50 mM KCl, and 1.25 U *Taq* DNA polymerase. *Taq* DNA polymerases from different suppliers have been used successfully.
4. Mineral oil.
5. Thermocycler apparatus.

2.2. Basic Procedure for Heteroduplex Analysis

1. Heteroduplex apparatus: A conventional vertical gel electrophoresis apparatus for sequencing or an automated DNA sequencer with the appropriate software for fragment analysis are required (*see* **Note 3**).
2. Power supply capable of reading 1200 V or more.
3. Mutation Detection Enhancement (MDE™) gel solution 2X concentrate (FMC Bioproducts, Rockland, ME). This is a polyacrylamide-like matrix that has a high sensitivity to DNA conformational differences (*see* **Notes 4** and **5**).
4. 10% ammonium persulfate.
5. N,N,N',N'-tetramethylethylenediamine (TEMED).
6. 10X TBE buffer: 0.89 *M* Tris-HCl, 0.89 *M* boric acid, and 20 m*M* EDTA, pH 8.0. For electrophoresis dilute 16.6-fold.
7. Electrophoresis buffer: 0.6X TBE.
8. Gel solution for one standard heteroduplex analysis: Prepare the volume of gel-forming solution appropriate for the corresponding apparatus. For a total volume of 100 mL: Add 50 mL of MDE™ gel to 44 mL of distilled water and 6 mL of 10X TBE buffer. Initiate the polymerization with 40 μL of TEMED and 400 μL of 10% ammonium persulfate (*see* **Note 6**).
9. Ethidium bromide: 1 mg/mL (*see* **Note 7**).

10. 10X loading buffer: For manual heteroduplex: 25% Ficoll 400, 0.25% orange G, 0.25% bromophenol blue, and 0.25% xylene cyanol. For automated heteroduplex: 25% Ficoll 400, and 0.5% blue dextran.
11. Thermostating bath at 95°C.
12. Thermostating bath at 37°C.
13. Computer and software for secondary editing and interpretation of the data (if automated sequencer is used).

2.3. Basic Procedure for Conformation Sensitive Gel Electrophoresis

The equipment and materials utilized are very similar to that used for manual heteroduplex, with the exception of the composition of the gel and the electrophoresis buffer, prepared as follows:

1. 5X TTE buffer: 0.44 M Tris-HCl, 0.145 M taurine, and 1 mM EDTA, pH 9.0. For electrophoresis dilute 10-fold.
2. Electrophoresis buffer: 0.5X TTE.
3. Polyacrylamide gel stock: A 25% polyacrylamide gel with a 99:1 ratio of acrylamide to 1,4-bis(acryloyl)piperazine.
4. Gel solution for one standard conformation sensitive gel: Prepare the volume of gel forming solution appropriate for the corresponding apparatus. For a total volume of 100 mL: Add 60 mL of the 25% polyacrylamide gel stock (99:1) to 4 mL of distilled water, 10 mL of 5X TTE buffer, 10 mL of ethylene glycol and 15 mL of formamide (*see* **Note 8**). Start the polymerization with 70 µL of TEMED and 1 mL of 10% ammonium persulfate.

3. Methods

3.1. PCR Reaction for Heteroduplex Analysis

It is critical to use PCR conditions that minimize unwanted side products, as these can result in artifacts that interfere with the identification of heteroduplex bands. It is difficult to define a single set of conditions that ensure optimal specific PCR amplification of the DNA target sequence. Conditions for amplification will depend on the particular PCR primers and will need to be established empirically. For optimization of the PCR conditions refer to **Notes 2** and **9**. Here we describe a basic protocol that has been successful for us in most cases.

1. Prepare the PCR reaction as follows: To a 0.5 mL Eppendorf tube add 5 µL of 10X PCR buffer, 5 µL of template DNA, and 33 µL of distilled water, for a total volume of 50 µL. Overlay the mixed reaction with 1–2 drops of mineral oil to prevent evaporation.
2. Transfer the tube to a thermocycler and heat at 95°C for 10 min. "Hot start" the reaction by the addition of the rest of the reagents, previously mixed in a master mix for all the samples: 1 µL of each primer, 5 µL of dNTP mix (2 mM), and 0.25 µL of *Taq* DNA polymerase (5 U/µL).

3. Perform 30 cycles of PCR using the following temperature profile: 95°C (denaturation) for 1 min, 55–60°C (primer annealing) for 1 min, 72°C (primer extension) for 1 min 30 s, and finally an additional step of 72°C for 10 min, to ensure that primer extension is completed.
4. Add 0.5 µL of loading buffer to 5 µL of PCR product and electrophorese on a 2% agarose gel to determine the yield and specificity of the PCR reaction.
5. If unspecific bands are also obtained, the PCR reaction should be run on a 2% low-melting-point agarose gel and the band of interest excised with a scalped blade. The resulting gel slices may be purified in different ways (*see* **Note 10**).

3.2. Basic Procedure for Heteroduplex Analysis

3.2.1. Manual Heteroduplex Analysis

We recommend adapting a DNA sequencing gel apparatus for use with 1.0-mm spacers and well-forming combs.

1. The glass plates should be clean and free of soap residue. To ensure this, spread some ethanol over the plate surface, and wipe dry with a paper towel.
2. Assemble the glass plates. Grease the spacers and position them on a glass plate. Clamp the sides and bottom of the plates to form a seal, as for a DNA sequencing gel.
3. Prepare the volume of gel solution appropriate for your apparatus (*see* **Subheading 2.2., step 8**). Place the reagents indicated into a beaker and mix gently by swirling.
4. Pour the gel solution into a syringe and carefully inject it at the lowered edge of the glass plates. Add slowly to avoid air bubbles.
5. Insert the well-forming comb, and lay the plates flat on the bench top for polymerization.
6. Allow the gel to polymerize for 60 min at room temperature before use.
7. Remove the comb and rinse each well with 0.6X TBE buffer.
8. Mount the gel casette on the electrophoresis apparatus and prepare sufficient 0.6X TBE to fill both the upper and the lower buffer chambers. Pre-electrophorese for 15 min at 800 V.
9. After the PCR reaction is finished, heat the reaction mixture at 95°C for 4 min, and slowly cool it to 37°C for 30 min (*see* **Note 11**).
10. Add 1 µL loading buffer for each 10 µL of sample and mix well by pipeting (*see* **Note 12**).
11. Rinse the wells with 0.6X TBE buffer and load the samples carefully.
12. Electrophorese at a maximum constant voltage of 20 V/cm of gel. For example, the maximum voltage for a 40 cm gel is 800 V.
13. The run time is directly proportional to PCR fragment size. On the first electrophoresis run, use the xylene cyanol dye as a marker to determine the run time for 30 cm of migration, which is the minimum distance recommended to ensure an optimal separation of heteroduplex and homoduplex bands.
14. The temperature of the gel should be controlled during the electrophoresis, and if it exceeds 40°C, a water-jacketed gel plate should be used (*see* **Note 13**).

15. After the run is finished, remove the gel cassette and separate the glass plates. Leave the gel adhered to one glass plate to facilitate handling during the staining and destaining.
16. Stain for 10–15 min in a solution of 0.6X TBE containing 1 µg/mL ethidium bromide. Destain for 5–10 min in 0.6X TBE to eliminate the background. Sometimes it is necessary to destain for longer times in order to detect faint bands (*see* **Note 14**).
17. To visualize the DNA fragments, invert the plate over a UV transilluminator. Remove the gel in the area of interest by cutting it for easier handling.

Figure 1 shows the results using the manual heteroduplex analysis to screen a 330 bp DNA fragment of the apo AI gene. Slower bands correspond to heteroduplex generated by a mutation in the apo AI gene that has been associated with familial hypoalphalipoproteinemia *(14)*.

3.2.2. Automated Heteroduplex Analysis

For this technique, an automated DNA sequencer is used. We have successfully used the ALFexpress™ DNA sequencer (Pharmacia Biotech) with the appropriate software to identify the DNA fragments with laser signals, but other automated DNA sequencers can be used. The advantage of this method is that small amounts of the PCR reaction can be detected when fluorescent primers are used. The laser detection gives narrow peaks (instead of broad bands as with ethidium bromide staining) corresponding to heteroduplex and homoduplex DNA fragments. The sensitivity of this method is higher compared to manual HA, as even a faint heteroduplex band is detected by the laser as a clear peak *(15)*.

1. Assemble the glass plates and proceed as **Subheading 3.2.1., steps 1–8**, except that you should not grease the spacers.
2. After the PCR reaction is finished, heat the reaction mixture at 95°C for 4 min, and slowly cool it to 37°C for 30 min.
3. Add 2 µL loading buffer for automated sequencer to 1 µL of PCR sample and mix well by pipeting.
4. Rinse the wells with 0.6X TBE buffer and load the samples carefully.
5. Run electrophoresis at a maximum constant voltage of 20 V/cm of gel.
6. The temperature of the gel should be controlled during the electrophoresis, and if it exceeds 40°C, a water-jacketed gel plate should be used. We usually perform the electrophoresis setting the bath at 25°C, to ensure a constant temperature during the run.
7. After the run is finished, analyze the peaks obtained with the appropriate software.

Figure 2 shows the results using the automated heteroduplex analysis to screen the exon 3 (A) and exon 11 (B) of the LDL receptor gene. The lower part in each case corresponds to a heterozygous subject for a mutation in this gene causing familial hypercholesterolemia.

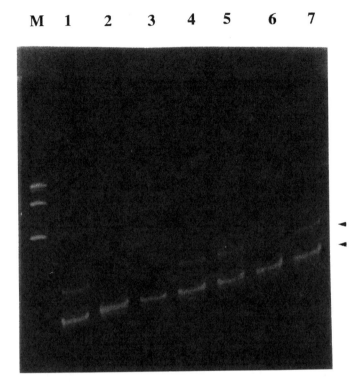

Fig. 1. PCR amplified fragments of apo AI gene subjected to manual heteroduplex analysis. **Lanes 1, 4, 5,** and **7** correspond to heterozygous subjects for a mutation in exon 4 of the apo AI gene. **Lanes 2, 3,** and **6** correspond to control subjects. M: ØX174-*Hae*III DNA size markers.

3.2.3. Conformation Sensitive Gel Electrophoresis (CSGE)

The method to carry out a CSGE is basically the same as a manual heteroduplex analysis with the differences indicated (*see* **Subheading 2.3.**).

Also, the gel must be pre-electrophoresed for 15 min at 45 W. The heteroduplexes are generated in the same way, by denaturation followed of renaturation at low temperature. After loading the samples, the gel is run for 9 h at 40 W.

4. Notes

1. If PCR fragments longer than 500 bp have to be analyzed, we recommend digesting them with the appropriate restriction enzyme to obtain the optimal fragment size.
2. The first step in designing a PCR reaction is the selection of the appropriate pair of primers. Some considerations that should be taken into account are the following:

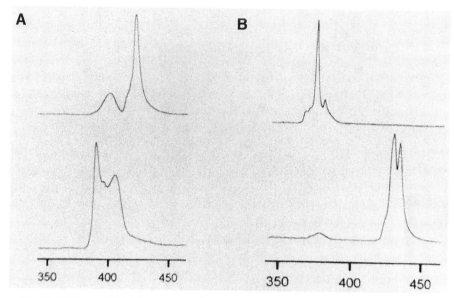

Fig. 2. PCR amplified fragments of exon 3 (**A**) and exon 11 (**B**) of the LDL receptor gene subjected to automated heteroduplex analysis. In both cases, the upper part corresponds to a control subject and lower part corresponds to a heterozygous subject for a mutation in the LDL receptor gene. Numbers below represent the time (in minutes) at which the laser detected the fluorescent DNA signal.

    a. Primers of 20–24 bp are long enough to produce specific amplification of the wanted region.
    b. Avoid primers that anneal in a repetitive or Alu sequence.
    c. Use primers with no mismatches in the target sequence, especially at the 3' ends.
    d. If it is possible, keep the GC to AT ratio of 50%, and try to avoid long stretches of the same base.
    e. Check that both primers are not complementary to each other, especially at the 3' ends, to avoid the "primer dimer" formation.
    f. To estimate the annealing temperature, we find very useful the following formula: $T(°C) = 4x (G + C) + 2x (A + T) -5$, being $G + C$ the content in G and C bases, and $A + T$, the content in A and T bases. Aim for a similar temperature for both primers.

3. Although HA can be performed in short gels, a long electrophoresis system may be necessary to resolve small mobility differences. Therefore, to avoid false-negative results, long track length is advisable.

4. The unpolymerized MDE™ gel solution is neurotoxic. Wear gloves when handling it.

5. It is also possible to use standard polyacrylamide gels, but we recommend the use of MDE™ gel, as the probability of detecting sequence differences is increased from 15% to approx 80% by using it.

6. Optionally, you can add 15 g of urea to the standard gel solution (15%). This helps to eliminate "doublets" that may form in some homoduplex negative controls and to minimize band broadening.
7. Ethidium bromide is mutagenic. Wear gloves when handling.
8. The recommended concentration of formamide for CSGE is 15%, but this could be optimized empirically, as different concentrations of formamide can improve separation between homoduplex and heteroduplex bands in each case.
9. Some considerations to take into account when designing a PCR reaction are the following:
   a. Mutations located within 50 bp of the ends of the PCR fragment produce minor changes in conformation that can be refractory to detection by heteroduplex. To avoid this inconvenience we recommend to amplify PCR products with some overlapping or to design primers 40–50 bp away of the target DNA.
   b. Use only highly purified, salt-free DNA.
   c. Optimize reagent and primer concentrations (0.2–1 mM) for each amplification reaction.
   d. Determine thermal cycle settings which eliminate nonspecific priming, especially the annealing temperature (as indicated in **Note 2f**). Use the minimum number of PCR cycles to obtain a sufficient quantity of DNA, usually 30 cycles or fewer.
   e. Improvements in specificity may also be achieved by varying the Mg^{2+} concentration, over the range 1–4 mM final concentration.
10. The following protocol for PCR purification from low melting point agarose has been successfully employed in our laboratory, but other methods are also effective:
    a. Excise the agarose gel fragments containing the DNA with a blade. Minimize exposure to UV radiation to avoid DNA damage. Place each gel slice into an Eppendorf tube.
    b. Melt gel slices at 67°C for 10 min. Determine the volume of liquid agarose.
    c. Add 4 vol of TE buffer (20 mM Tris-HCl, 1 mM EDTA, pH 8.0) warmed to 67°C. Mix and maintain the samples at 67°C until phenol extraction.
    d. All subsequent steps are carried out at room temperature. Mix the diluted agarose with an equal volume of phenol saturated with TE buffer. Mix and centrifuge at 12,000g for 10 min. Transfer the top aqueous phase to a clean Eppendorf tube. Reextract with phenol/chloroform and then with chloroform alone as described above.
    e. Add 1/10 vol 3 M potassium acetate and 2.5 vol of 100% ethanol to the aqueous phase. Leave at –20°C for 20 min, and centrifuge at 12,000g for 15 min. Remove the supernatant and wash pellet with 200 µL of 70% ethanol. Dry the pellet and resuspend in the desired volume of TE or distilled water.
11. Heteroduplex DNA is generated during the PCR amplification by the annealing of complementary strands with some sequence difference *(16)*. However, to obtain the maximum yield of heteroduplex DNA, we recommend denaturing at 95°C and renaturing at 37°C after the PCR reaction is finished. It is important to cool slowly after denaturation, because it can result in nonspecific reannealing.

This step is also important when no wild-type copy of the target is present in the sample analyzed, as it can be added exogeneously to generate the heteroduplexes.

12. Approximately 5–10% of the total PCR volume should be loaded per lane in the manual heteroduplex. Loading too much sample onto the gel results in a failure to see heteroduplex bands, as heteroduplex and homoduplex bands merge.

13. It is important to ensure a homogeneous temperature distribution during the gel electrophoresis. If this does not exceed 40°C and a water-jacketed gel plate is not available, an aluminium plate attached to the glass plate with the gel can be used for this purpose.

14. The heteroduplex DNA staining is about 25% as intense as the homoduplex DNA. For this reason, when using ethidium bromide staining, heteroduplex bands are visualized as faint bands, even if sufficient DNA has been loaded on the gel.

References

1. Cotton, R. G. H. (1993) Current methods of mutation detection. *Mutat. Res.* **285,** 125–144.
2. Keen, J., Lester, D., Inglehearn, C., Curtis, A., and Bhattacharya S. (1991) Rapid detection of single base mismatches as heteroduplexes on HydroLink gels. *Trends Genet.* **7,** 5.
3. Perry, D. J. and Carrell, R. W. (1992) HydroLink gels: A rapid and simple approach to the detection of DNA mutations in thromboembolic disease. *J. Clin. Pathol.* **45,** 158–160.
4. White, M. B., Carvalho, M., Derse, D., O'Brien, S. J., and Dean, M. (1992) Detecting single base substitutions as heteroduplex polymorphisms. *Genomics* **12,** 301–306.
5. Glavac, D. and Dean, M. (1995) Applications of heteroduplex analysis for mutation detection in disease genes. *Hum. Mutat.* **6,** 281–287.
6. Mashal, R. D. and Sklar, J. (1996) Practical methods of mutation detection. *Curr. Opin. Genet. Develop.* **6,** 275–280.
7. Cenarro, A., Jensen, H. K., Casao, E., Civeira, F., González-Bonillo, J., Pocoví, M., and Gregersen, N. (1996) Identification of a novel mutation in exon 13 of the LDL receptor gene causing familial hypercholesterolemia in two Spanish families. *Biochim. Biophys. Acta* **1316,** 1–4.
8. Soto, D. and Sukumar, S. (1992) Improved detection of mutations in the p53 gene in human tumors as single-stranded conformation polymorphisms and double-stranded heteroduplex DNA. *PCR Meth. Appl.* **2,** 96–98.
9. Ganguly, A., Rock, M. J., and Prockop, D. J. (1993) Conformation-sensitive gel electrophoresis for rapid detection of single-base differences in double-stranded PCR products and DNA fragments: Evidence for solvent-induced bends in DNA heteroduplexes. *Proc. Natl. Acad. Sci. USA* **90,** 10,325–10,329.
10. Bhattacharya, A. and Lilley, D. M. (1989) The contrasting structures of mismatched DNA sequences containing looped-out bases (bulges) and multiple mismatches (bubbles). *Nucleic Acids Res.* **17,** 6821–6840.

11. Williams, C. J., Rock, M., Considine, E., McCarron, S., Gow, P., Ladda, R., et al. (1995) Three new point mutations in type II procollagen (COL2A1) and identification of a fourth family with the COL2A1 Arg519->Cys base substitution using conformation sensitive gel electrophoresis. *Hum. Mol. Genet.* **4,** 309–312.

12. Körkko, J., Annunen, S., Puilajamaa, T., Prockop, D. J., and Ala-Kokko, L. (1998) Conformation sensitive gel electrophoresis for simple and accurate detection of mutations: Comparison with denaturing gradient gel electrophoresis and nucleotide sequencing. *Proc. Natl. Acad. Sci. USA* **95,** 1681–1685.

13. Williams, I. J., Abuzenadah, A., Winship, P. R., Preston, F. E., Dolan, G., Wright, J., et al. (1998) Precise carrier diagnosis in families with haemophilia A: use of conformation sensitive gel electrophoresis for mutation screening and polymorphism analysis. *Thromb. Haemost.* **79,** 723–726.

14. Recalde, D., Cenarro, A., Civeira, F., and Pocoví, M. (1998) Apo A-I Zaragoza (L144R): A novel mutation in the apolipoprotein A-I gene associated with familial hypoalphalipoproteinemia. *Hum. Mutat. Mutation and Polymorphism Report* **11,** 416.

15. Makino, R., Yazyu, H., Kishimoto, Y., Sekiya, T., and Hayashi, K. (1992) F-SSCP: Fluorescence-based polymerase chain reaction-single-strand conformation polymorphism (PCR-SSCP) analysis. *PCR Meth. Appl.* **2,** 10–13.

16. Nagamine, C. M., Chan, K., and Lau, Y-F. C. (1989) A PCR artifact: Generation of heteroduplexes. *Am. J. Hum. Genet.* **45,** 337–339.

3

Radiation Hybrid (RH) Mapping of Human Smooth Muscle-Restricted Genes

Joseph M. Miano, Emilio Garcia, and Ralf Krahe

1. Introduction

Recent molecular genetic studies in cardiac and skeletal muscle have revealed mutations in a battery of sarcomeric muscle-restricted genes that appear to be associated with various myopathies *(1,2)*. In sharp contrast, no mutations in smooth muscle cell (SMC)-restricted genes have been linked to a SMC disease phenotype, although a review of the literature indicates that many SMC diseases with a presumed genetic basis are present in human populations *(3–13)*. An important first step in linking a disease phenotype to a mutation within a specific gene is the accurate physical mapping of the candidate gene to a specific chromosomal region within the context of other genetic markers, such as highly polymorphic microsatellite markers now routinely used for recombination-based linkage analysis of families segregating a particular disease phenotype. Several methods exist for the physical mapping of genes, including fluorescent in situ hybridization (FISH) *(14)* and interspecific mouse back-crossing *(15)*. FISH analysis is relatively fast, but often requires large genomic clones and does not afford the high-resolution mapping required to link a gene locus to a disease phenotype. Interspecific mouse back-crossing can be quite powerful with respect to resolution, but studies are necessarily limited to the mouse genome. Thus, a broadly applicable, fast and simple method of gene mapping would be desirable to aid investigators in localizing potential candidate disease genes, especially those pertaining to SMC-associated diseases.

Radiation hybrid (RH) mapping can be used to rapidly map genes; it is based on the now more or less ubiquitous method of PCR amplification of DNA *(16)*. Highly informative panels of RH cell lines exist for various genomes, includ-

From: *Methods in Molecular Medicine, vol. 30: Vascular Disease: Molecular Biology and Gene Therapy Protocols*
Edited by: A. H. Baker © Humana Press Inc., Totowa, NJ

ing the human *(16,17)*, and the mouse *(18)*, as well as for a wide variety of other species and model systems for human disease (Research Genetics, Huntsville, AL; http://www.resgen.com). RH mapping is essentially a somatic cell genetic approach and is well suited for the construction of high-resolution, long-range contiguous maps of the genome under study. For the human RH panels, human diploid cells have been lethally irradiated with different doses of radiation and then rescued by fusion with nonirradiated, recipient hamster cells under conditions where only somatic cell hybrids between the irradiated and nonirradiated cells can form viable colonies *(19)*. The approach is the same for RH panels of other species. The resulting hybrid cell lines contain the normal diploid hamster genome and fragments of human chromosomes often inserted into the middle of hamster chromosomes. The frequency of irradiation-induced breakage between two markers on the same chromosomes is a function of the radiation dosage used and the distance between the two markers *(17)*: 1 centiRay (cR) corresponds to a 1% frequency of breakage between two markers after X-ray irradiation. Thus, the frequency of breakage can be used as a measure of distance, and marker order can be determined in a manner analogous to meiotic, recombination-based linkage analysis *(17)*. Similar to meiotic linkage analysis, marker order and relative confidence in that order are determined using standard maximum likelihood statistical methods. In contrast to meiotic linkage mapping which is dependent on polymorphic markers for map construction, RH mapping can integrate polymorphic and nonpolymorphic markers, such as STSs generated from expressed sequences, i.e., genes. The analysis is simplified by the availability of various analysis tools, so-called RH mapping servers, which support the mapping with the different RH panels.

Currently, three different hamster–human whole genome RH panels are available (Research Genetics; http://www.resgen.com). Based on the radiation dosage used for the irradiation, each panel offers different levels of resolution such that these panels provide complementary resources that can be used to construct RH-based maps over a wide range of resolution, depending on the specific needs of the researcher. The GeneBridge 4 (GB4) panel was generated at *Gene*thon and Cam*bridge* University (hence the name) with a relatively low dose of 3,000 rads of X-rays and consists of 93 RH clones: $1cR_{3,000}$ corresponds to roughly 300 kb *(16,20)*. The GB4 panel, therefore, provides a low resolution panel with approx 1-Mb resolution and constitutes a good first pass panel for fast regional mapping. The G3 panel, generated with 10,000 rads of irradiation at the Stanford Human Genome Center (SHGC), consists of 83 RH clones and provides medium resolution of about 240 kb; 1 $cR_{10,000}$ corresponds to about 29 kb. The GB4 and G3 panels have been used to integrate genes with markers on the human meiotic map *(21*; http://www.ncbi.nlm.nih.gov/SCIENCE96/). A third panel, the TNG panel, also generated at SHGC, is the result of irradiation with 50,000 rads and consists of 90 RH clones *(17)*. The TNG panel provides the highest resolution of up to 50 kb and can be used to generate high-confidence 100 kb maps. All three panels can be used for chromosomal assignments, ordering of markers in a region of interest, as well as the establishment of the physical distance between markers in a candidate region. An integrated map based on all three panels has just been released *(22*; http:// www.ncbi.nlm.nih.gov/genemap). The advantage of the low- and medium-resolution panels is the ready placement of a particular gene under study within a relatively dense framework map of markers mapped with high accuracy. The disadvantage is the lower resolution in cases where higher resolution is required or desired. For reliable assignment and regional localization, the use of at least two of the described panels is suggested. Another major advantage of RH mapping is the integration of the respective RH maps with other genomic maps, namely, the YAC-based STS-content map. This integration allows the easy and fast identification of genomic clones for the region and hence the gene of interest, which in turn can be used for FISH or the further genomic characterization of the gene. Additional valuable information on the generation of the panels and the construction of the respective maps is available directly from the panel-specific RH mapping servers: for the GB4 panel at http://www-genome.wi.mit.edu/cgi-bin/contig/rhmapper.pl; for the G3 panel at http:www-shgc.stanford.edu; and for the TNG panel at http://www-shgc.stanford.edu/RH/TNGindex.html.

In RH mapping, genomic DNA from each of the hybrid cell lines is subjected to PCR amplification using human-specific primers. It is important to discriminate between the human gene and the corresponding homologue in the hamster (the same is, of course, true for any of the other available RH panels for other species). Thus, care must be taken in the design and optimization of PCR primers (**Subheading 3.1.**). Once such species-specific primers are in hand, PCR reactions are carried out on each of the RH cell lines (**Subheading 3.2.**). The PCR reactions are then resolved through an agarose (or polyacrylamide) gel and scored to generate a "linear vector" of numbers based on the presence or absence of a positive PCR result (**Subheading 3.3.**; **Fig. 1**). The last step in RH mapping is the analysis of the vector, which is based on preexisting markers whose position in the genome was determined at high accuracy, so-called framework markers—either polymorphic or nonpolymorphic STSs or ESTs *(23)*. Though the theory of deducing the position of a human gene based on the presence of established genetic markers is beyond the scope of this chapter, **Subheading 3.4.** briefly describes the necessary analysis of the vector, using one of the available RH mapping servers available through the aforementioned internet addresses. We have recently used the RH mapping approach described below with the GB4 panel to localize the human smooth muscle calponin gene on chromosome 19p13.2 *(24)*.

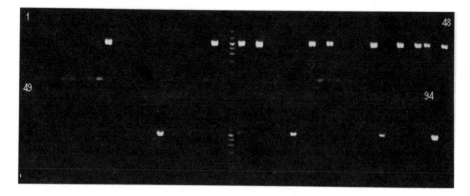

Fig. 1. A typical agarose gel of PCR amplified DNA from an RH panel of cell lines. A duplicate experiment revealed 100% concordancy in amplified signals. The positive signals above were scored "1" and the negatives scored "0" to generate the following vector of data to ascertain the map: 0000000010000000000010101000001 010000100101101000000000000000010000000010000010000000000100000. The vector was generated by reading from the top left of the gel (hybrid 1) to the bottom right (hybrid 94). The positive signal in lane 95 represents human genomic DNA.

2. Materials

2.1. Optimization of PCR Primers

1. cDNA or genomic sequences of human gene and hamster (if available) gene (*see* **Note 1**).
2. Software program for the design of oligonucleotide primers (*see* **Note 2**).
3. Deionized/autoclaved water for resuspending oligonucleotide primers (100 ng/µL working stock for a 21-mer with 50% G/C content).
4. Hamster and human genomic DNA (5 ng/µL working stock) to be used for testing oligonucleotide primers and as controls for PCR of the RH panel (*see* **Note 3**).
5. Qiagen- or CsCl-prepared plasmid DNA containing human cDNA of interest to be used as a positive control in PCR amplification studies (25 ng/µL working stock). Keep at 4°C.
6. PCR Supermix (GibcoBRL).
7. Aerosolized pipet tips.
8. 0.5-mL PCR tubes.
9. Mineral Oil if a PCR machine without a heated lid is used.
10. Standard PCR machine (e.g., Perkin Elmer Cetus Model 480, MJ-Research PTC-200 with heated lid and 96-well alpha unit for higher throughput mapping).
11. SeaKem LE Agarose (FMC, Rockland, ME).
12. Ethidium bromide: dissolve 500 mg in 50 mL of 1x TE buffer, vortex to dissolve and sterile filter as a 10 mg/mL stock. Store stock solution in 50-mL conical tube wrapped in aluminum foil at 4°C or room temperature (*see* **Note 4**).

13. 10x Tris-Acetate-EDTA: dissolve 48.4 g Tris in deionized water and add 11.4 mL glacial acetic acid and 20 mL 0.5 *M* EDTA. Bring total volume to 1 L and store at room temperature.
14. Agarose gels: for a standard 13 × 10 cm gel former, mix 3 g SeaKem LE agarose in 200 mL of 1x TAE, microwave for 2 min and swirl to dissolve.

2.2. PCR Amplification of RH Panel

1. RH panel of choice (Research Genetics, GB4 Cat. No. RH02.02, G3 Cat. No. RH01.02, TNG RH03.02). Each vial representing a hybrid cell line should be diluted in water to 5 ng/μL and stored at 4°C.
2. Motorized Microliter Pipet (Rainin [Woburn, MA], Model ED-250).
3. PCR Machine (*see* **Note 5**).

2.3. Gel Electrophoresis of PCR Results

1. Agarose gel electrophoresis box with 50-tooth combs (Owl Scientific, Model A3-1).
2. Sybr Green DNA stain (*see* **Note 4**).
3. 6X gel loading dye: 0.25% bromophenol blue, 0.25% xylene cyanol FF, and 30% glycerol.
4. 100-base pair DNA ladder (Pharmacia). Store at 4 °C.
5. Thin-wall polycarbonate 192-well (12 rows × 16 columns) plate (Costar, Cambridge, MA).
6. 12-channel Hamilton multiplex gel loading syringe (Fischer Scientific).

2.4. Analysis of PCR Data From RH Panels

1. Gel documentation system (light box with Polaroid land camera or other system).
2. A suitable spreadsheet and word processor (e.g., Microsoft Excel and Word software programs); set up the spreadsheet in advance according to the layout required (*see* addresses in **step 3**) by the RH mapper server. This will ease the management of the obtained data.
3. Internet access to RH mapper servers to analyze the vector: for the GB4 panel at http://www-genome.wi.mit.edu/cgi-bin/contig/rhmapper.pl, for the G3 panel at http:www-shgc.stanford.edu, and for the TNG panel at http://www-shgc.stanford.edu/RH/TNGindex.html.

3. Methods

3.1. Optimization of PCR Primers

1. Generate human-specific primers with at least one of the primers in the noncoding region, either the 5' end or preferentially the 3' UTR (which generally shows greater variation), using GCG (*see* **Note 1**).
2. Label four PCR tubes as follows: human, hamster, positive (for human plasmid, if available) and negative (water control).
3. Make a master PCR mix containing 45 μL of Supermix and 1 μL of each primer (diluted to 100 ng/μL) per reaction tube (or a total of 202.5 μL of Supermix and

4.5 µL of each primer, *see* **Note 6**). Be sure to use aerosolized tips for all PCR applications.

4. Dispense master mix into each of the four labeled tubes (47 µL/tube) followed by 3 µL of each diluted DNA sample.
5. Add 2–3 drops of mineral oil to each tube, gently tap with finger, "pico-spin" and load into PCR machine.
6. Set up PCR parameters as follows: a 3–10-min "hot start" at 94°C linked to 30 cycles of denaturation (94°C for 30 s), annealing (3–4°C below Tm of each primer; *see* **Note 7**) and extension (72°C for 30 s). A final 5–10-min extension at 72°C should be performed to "polish" incompletely amplified products.
7. While PCR reaction is in progress, pour a 1.5% agarose gel in 1X TAE buffer (*see* **Note 8**).
8. When agarose has cooled to approx 55°C (flask can be safely placed on forearm), add 3.5 µL of 10 mg/mL ethidium bromide (*see* **Note 4**), swirl and pour in sealed gel former. Add 1X TAE running buffer to cover gel.
9. Following PCR, remove tubes from machine and add 10 µL of 6X loading dye to each tube (*see* **Note 9**).
10. Load 15–20 µL of each reaction in well of gel alongside a 100-base pair ladder and run the samples until the bromophenol blue dye front (approx 300 base pairs) has migrated the length of the gel. Visualize samples under standard UV illumination box (*see* **Note 10**).

3.2. PCR Amplification of RH Panel

1. Label PCR tubes with the number of each hybrid cell line DNA from the RH panel of choice as well as the hamster and human genomic DNA controls. Alternatively set up a 96-well micro-titer plate (*see* **Note 11**).
2. Using aerosolized tips, transfer 3 µL of each DNA sample to its respective PCR tube and cap each tube to prevent cross-contamination.
3. Make a master mix of the PCR Supermix reagent plus primers in a 15-mL conical tube as follows: combine the PCR Supermix (at 20 µL per tube) and primer (at 1 µL of 100 ng/µL stock) in the tube and gently vortex to mix (*see* **Note 12**).
4. Dispense the master mix to each of the labeled PCR tubes containing DNA using a Rainin motorized repeat pipetter adjusted to a volume of 22 µL.
5. Add 30 µL of mineral oil to each of the tubes using the repeat pipeter as above.
6. Cap all tubes, gently flick with finger, "pico-spin" and then load in PCR machine.
7. Run optimized PCR parameters that were ascertained in **Subheading 3.1.** (*see* **Note 13**).
8. While first reactions are running, pour the gel and begin assembling the duplicate PCR reactions.
9. Store first reactions at room temperature while duplicate reactions are running.

3.3. Gel Electrophoresis of PCR Results

1. While the last of PCR reactions are running, pour a 1.5% agarose gel in large gel apparatus (**Subheading 2.3.**). Insert four 50-tooth combs spaced evenly apart in

gel box. Add 15 μL of Sybr Green DNA stain (*see* **Note 4**) to cooled molten agarose and pour. Add 1X TAE running buffer (approx 4 L for the gel box used here).

2. Combine 30 μL of water to 15 μL of 100-base pair ladder in a tube (set on ice).
3. After PCR, add 5 μL of loading dye to each of the tubes using a repeat pipeter.
4. "Pico-spin" the samples and then assemble the samples in a staggered array for transfer to the microtiter plate (*see* **Note 14**).
5. Manually transfer 15 μL of each staggered sample to a 192-well microtiter plate. Remember to ensure that the staggered tubes are arrayed in the same manner on the plate.
6. Once the staggered array is in place, use a 12-channel Hamilton multiplex gel loading syringe to dispense 10 μL of each row to the gel. Each of the 12 syringes is spaced apart enough to allow every other well to be loaded. In this manner, the odd numbered samples are dispensed into the corresponding odd-numbered wells of the gel, leaving every other well empty. These empty, even-numbered wells will be filled with the even-numbered samples arrayed in the second row of the microtiter plate. It is best to run the gel in a staggered fashion (10–15 min apart depending on the size of the PCR product) to discern possible leakage of samples into neighboring wells, which could result in false positives.
7. Skip the 25th well (it will be used for a 100-base pair ladder) and load the next two rows of staggered samples. Leave the 50th well blank and load the next set of wells with the next staggered samples on the microtiter plate. Note that the last two samples of each PCR run should correspond to the hamster and human genomic DNA controls.
8. Once all samples are loaded, add 10 μL of ladder to each of the middle lanes of each row of wells.
9. Run the electrophoresis for approx 1 h (*see* **Notes 15** and **16**; **Fig. 1**).

3.4. Analysis of PCR Data From RH Panels

1. Take picture of gel and examine for concordancy between duplicate samples.
2. Score each lane as follows: a 0, for no PCR product, a 1, for a positive PCR signal, and a 2, for an ambiguous PCR signal (*see* **Fig. 1** for example).
3. Create spreadsheet in Microsoft Excel with columns labeled according to each hybrid cell line. Record the data for each cell line in spreadsheet; make sure that the results for the positive (human) and negative (hamster) controls are deleted prior to further processing. Save the Excel file as a tab-delimited file to be processed with the word processor.
4. Open the vector file with Word and remove all tabs and save as a text file.
5. The content of the text file can now be copied and pasted directly into the graphical user interface of the respective RH mapping server (*see* **Subheading 2.4.**).
6. Specify output format; the requested parameters for the analysis (lod thresholds and requested map), provide the return e-mail address, and submit. Multiple results can be submitted at the same time; however, each vector entry should be clearly identified with a specific identifier.

3.5. Applications of RH Mapping Results

The results gained in the above experiments can be used to further define individual genes using techniques such as:

1. Screening bacterial artificial chromosome (BAC) libraries to obtain large genomic fragments of the DNA (http://www.resgen.com).
2. Determination of the genomic organisation of the gene within the BAC using specific primers to the cDNA sequence (*see* **ref.** *24* for details).
3. Making transgenic cell lines and mice with the BAC to delineate distal regulatory elements controlling the gene's expression profile. The same BAC transgenic cells and mice may be used to study the effects of "gain of function" mutations on the cell/animal's physiology or pathology.
4. Use the BAC to screen for polymorphisms (single nucleotide or simple sequence repeats) that could be used to ascertain genetic lesions linked to a specific disease phenotype.

4. Notes

1. We use the Genetics Computer Group's (GCG) suite of software programs to analyze nucleic acid sequences (http://www.gcg.com). Accession numbers to all GenBank sequences related to your gene of interest can be obtained by using the "stringsearch" command in GCG. Specific accession numbers corresponding to a species-specific sequence can then be selected from the stringsearch result using the "fetch" command. A "fasta" or "gap" command can then be executed to compare the sequence homologies between human and hamster sequences when both are present. It is imperative that great care be taken in the design of the PCR primers. We recommend that two sets of primers be made with at least one of the sets designed to amplify the 5' or 3' untranslated region of the human cDNA of interest. Alternatively, if genomic DNA sequence is available and the intron-exon structure of the gene is known, intronic sequence can also be used to design a species-specific primer. The PCR product should ideally be between 200–400-base pairs in length. We store our stock primers at –20°C and working stocks at 4°C. The first author has found that primers can be stored at 4°C for several years without degradation.
2. Several oligonucleotide primer design programs exist (e.g., Oligo 4.0). However, Operon Technologies, Inc. offers free software on the internet (http://web712d0.ntx.net/cgi-bin/ss2b1/toolkit.cgi). This same web site calculates the price and provides a link for easy ordering of the oligonucleotide.
3. Hamster (Cat. No. RH02controlA23) and human (RH02controlHFL) genomic DNA are obtained from Research Genetics (http://www.resgen.com).
4. Ethidium bromide is classified as a carcinogen. A safer and superior stain for visualizing PCR products is Sybr Green (FMC).
5. Genome labs often possess "waffle iron" PCR machines (Tetrad 16-plate format, IAS Products, Inc.) that accommodate 192- or 384-well plates. Although these high throughput machines simplify RH panel mapping greatly, they often lead to

erroneous PCR results. Thus, we use standard 48- or 96-well PCR machines (Perkin Elmer Models 480 and 9600, respectively) that accommodate tubes rather than plates; if the 9600 machine is used, then 0.2-μL tubes are needed (Perkin Elmer, Cat. No. N801-0540). While such machines add more labor in terms of pipetting, results are much more consistent and clean.

6. We typically multiply by the number of tubes plus 0.5 (4.5 in example) to correct for errors in pipeting.

7. We recommend two PCR reactions be tested with annealing temperatures varying by 3–5°C.

8. Microwaving agarose causes superheating and can dangerously result in boilover with resultant burning of skin. To minimize this hazard, we microwave 200 mL of agarose in a 1-L flask and hold the flask at its neck with a folded paper towel on removal from the microwave.

9. Mineral oil can be "phased" to the bottom of the tube by adding 50 μL of TE-saturated chloroform; however, this is unsafe and impractical following PCR of the RH cell lines.

10. Most UV boxes emit shortwave UV light (300–310 nm). Thus, proper eye protection should be worn during visualization of gel.

11. PCR of the RH panel should be performed in duplicate to confirm positive signals. Thus, for a typical RH panel of 94 hybrid lines, one will need to label 188 tubes plus two hamster and two human genomic DNA control tubes.

12. We have demonstrated adequate PCR products with as little as 20 μL of PCR Supermix. For 192 tubes, we mix 4 mL of Supermix with 200 μL of each diluted primer.

13. If PCR is performed in a Perkin Elmer Model 480, then it will be necessary to divide the samples in half and use a second machine. This is fine so long as the machines are within a few degrees error of one another.

14. The samples should be assembled in a manner that will allow rapid loading into the gel. We recommend that the tubes be staggered in a linear array (e.g., tube 1, 3, 5, 7, 9, etc.) 12 across per row. This allows for easy access and dispensing with the 12-channel Hamilton multiplex gel loading syringe. For example, we typically array a row of odd numbered tubes (1, 3, 5, etc.) followed by even numbered tubes (2, 4, 6, etc.) in the microtiter plate.

15. The samples only need to run far enough in the gel to discern a positive signal.

16. If due to high homology between the human and hamster genes, PCR amplification of DNA from both species provides positive results, it is often possible to separate the PCR fragments by PAGE electrophoresis on 6–8% denaturing polyacrylamide gel electrophoresis. For detection, PAGE gels can be silver-stained. Even if the genes are highly conserved there usually is a slight size difference which allows for distinction of the two products by PAGE.

References

1. Bonne, G., Carrier, L., Richard, P., and Hainque, B., Schwartz, K. (1998) Familial hypertrophic cardiomyopathy: from mutations to functional defects. *Circ. Res.* **83**, 580–593.

2. Brown, S. C. and Lucy, J. A. (1993) Dystrophin as a mechanochemical transducer in skeletal muscle. *BioEssays* **15**, 413–419.
3. Smolarek, T. A., Wessner, L. L., McCormack, F. X., Mylet, J. C., Menon, A. G., and Henske, E. P. (1998) Evidence that lymphangiomyomatosis is caused by TSC2 mutations: chromosome 16p13 loss of heterozygosity in angiomyolipomas and lymph nodes from women with lymphangiomyomatosis. *Am. J. Hum. Genet.* **62**, 810–815.
4. Zhou, J., Mochizuki, T., Smeets, H., Antignac, C., Laurila, P., de Paepe, A., et al. (1993) Deletion of the paired a5(IV) and a6(IV) collagen genes in inherited smooth muscle cell tumors. *Science* **261**, 1167–1169.
5. Fukai, N., Aoyagi, M., Yamamoto, M., Sakamoto, H., Ogami, K., Matsushima, Y., et al. (1994) Human arterial smooth muscle cell strains derived from patients with moyamoya disease: changes in biological characteristics and proliferative response during cellular aging in vitro. *Mech. Ageing Dev.* **75**, 21–33.
6. Kalaria, R. N. (1997) Cerebrovascular degeneration is related to amyloid-β protein deposition in Alzheimer's disease. *Ann. NY Acad. Sci.* **826**, 263–271.
7. Fromont-Hankard, G., Lafer, D., and Masood, S. (1996) Altered expression of alpha-smooth muscle isoactin in Hirschsprung's disease. *Arch. Pathol. Lab. Med.* **120**, 270–274.
8. Vermillion, D. L., Huizinga, J. D., Riddell, R. H., and Collins, S. M. (1993) Altered small intestinal smooth muscle function in Crohn's disease. *Gastroenterology* **104**, 1692–1699.
9. Molenaar, W. M., Rosman, J. B., Donker, A. J., and Houthoff, H. J. (1987) The pathology and pathogenesis of malignant atrophic papulosis (Degos' disease). A case study with reference to other vascular disorders. *Pathol. Res. Pract.* **182**, 98–106.
10. Slavin, R. E. and de Groot, W. J. (1981) Pathology of the lung in Behcet's disease. Case report and review of the literature. *Am. J. Surg. Pathol.* **5**, 779–788.
11. Goldfischer, S., Coltoff-Schille,r B., Biempica, L., and Wolinsky, H. (1975) Lysosomes and the sclerotic arterial lesion in Hurler's disease. *Hum. Pathol.* **6**, 633–637.
12. Joutel, A., Corpechot, C., Ducros, A. Vahedi, K., Chabriat, H., Mouton, P., et al. (1996) *Notch 3* mutations in CADASIL, a hereditary adult-onset condition causing stroke and dementia. *Nature* **383**, 707–710.
13. Ohshiro, K. and Puri, P. (1998) Pathogenesis of infantile hypertrophic pyloric stenosis: recent progress. *Pediatr. Surg. Int.* **13**, 243–252.
14. Gerhard, D. S., Kawasaki, E. S., Bancroft, F. C., and Szabo, P. (1981) Localization of a unique gene by direct hybridization *in situ*. *Proc. Natl. Acad. Sci. USA* **78**, 3755–3759.
15. Copeland, N. G. and Jenkins, N. A. (1991) Development and applications of a molecular genetic linkage map of the mouse genome. *Trends Genet.* **7**, 113–118.
16. Gyapay, G., Schmitt, K., Fizames, C., Jones, H., Vegaczarny, N., Spillett, D. J., et al. (1996) A radiation hybrid map of the human genome. *Hum. Mol. Genet.* **5**, 339–346.
17. Stewart, E. A., McKusick, K. B., Aggarwal, A., Bajorek, E., Brady, S., Chu, A., et al. (1997) An STS-based radiation hybrid map of the human genome. *Genome Res.* **7**, 422–433.

18. Flaherty, L. and Herron, B. (1998) The new kid on the block—a whole genome mouse radiation hybrid panel. *Mamm. Genome.* **9,** 417,418.
19. Walter, M. A., Spillett, D. J., Thomas, P., Weissenbach, J., and Goodfellow, P. N. (1994) A method for constructing radiation hybrid maps of whole genomes. *Nat. Genet.* **7,** 22–28.
20. Hudson, T. J., Stein, L. D., Gerety, S. S., Ma, J., Castle, A. B., Silva, J., Slonim, D. K., Baptista, R., Kruglyak, L., Xu, S. H., et al. (1995) An STS-based map of the human genome. *Science* **270,** 1945–1954.
21. Schuler, G. D., Boguski, M. S., Stewart, E. A., Stein, L. D., Gyapay, G., Rice, K., et al. (1996) A gene map of the human genome. *Science* **274,** 540–546.
22. Deloukas, P., Schuler, G. D., Gyapay, G., Beasley, C., Soderlund, P., Rodriguez-Tome, P., et al. (1998) A physical map of 30,000 human genes. *Science* **282,** 744–746.
23. Kruglyak, L. and Lander, E. S. (1995) High-resolution genetic mapping of complex traits. *Am. J. Hum. Genet.* **56,** 1212–1223.
24. Miano, J. M., Krahe, R., Garcia, E., Elliott, J. M., and Olson, E. N. (1997) Expression, genomic structure and high resolution mapping to 19p13.2 of the human smooth muscle cell calponin gene. *Gene* **197,** 215–224.

II

Isolation of Genes Expressed in Vascular Tissue

4

Efficient Extraction of RNA from Vascular Tissue

Catherine F. Townsend, Christopher M. H. Newman,
and Sheila E. Francis

1. Introduction

The development of new and effective techniques to study differential gene expression has revolutionized biomedical research during the last decade. Such techniques include differential display reverse transcription polymerase chain reaction (*dd*RTPCR) (*see* Chapter 9), first described in 1992 *(1)*, cDNA representational difference analysis (cDNA RDA) (*see* Chapter 8), first described in 1994 *(2)*, and serial analysis of gene expression (SAGE), first described in 1995 *(3)*. All have the potential to be powerful tools in the study of gene expression in healthy and diseased vascular tissue. The starting material in all these gene expression studies is high quality RNA. However, it is widely realized that the efficient extraction of such RNA from vascular tissue is difficult, for reasons that will be described later. The majority of studies on gene expression in vascular disease to date have used cultured vascular cells *(4–6)*, as the RNA extraction is easier and the yield greater than from solid tissue. However, cell culture *per se* induces changes in gene expression, and so the use of the intact tissue would be a more valid approach for studying gene expression in vascular disease.

The successful extraction of RNA from solid vascular tissue is difficult. This material is rich in connective tissue and, in many cases, is relatively hypocellular, and RNA yields per mg of vascular tissue are generally low (0.2–0.3 µg/mg tissue, *see* **Fig. 1**), in comparison to approx 5 µg/mg for liver tissue *(7)*. The "fibrous" nature of vascular tissue also makes it extremely difficult to homogenize efficiently. The presence of calcified atherosclerotic plaque in diseased human samples causes increased hardening of the intrinsically fibrous

From: *Methods in Molecular Medicine, vol. 30: Vascular Disease: Molecular Biology and Gene Therapy Protocols*
Edited by: A. H. Baker © Humana Press Inc., Totowa, NJ

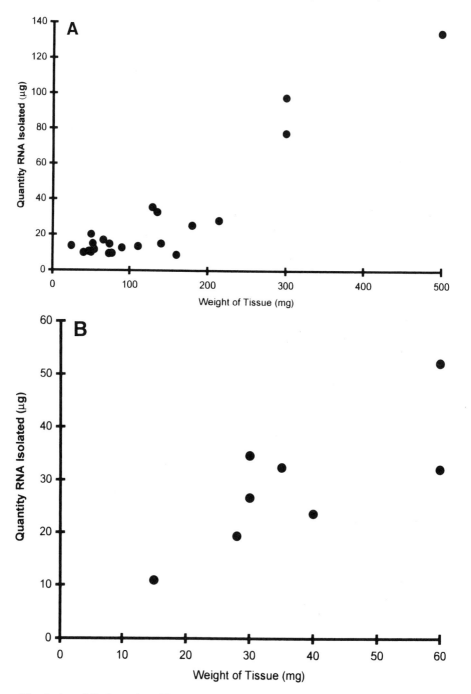

Fig. 1. A and B show the efficiency of RNA extraction from human (**A**) and porcine (**B**) vascular tissue, per mg starting weight of tissue, using the protocols described here.

tissue, increasing the difficulties of homogenization and further reducing RNA yields. Moreover, human vascular tissue samples desirable for use in studies of gene expression are often small, e.g., atherectomy specimens, atherosclerotic lesions etc., exacerbating these problems. The method of RNA extraction used in our laboratory uses RNAzol B, an RNA extraction reagent based on the one-step guanidinium thiocyanate method of RNA isolation *(8)* and a commercially available hand-held homogenizer, allowing efficient disruption of the tissue. We have optimized the "standard" protocol supplied with RNAzol B *(9)* for RNA extraction from particularly small samples of diseased human vascular tissue. These modifications include keeping the tissue on dry ice throughout the homogenization procedure to avoid degradation of RNA, the removal of insoluble material (i.e., calcified material) from the homogenate by an additional centrifugation step, and the use of a double volume of chloroform for extraction to remove excess lipids and proteins. Separate homogenization procedures are described for the isolation of very small and larger samples, due to the necessary differences in handling of these two types of samples. An example of the high quality RNA which can be obtained from small quantities of diseased human vascular tissue using the protocol described in **Subheading 2.2.1.** is shown in **Fig. 2**.

2. Materials

2.1. Tissue

Our laboratory uses human saphenous vein tissue obtained during coronary artery bypass surgery, coronary arteries obtained from cardiac transplant recipient hearts at the time of transplantation, and atherectomy specimens. We also use porcine vessels, but the protocols that follow could be used for isolation of RNA from any vascular material. The use of post-mortem tissue is not usually possible as tissue is often not available until several days following death, during which time extensive RNA degradation will usually have occurred.

2.2. Homogenization

2.2.1. Tissue Homogenization (< 65 mg samples) (see to **Note 1**)

1. "Pellet Pestle" hand held homogenizer (Burkard Scientific, Uxbridge, UK).
2. Autoclaved Pestle inserts and 1.5 mL homogenization tubes (Burkard Scientific).
3. Sterile (autoclaved) plastic 50-mL beaker.
4. Sterile scalpel blade and 21-gage needle.
5. RNAzol B (Biogenesis Ltd, Poole, Dorset, UK), store in the dark at 4°C.
6. Aluminum thermoblock suitable for 1.5-mL microcentrifuge tubes (removable, of the type used in heatblocks).
7. Dry ice.
8. RNase away (Promega, Madison, WI) to remove RNases from Gilsons, work surfaces, etc.

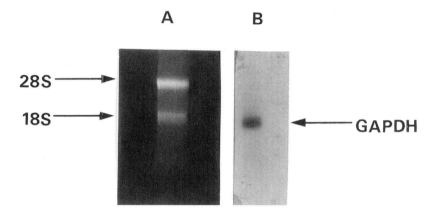

Fig. 2. (**A**) shows a 1.1% denaturing agarose gel on which 10 μg of high quality RNA extracted from 54 mg of diseased human coronary artery (using the protocol described here for tissue homogenization of samples <65 mg in weight, **Subheading 2.2.1.**) has been electrophoresed. The 28S and 18S ribosomal bands are clearly visible and have been marked. (**B**) shows a Northern Blot of the same sample, probed with ^{32}P labeled GAPDH (glyceraldehyde-3-phosphate dehydrogenase) cDNA.

2.2.2. Tissue Homogenization (> 200 mg)

1. Baked ceramic pestle and mortar (preferably a relatively large pestle with small mortar).
2. Liquid nitrogen.
3. Polypropylene 15-mL Falcon tubes (Becton Dickinson, Franklin Lakes, NJ) (*see* **Note 2**).
4. Screw-top microcentrifuge tubes (Sarstedt): RNase and DNase free, with gasket to prevent leakage. Will withstand >13,000*g*.

2.3. RNA Isolation

1. Chloroform (Sigma): purity 99+%.
2. 100% isopropanol (molecular biology grade).
3. 75% (v/v) ethanol: Make up using RNase-free H_2O, which has been treated with DEPC (diethylpyrocarbonate) (*see* **Note 3**) (*10*).
4. DEPC treated H_2O.
5. Wet ice.
6. A refrigerated microcentrifuge, if available, is very useful.

3. Methods
3.1. Tissue

1. Snap freeze tissue samples in liquid nitrogen in cryovials immediately following surgery.

2. Store in the liquid or vapor phase of liquid nitrogen (where they are stable for several years) until use. Cut very large samples into sections of approx 5 mm in length prior to freezing, to maximise the efficiency of homogenization. To avoid RNA degradation we aim to freeze vascular samples within 30 min following explantation *(11)*.

3.2. Homogenization

Alternative protocols are given for the homogenization of small (< 65 mg) and larger (> 200 mg) samples. Firstly the frozen tissue sample must be rapidly weighed and returned to liquid nitrogen to prevent thawing, and the appropriate homogenization protocol followed (*see* **Note 1**).

3.2.1. Protocol 1: Tissue Homogenization (< 65 mg Samples)

Extraction of total RNA using this method takes approx 2.25 h for one sample, including a 30-min equipment cooling time.

1. Pre-cool the aluminum thermoblock and sterile plastic 50-mL beaker on dry ice for 30 min prior to homogenization.
2. Macerate the tissue sample into very small pieces (< 0.5 × 0.5 × 0.5 mm), using the sterile scalpel blade and 21-gauge needle, in the sterile beaker on dry ice.
3. Remove the beaker from dry ice and add 1.5 mL of RNAzol B to the tissue fragments in the beaker (*see* **Note 4**).
4. Cut off the end of a sterile 1-mL Gilson tip, and pipette the tissue suspension into the 1.5 mL homogenization tube, and centrifuge for 20–30 s to settle the contents of the tube.
5. Aspirate 1 mL of the RNAzol B supernatant in the homogenization tube, and transfer to the original beaker, on dry ice. Any tiny fragments of tissue left in the beaker will thereby be conserved.
6. Transfer the homogenization tube to the pre-cooled thermoblock, and homogenize on dry ice using the hand held homogenizer for approx 10 min, or until a very fine suspension is formed (*see* **Notes 5** and **6**).
7. Thaw the 1 mL RNAzol B in the beaker, and return to the homogenate.
8. Centrifuge at 20,000*g* for 10 min at 4°C to sediment insoluble material, and aliquot supernatant into two 2-mL screw-top microcentrifuge tubes.
9. Add 0.2 volumes of chloroform (i.e., approx 150 µL) to each tube and shake vigorously for 15–30 s to mix.
10. Continue with **Subheading 3.2., step 1**.

3.2.2. Protocol 2: Tissue Homogenization (> 200 mg Samples)

Extraction of total RNA using this method takes approx 1.5 h.

1. Pre-cool a baked pestle and mortar with liquid nitrogen, until effervescence ceases (*see* **Note 7**).
2. Add tissue sample, and crush in liquid nitrogen until a very fine powder is achieved. The tissue should not be allowed to thaw. If more time is required for

homogenization, more liquid nitrogen should be added. Allow the liquid nitrogen to evaporate off, and quickly transfer tissue powder without thawing to a 15-mL polypropylene Falcon tube containing RNAzol B (2 mL/100 mg starting weight of tissue).

3. Add 0.1 volume of chloroform and shake vigorously for 15–30 s to mix, and aliquot into 2-mL screw-top RNase free microcentrifuge tubes.

3.3. RNA Isolation

1. Incubate homogenate/chloroform mixture on wet ice for 15 min.
2. Spin at 20,000*g* at 4°C for 15 min. Three "phases" can be seen, a colorless upper "aqueous" phase containing RNA, a white "interphase" containing DNA, and a blue lower phase containing proteins.
3. Carefully transfer upper aqueous phase into fresh 2-mL microcentrifuge tubes (avoiding contamination with the interphase) and add 1 volume of 100% isopropanol.
4. Incubate on ice for at least 15 min to precipitate the RNA.
5. Spin at 20,000*g* at 4°C for 15 min. The RNA forms a white pellet on the bottom and sides of the tube.
6. Carefully decant the isopropanol by tipping off most of the volume, and pipetting off any residual liquid, and add 1 mL of 75% ethanol to the RNA pellet. Gently tap the tube to dislodge the pellet. Centrifuge again at 20,000*g* at 4°C for 5 min.
7. Decant the ethanol, and carefully aspirate off any residual fluid without disturbing the RNA pellet.
8. Air dry for 5 min, and re-dissolve in 5–20 mL of DEPC treated H_2O, depending on the size of the pellet. RNA should be stored at –80°C (*see* **Notes 8–10**).

4. Notes

1. The use of a homogenization procedure adapted specifically for a given vascular tissue quantity greatly increases the efficiency of RNA isolation. The tissue sample should be weighed as described, and the appropriate protocol followed. For tissue samples of between 65 and 200 mg, we have found it most efficient to split the sample into several sections weighing approx 65 mg each, and follow the homogenization procedure for small samples. This does increase the time span for RNA isolation, but it is beneficial in that small quantities of tissue are not left behind in the mortar, as would be the case if using the protocol adapted for larger tissue samples.
2. Polystyrene tubes are dissolved by RNAzol B.
3. Treatment with diethylpyrocarbonate (DEPC) is necessary to remove contaminating RNases present in water which is used to make up solutions for use in RNA work. 0.2 mL of DEPC is added per 100 mL water, in a fume hood, and the bottles left open-topped over night. The water is then autoclaved to inactivate the DEPC. A commentary on the basic principles of RNA extraction, including the use of DEPC to inactivate ribonucleases, can be found in **ref. *10***.

4. RNazol B is a commercially available RNA extraction solution that we have found to give good results in the isolation of RNA from vascular tissue. It is based on the single step method of RNA isolation by acid guanidinium thiocyanate-phenol-chloroform extraction method *(7,8)*. The guanidinium thiocyanate denaturing solution published by Chomczynski and Sacchi *(8)*, which could be used as an alternative to RNAzol B if this is not available, is 4 *M* guanidinium thiocyanate, 25 m*M* sodium citrate, pH 7, 0.5% sarcosyl, 0.1 *M* 2-mercaptoethanol.

5. We have found it necessary to use dry ice while homogenizing to avoid RNA degradation caused by temperature increase during the prolonged homogenization procedure. However, the extremely cold temperatures cause the RNAzol to freeze during homogenization. It is therefore necessary to gently thaw the RNAzol with gloved hands or on the bench when freezing occurs.

6. RNAzol B is hazardous: use eye protection whilst homogenizing.

7. Liquid nitrogen is hazardous. Wear insulating gloves and eye protection.

8. If RNA is to be stored for long periods of time (>1 wk), we recommend storage in 75% ethanol at –80°C or colder. When needed, the RNA should be centrifuged at 20,000*g* for 5 min at 4°C to pellet the RNA, which should then be dissolved as in **Subheading 3.2., steps 7** and **8**.

9. For gene expression studies where mRNA is required as the starting material, we routinely use Dynal Oligo dT (25) Dynabeads or a Qiagen Oligotex Kit to poly A select mRNA from total RNA obtained by the above protocol. For extracting mRNA using this method, we would not recommend beginning with less than 40 µg total RNA.

10. Using the outlined methods, we have not found it necessary to remove contaminating genomic DNA from our RNA preparations for reverse transcription polymerase chain reaction, and Northern Analysis. However, if the RNA is to be used with primers that do <u>not</u> discriminate between products from genomic DNA and RNA, or for differential display, we recommend DNase treatment prior to use. In our laboratory, the MessageClean kit (Genhunter, Nashville, TN) is used for this purpose.

References

1. Liang, P. and Pardee, A. B. (1992) Differential display of eukaryotic messenger RNA by means of the polymerase chain reaction. *Science* **257,** 967–971.
2. Hubank, M. and Schatz, D. G. (1994) Identifying differences in mRNA expression by representational difference analysis of cDNA. *Nucleic Acids Res.* **22,** 5640–5648.
3. Velculescu, V. E., Zhang, I., Vogelstein, B., and Kinzler, K. W. (1995) Serial Analysis of Gene Expression. *Science* **270,** 484–487.
4. Hultgårdh-Nilsson, A., Lövdahl, C.. Blomgren, K., Kallin, B., and Thyberg, J. (1997) Expression of phenotype- and proliferation-related genes in rat aortic smooth muscle cells in primary culture. *Cardiovasc. Res.* **34,** 418–430.
5. Koike, H., Karas, R. H., Baur, W. E., O'Donnell Jr., T. F., and Mendelsohn, M. E. (1996) Differential display polymerase chain reaction identifies nucleophosmin

as an estrogen-regulated gene in human vascular smooth muscle cells. *J. Vasc. Surg.* **23,** 477–482.

6. Kirschenlohr, H. L., Metcalfe, J. C., Weissberg, P. L., and Grainger, D. J. (1993) Adult human aortic smooth muscle cells in culture express active TGFβ. *Am. J. Physiol.* **265,** C571–C576.

7. Gauthier, E. R., Madison, S. D., and Michel, R. N. (1997) Rapid RNA isolation without the use of commercial kits: application to small tissue samples. *Pflugers Arch.- Eur. J. Physiol.* **433,** 664–668.

8. Chomczynski, P. and Sacchi, N. (1987) Single step method of RNA isolation by acid guanidinium thiocyanate-phenol-chloroform extraction. *Anal. Biochem.* **115** 419-423.

9. Biogenesis (1991) *Tel-Test Bulletin* No. 2.

10. Jones, P., Qiu, J., and Rickwood, D. (1994) *RNA Isolation and Analysis,* Bios Scientific Publishers, Oxford, UK.

11. Galea, J., Armstrong, J., Gadson, P., Holden, H., Francis, S. E., Holt, C. M. (1996) Interleukin-1β in coronary arteries of patients with ischemic heart disease. *Arterioscler. Thromb. Vasc. Biol.* **16,** 1000–1006.

5

Preparation of cDNA Libraries from Vascular Cells

Mark E. Lieb and Mark B. Taubman

1. Introduction

The vast majority of past and present efforts in the molecular cloning of expressed sequences involve isolation of clones from cDNA libraries constructed in bacteriophage lambda *(1,2)*. As discussed in Chapter 6, screening these cDNA libraries using labeled probes remains the most straightforward method to isolate full length cDNAs for which some partial sequence information is known. Although the availability of high quality reagents and kits over the past decade has made the process of library construction increasingly straightforward, generation of high-quality libraries is a task that still requires a fair amount of dedicated effort. Because alternative PCR-based cloning strategies have become increasingly popular alternatives to cDNA library screening, it is useful to consider the advantages and disadvantages of each strategy before embarking on a project to construct a cDNA library (**Table 1**). In our opinion, it is worthwhile to construct a cDNA library when the transcript of interest is not exceedingly rare (i.e., can readily be detected by Northern blot analysis of total RNA), when multiple cDNAs will need to be cloned over a period of time, and in situations where occasional mutations can not be tolerated (for example, if the cDNA is to be expressed in mammalian cells to examine function). In situations where the transcript of interest is expressed at exceedingly low levels, or when only a single cDNA needs to be cloned, a PCR-based strategy should be considered. When the tissue source is precious (such as a unique clinical specimen), successful construction of a phage library provides a resource that can be amplified and used for multiple cloning projects over many years, but runs the risk of consuming the available RNA if the library construction fails.

From: *Methods in Molecular Medicine, vol. 30: Vascular Disease: Molecular Biology and Gene Therapy Protocols*
Edited by: A. H. Baker © Humana Press Inc., Totowa, NJ

Table 1
Comparison of Relative Advantages of cDNA Cloning from Lambda
Phage Libraries by Plaque Hybridization Compared to Newer PCR-
Based Strategies

	Lambda phage cDNA library	PCR-based strategy
Freedom from error	++	+/–
Able to detect very rare transcripts	–	++
Reusable	++	–
Useful for rare/precious tissue samples	–	++

Although any collection of cDNA that includes representative copies of all the mRNAs expressed in a particular tissue or cell could be referred to as a cDNA library, for the purpose of this chapter we will discuss the construction of libraries that are suitable for screening with the techniques outlined in Chapter 6. Conceptually, the construction of a cDNA library is straightforward and is outlined in **Fig. 1**. After total RNA is isolated from the tissue or cells of interest, mRNA is separated from the total RNA. mRNA then serves as a template for the enzyme reverse transcriptase, which makes a single stranded DNA copy of each mRNA strand in the purified preparation. After the reverse transcriptase reaction, the library consists of double-stranded RNA:DNA hybrids of the original mRNA paired to the complementary cDNA. In the second strand reaction, the enzyme RNAse H is used to create a series of nicks in the original mRNA and the remaining pieces of mRNA in the RNA:DNA hybrid serve as primers for the enzyme DNA polymerase I. The polymerase synthesizes the second stand of cDNA in a reaction that also removes the RNA primers. The double-stranded cDNA is inserted into the bacteriophage lambda genome through the use of DNA ligase, which also repairs the "nicks" that remain in the second strand after the second strand reaction. Phage DNA is then "packaged" to produce intact bacteriophage particles that are then used to infect *Escherichia coli*. The phage multiply in the bacteria to produce "clones" each one containing many copies of a single-phage particle. When the library is constructed properly, each phage particle will contain a single cDNA insert and the relative abundance of phage containing cDNA corresponding to a particular gene product will be directly proportional to its mRNA level in the tissue from which the RNA was isolated.

In most vascular tissues, mRNA makes up about 1% of total cellular RNA and therefore must be purified prior to library construction, so that the library can be efficiently screened. Purification of intact, high-quality mRNA is the single most important step in creating a library, which will have a high per-

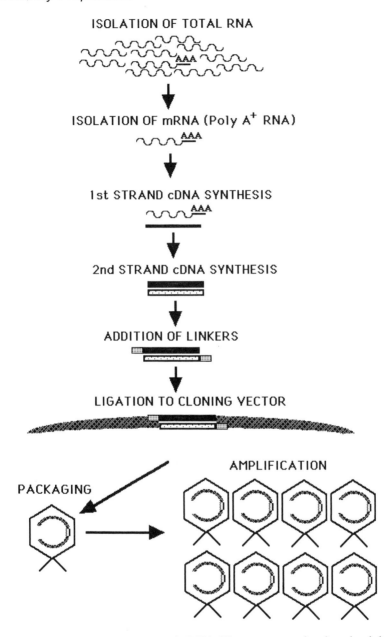

Fig. 1. Schematic representation of cDNA library preparation in a lambda phage cloning vector.

centage of full-length transcripts. It is critical that the RNA isolated from the cells or tissues of interest is free from contaminating nucleases before purification of mRNA, because any contaminating RNAse will have ample opportunity to degrade the RNA in the subsequent steps. Because vascular tissues can be difficult to use as sources of nuclease-free RNA, it is important to verify that the technique used for isolation of total RNA is effective in the vascular tissue of interest (*see* Chapter 4). Once intact mRNA is isolated, the original source of the mRNA does not influence the remaining steps in the construction of a cDNA library. Therefore, the isolation of high quality RNA is the only step in the process of library construction which has unique considerations vis-à-vis vascular cells.

In order for the cDNA library to be truly representative of the original population of mRNA, the method used to introduce the cDNA into the cloning vector must be highly efficient, must not introduce systematic bias for or against a particular cDNA ,and must ensure that only a single cDNA species is introduced into each phage. The double-stranded cDNA produced in the previous steps will have blunt ends, which would be difficult to efficiently join to other DNA molecules. There are numerous ways of addressing this issue and the major differences between published techniques is in how they tackle the problem of efficiently ligating cDNA into the cloning vector. The greater the efficiency of this process, the greater the chance that rare transcripts will be represented in the library. We employ the use of commercially available synthetic linkers that are blunt on one end and have protruding termini that are compatible with the protruding termini of the cloning vector. They lack a 5' phosphate on their protruding termini and are phosphorylated on their blunt end. The use of a large molar excess of linkers allows their blunt ends to efficiently ligate to the cDNA while the lack of a 5' phosphate on the overhanging ends prevents the overhanging ends from ligating to other linkers in the reaction mix. The ligase is then inactivated and a 5' phosphate is added to the protruding termini by T4 DNA kinase. Excess linkers and linker-dimers are removed by spun column chromatography and the cDNA is joined to the compatible overhanging ends of a predigested, dephosphorylated cloning vector in a second ligation reaction.

Although the methods below (modified from **ref. *1***) have worked well in our laboratory for constructing libraries from vascular smooth muscle cells, any technique which has been used successfully in other tissues should be expected to have equal efficacy when applied to purified mRNA from vascular tissues. It is worth mentioning that a number of vendors offer cDNA synthesis "kits" that include all of the reagents to synthesize double stranded cDNA from poly A+ RNA. If one is in the position of having to purchase all of the reagents for cDNA synthesis, the kits are usually a good value and in addition they offer various innovations to streamline the synthesis process. Although we encourage the use of these kits, it is important to remember that each step in the construction of a cDNA library is dependent upon the preceding steps and therefore we recommend following the quality control steps described in the Notes section, regardless of which specific protocol is employed.

2. Materials

All solutions should be prepared from sterile deionized or distilled water and any solutions which will come in contact with RNA should be prepared from water treated with 0.01% diethyl pyrocarbonate (DEPC) overnight at room temperature and then autoclaved to remove traces of DEPC. All glassware that will come in contact with RNA should be baked at > 180°C for 8 h. Disposable plasticware can generally be assumed to be RNAse free and should be used wherever possible.

2.1. Isolation of Poly A⁺ RNA from total RNA (see Note 1)

1. Oligo dT cellulose: type 3, 0.5 g column (Becton Dickinson and Co., Franklin Lakes, NJ). Prepare with binding and elution buffers according to manufacturers protocol.
2. 2X Binding buffer (high salt): 20 mM Tris-HCl, pH 7.5, 1 M NaCl, 1% SDS, 2 mM EDTA.
3. Elution buffer (low salt): 10 mM Tris-HCl, pH 7.5, 0.5% SDS, 1 mM EDTA. Following elution of poly A⁺ RNA, the column may be stored at 4°C in elution buffer with the addition of 0.02% Sodium Azide (Toxic).
4. 0.1 N NaOH. Prepare from 10 N NaOH.
5. 3 M NaAc, pH 5.2. Store at room temperature.
6. Ethanol and 70% ethanol (v/v in water).

2.2. Preparation of Single-Stranded cDNA (see Note 2)

1. Superscript™ reverse transcriptase (Gibco BRL).
2. 5X first strand buffer (Gibco BRL).
3. 0.1 M DTT (Gibco BRL).
4. dNTP mix: mix equal volumes of 25 mM dGTP, dATP, dCTP and dTTP (Boehringer Mannheim).
5. RNAse inhibitor (20–40 U/μL) (Promega).
6. [α-^{32}P]dCTP (3000 Ci/mmol) (NEN™ Life Science Products , Boston, MA).
7. Oligo dT$_{12-18}$: 1 mg/mL (Pharmacia) (*see* **Note 3**).
8. TE: 10 mM Tris-HCl, pH 7.5, 1 mM EDTA. Autoclave and store at room temperature (*see* **Note 4**).
9. Phenol:chloroform. Mix equal volumes of TE saturated phenol, pH 8.0 (Fisher Scientific) and chloroform. Store under excess TE in a dark glass bottle.

2.3. The Second-Strand Reaction

1. *E. coli* DNA Polymerase I (10 U/μL) and 10x reaction buffer (NEBiolabs).
2. RNAse H (approx 1 U/μL) (Pharmacia).

3. DNA Polymerase I, Large (Klenow) Fragment (NEBiolabs).
4. cDNA spun columns (Pharmacia).

2.4. Introduction of cDNA into a Cloning Vector

1. *Eco*RI/*Not*I Cohesive-End adaptors: 0.01 A_{260} U/µL (Pharmacia).
2. T4 DNA ligase (NEBioLabs). Store at –20°C.
3. T4 polynucleotide kinase (NEBioLabs). Store at –20°C.
4. ATP 20 mM solution. Make fresh dilution with water from 100 mM stock (Pharmacia).
5. Lambda Zap® II *(3) Eco*RI/CIAP-treated vector (Stratagene) (*see* **Note 5**).

2.5. Packaging, Amplification, and Titering

1. Gigapack® High efficiency packaging extract (Stratagene).
2. LB broth: 1% tryptone, 0.5% yeast extract, 1% NaCl (all available from Gibco BRL). Adjust the pH to 7.5 with NaOH. Autoclave and store at room temperature.
3. NZY broth (1 L): 21 g of NZY powder (Gibco BRL), 2 g of $MgSO_4.7H_2O$. Adjust the pH to 7.5 with NaOH. Use immediately to make NZY top or bottom agar or autoclave and store at room temperature.
4. NZY top agarose: NZY broth with 0.7% agarose. Autoclave and cool to 50°C in water bath prior to use.
5. NZY bottom agar: NZY broth with 1.5% agar. Autoclave and cool to 50°C in water bath prior to pouring plates. Hold plates 2–3 d at room temp before use. Store at 4°C in sealed plastic bag.
6. SM buffer: 100 mM NaCl, 8 mM $MgSO_4$, 50 mM Tris-HCl pH 7.5, 0.01% gelatin. Autoclave and store at room temperature.
7. *E. coli* strain XL1-blue MRF' (Stratagene) (*see* **Note 6**).
8. Isopropylthio-β-D-galactoside (IPTG): 0.5 M in water. Store at –20°C (Boehringer Mannheim).
9. 5-bromo-4-chloro-3-indolyl-β-D-galactopyranoside (X-gal): 250 mg/mL in dimethylformamide (DMF). Store at –20°C in dark (Boehringer Mannheim).

3. Methods

3.1. Isolation of PolyA⁺ RNA from Total RNA (see Note 1)

1. Prepare the column according to manufacturer's instructions and equilibrate in 1X binding buffer.
2. Suspend the RNA sample in water at a concentration of approx 1–2 mg/mL.
3. Heat to 70°C for 3 min then quick cool on ice.
4. Add an equal volume of 2X binding buffer (at room temperature).
5. Immediately apply sample to column. Collect effluent in a 15-mL polypropylene tube. Reapply at least three times.
6. Wash with approx 20 column volumes of 1X binding buffer. Monitor the effluent until the OD_{260} blanked against binding buffer returns to zero.
7. Elute polyA⁺ RNA elution buffer and collect 1 ml fractions in siliconized microfuge tubes. Measure OD_{260} of each fraction (or a small aliquot of each sample).

8. Pool three peak fractions.
9. Heat pooled fractions to 70°C then quick cool on ice.
10. Repeat **steps 4–8** with the pooled fractions, then proceed to **step 12**.
11. Column may be regenerated by washing with two bed volumes of 0.1 *M* NaOH followed by >10 volumes 1X binding buffer (until pH of effluent returns to 7.5).
12. Measure the OD_{260} of the pooled fractions blanked against elution buffer. Calculate the concentration of poly A⁺ RNA and transfer to a 1.5-mL microfuge tubes in approx 5-mg aliquots.
13. Precipitate with 0.1 volume of 3 *M* sodium acetate, pH 5.2 and 2 volumes of 100% ethanol.
14. Place at –20°C for 1 h then spin at >10,000*g* for 30 min in a 4°C microcentrifuge.
15. Discard the supernatant.
16. Wash with 1 mL of 70% ethanol (may be stored in 70% ethanol at –80°C for prolonged periods of time until ready for next step).

3.2. Preparation of Single-Stranded cDNA (see Note 2)

1. Carefully remove the ethanol from 5 µg of poly A⁺ RNA with a pipet and allow the pellet to air dry at room temperature (approx 5–10 min).
2. Resuspend the RNA pellet in 10 µL water.
3. Prepare a first strand reaction mix by combining (on ice): 5 mL of 5X reaction buffer, 1 µL of RNAse inhibitor, 2 µL of dNTP mix, 1 µL of oligo dT primer, 2 µL of [α-^{32}P] dCTP (diluted in 1 µL water), 1.5 µL of 0.1 *M* DTT, water to 15 mL.
4. Heat the resuspended RNA to 70°C for 3 min, quick-cool on ice (30 s) and add to the first strand reaction mix. Stir gently with pipet tip.
5. Add 1 µL of M-MuLV reverse transcriptase. Stir. Incubate at 42°C for 1 h. Near the end of the 1 h incubation, prepare the second strand reaction mix (*see* **Subheading 3.3., step 1**).
6. Heat to 70°C for 15 min. Place on ice. Remove 2 µL for analysis of incorporation (*see* **Note 7**).

3.3. The second-Strand Reaction

1. Second strand reaction mix: 10 µL of 10x DNA Polymerase buffer, 1 µL of undiluted [α-^{32}P] dCTP, 1 µL of RNAse H, 5µL DNA polymerase I, and water to final volume of 76 µL. Hold on ice.
2. Add the completed first strand mix directly to the second strand mix.
3. Incubate at 12°C for 60 min, and 22°C for 60 min. Remove 1 µL for analysis of incorporation.
4. Add 1 µL of DNA Polymerase I Large (Klenow) fragment and incubate for 15 min at room temperature to fill in recessed ends.
5. Heat to 75°C for 10 min. Add an equal volume of phenol chloroform. Vortex. Spin in a microcentrifuge for approx 1 min.
6. Transfer the upper (aqueous) layer to a cDNA spun column equilibrated in TE according to the manufacturer's instructions.

7. Recover the eluted DNA and add 1/10th volume of 3 *M* sodium chloride (pH 5.2) and 2 volumes of ethanol. Mix well and chill at 20°C for 1 h. Spin at >10,000g for 30 min at 4°C.

8. Carefully pipet away the ethanol (*see* **Note 8**). Allow the pellet to air dry.

9. Resuspend the DNA pellet in 10 µL of 10 m*M* Tris-HCl (pH 7.5).

3.4. Introduction of cDNA into a Cloning Vector

1. Add the following directly to the resuspended cDNA: 2 µL of 10x ligation buffer, 1 µL of adaptors (per 5 µg of poly A$^+$ starting material), 1 µL of T4 DNA ligase. Water to final volume of 20 µL. Incubate overnight at 16°C.

2. The next morning, heat to 65°C to inactivate the enzyme. Chill on ice.

3. Add 1 µL of ATP solution and 1 µL of T4 polynucleotide kinase and incubate at 37°C to phosphorylate the cohesive ends.

4. Heat the reaction to 65°C for 10 min. Add TE to a final volume of 100 µL and extract with an equal volume of phenol:chloroform. Ethanol precipitate as described in **steps 7** and **8** above.

5. Resuspend the cDNA in 20 µL of TE. Remove 2 µL for performing test ligations and store the remaining material at –70°C until the results of the test ligations are determined.

6. Dilute the 2-µL aliquot to 5 µL with water and set up three parallel ligation reactions using 2 µL, 1 µL, and 0.5 µL of cDNA according to the following recipe: 0.5 µL of 10x ligase buffer, 0.5 µL of T4 DNA ligase, 1.0 µL of lambda Zap II predigested arms, aliquot of cDNA, and water to 5 µL.

7. Incubate overnight at 14°C.

8. Proceed directly to packaging step, below.

9. When the most efficient ratio of cDNA to phage has been determined, scale up and repeat the ligation and packaging using the rest of the cDNA

3.5. Packaging, Amplification, and Titering

1. Package each of the three ligation mixtures using the manufacturer's instructions. This takes approx 2–3 h. Store at 4°C.

2. Make serial dilutions of an aliquot of the freshly packaged phage in SM buffer. Mix 2 µL of each dilution with 200 µL of host cells OD 0.5 in a 15-mL conical and incubate at 37°C 15–30 min.

3. Add 4 mL of 50°C top agarose to which 20 µL IPTG and 60 µL X-gal has been added. Quickly cap and invert the tube twice then smoothly pour onto a prewarmed 100 mm NZY plate and cover.

4. Allow the agar to solidify approx 20 min. Remove condensation from the lid of the plate with a clean Kim-wipe, invert the plate and place in a 37°C incubator for approx 8 h.

5. When plaques become clearly visible, move the plates to 4°C.

6. Determine the ratio of white (recombinant) to blue (background) plaques for each ligation reaction (*see* **Note 9**).

7. Repeat **steps 2–5** with the packaged library to determine the titer (*see* **Note 10**).

8. To amplify the library, determine size of the aliquot needed to generate 10^5 plaques per plate. Repeat *steps 2–5* to make five 100-mm plates with 10^5 plaques per 100-mm plate. If the library does not contain this many plaques, then just amplify what is available. Once plaques become clearly visible, add several milliliters of SM buffer to each plate leave at 2 h at room temperature or overnight at 4°C with occasional rocking.
9. Pipet the SM buffer into a clean centrifuge tube.
10. Rinse the plates with another 1–2 mL SM buffer and add to the elute in the centrifuge tube.
11. Centrifuge at 7000g for 30 min at 4°C to pellet debris.
12. Transfer into clean microfuge tubes in 0.5–1-mL aliquots with a drop of chloroform in each tube.
13. Check the titer; it should be > 1×10^9 pfu/mL. The library is ready for screening, as described in Chapter 6. It may be stored for months to years at 4°C; however, the titer will drop with time. For prolonged storage, add DMSO to 7% and keep at –70°C indefinitely. Store defrosted aliquots at 4°C. Do not refreeze.

4. Notes

1. A variety of vendors now offer mRNA isolation kits which generally include RNAse free disposable chromatography columns, buffering agents and detailed instructions. These are particularly helpful for avoiding RNAse contamination in laboratories where RNA work is not routinely performed and could probably be used to substitute for the method detailed here. A word of caution: a number of "single-step" kits are available that isolate poly A$^+$ mRNA by incubating cell lysates generated by proteinase K digestion directly with an oligo dT resin and then rapidly washing away contaminants. Although these "single-step" techniques can vastly reduce the amount of time needed to isolate mRNA for use in a variety of applications, in our experience the poly A$^+$ mRNA isolated from vascular cells and tissues using these methods has not been of sufficiently high quality for use in cDNA library construction. Because most vascular tissues contain significant amounts of extracellular matrix, we find that rapid disruption of the tissue in guanidinium thiocyanate is still the preferred method for obtaining high quality RNA. Prior to isolation of poly A$^+$ RNA, the total RNA should be examined by agarose electrophoresis through formaldehyde containing gels followed by staining with ethidium bromide.
2. Pharmacia manufactures a cDNA synthesis kit which includes all of the reagents for synthesis of cDNA, including *Eco*RI/*Not*I adaptors that are ready to be ligated into the cloning vector. We find this to be a tremendous convenience, particularly because it eliminates the need for several of the ethanol precipitation steps, streamlining the method to a two day procedure. A number of vendors manufacture kits with protocols for the production of blunt-end cDNA. Although we have no experience with them, it is reasonable to assume that the blunt-end cDNA generated from these protocols could be incorporated into this protocol at **step 3.4**.

3. A potential problem with libraries constructed from oligo dT-primed cDNA is that certain mRNAs contain significant secondary structure (such as stem loops which may form between complementary stretches of nucleotides in the single stranded mRNA), which prevent the enzyme from generating full-length cDNA transcripts that extend all the way to the 5' end of the mRNA. To circumvent this problem, random hexamers can be added to or used as a substitute for oligo dT primers in the reverse transcription reaction. Although a random-primed cDNA library will most likely lack full-length clones, it will not have the 3' bias of an oligo dT-primed library. With the availability of highly purified reverse transcriptase, cDNA libraries which contain numerous full-length transcripts can be routinely constructed by oligo dT-primed synthesis of cDNA. However, when sufficient mRNA is available, it is still a reasonable precaution to construct both oligo dT- and random-primed libraries from the same RNA sample. We recommend that the oligo dT library be screened first. If full length clones are not obtained, the clone with the largest insert obtained from this screening can then be used as a probe to screen the random-primed library to isolate clones that might extend to the 5' end.

4. DEPC can not be used in solutions that contain Tris.

5. The appropriate choice of vector is dependent on the intended downstream application. A variety of modifications have been introduced into lambda phage to facilitate cDNA cloning. Vectors such as lambda *Zap*II (Stratagene) allow overnight conversion of the phage to a circular phagemid containing the cloned insert. This can save countless hours of subsequent work by eliminating the need to propagate large amounts of phage in order to subclone cDNAs of interest into plasmid vectors. Additional features that have been engineered into various cloning vectors include promoters for expressing the cloned insert in bacteria or mammalian cells.

6. For the bacteria, inoculate 25 mL of LB supplemented with 0.2% maltose and 10 mM MgSO$_4$ in a sterile 50-mL conical and grow overnight at 30°C with shaking. Pellet the bacteria by centrifugation at approx 3000g at 4°C and resuspend in 1/2 column ice cold 10 mM MgSO$_4$. Measure OD$_{600}$ and adjust to 0.5 with 10 mM MgSO$_4$.

7. An essential quality control step is the addition of a small amount of radiolabeled nucleotide to the cDNA synthesis reaction (or to a small scale, parallel reaction). An aliquot of cDNA is then removed in **step 6** and set aside. While proceeding with the second strand reaction and ethanol precipitation, the aliquot is examined by agarose gel electrophoresis and autoradiography and compared to molecular weight standards. A clearly visible smear with a maximum size of greater than 5 kb is characteristic of successful cDNA synthesis from intact poly A$^+$ mRNA. The bulk of the signal should be greater than 1 kb. If this is not the case, it most likely represents a problem with poly A$^+$ mRNA. Rather than proceed with library construction, it is worthwhile to either repeat the poly A$^+$ purification and/or to perform northern blot analysis using 1–2 μg of the poly A$^+$ RNA and probe the blot for either the gene of interest or a housekeeping gene such as alpha-actin to verify that full length transcripts are present.

Most workers monitor the efficiency of the first and second strand reactions by spotting 1 µL of each reaction on DE81 paper before and after the synthesis reactions, washing the "after" filters with phosphate buffer and then scintillation counting *(1)*. Whereas this does provide an accurate measure of the efficiency of the reactions, it does not provide the more relevant information provided by electrophoresis—namely: the prevalence of full-length (or near full-length) transcripts.

8. All of the radioactivity remaining in the tube should be incorporated into the cDNA. Because the DNA pellet may not be visible, it is useful to "track" the DNA with a Geiger counter in the ethanol precipitation steps.

9. Successful ligation of the cDNA into the phage should result in a 10- to 100-fold increase of white colonies compared to background. If this is not achieved, it may be necessary to perform additional test ligations. The ratio of cDNA to phage which results in the highest ratio of white plaques is the ratio to chose for the subsequent scaled-up ligation. It is common for one of the test ligations to have sufficient titer to create a fully representative library

10. The blue/white color selection scheme provides information about the percentage of recombinant clones. We find that prior to amplification, it is worthwhile to determine if a significant percentage of the clones contain potentially full-length transcripts. First, select 10–20 plaques from one of the titering plates and follow the manufacturer's procedure for in vivo excision of the pBluescript phagemid. Prepare mini-prep DNA and digest each sample with *Not*I or *Eco*RI and examine by agarose gel electrophoresis. If many of the plaques contain inserts > 1 kb, then it is worth amplifying the library.

References

1. Sambrook, J., Fritsch, E., and Maniatis, T. (1989) *Molecular Cloning: A Laboratory Manual*, Cold Spring Harbor Laboratory Press, Cold Spring Harbor, NY.
2. Gubler, U. and Hoffman, N. (1983) A simple and very efficient method for generating cDNA libraries. *Gene* **25,** 263–269.
3. Short, J. M., Fernandez, J. M., Sorge, J. A., and Huse, W. D. (1988) Lambda ZAP: a bacteriophage lambda expression vector with in vivo excision properties. *Nucleic Acids Res.* **16(15),** 7583–7600.

6

Screening cDNA Libraries Using Partial Probes to Isolate Full-Length cDNAs from Vascular Cells

Csilla Csortos, Virginie Lazar, and Joe G. N. Garcia

1. Introduction

The purpose of screening cDNA libraries is to isolate a particular cDNA clone encoding a mRNA and by implication, a protein, of interest. The screening is based on identification of the desired clone among a large number of recombinant clones within the library selected *(1,2)*. As an example of both the utility and power of library screening, we will relate our own library screening efforts utilized to isolate the nonmuscle high molecular weight myosin light chain kinase isoform from a human umbilical vein endothelial cell cDNA library *(3)*. This unique nonmuscle myosin light chain kinase isoform phosphorylates myosin light chains, thereby playing an essential role in agonist-mediated endothelial cell contraction, paracellular gap formation and increased vascular permeability. We are hopeful that this step-by-step approach will help the reader to understand the discussed methods.

The following scheme represents a synopsis of the main steps utilized to perform cDNA library screening:

Obtain or generate the cDNA library (*see also* Chapter 5)
↓
plate the library
↓
transfer the library to filter membranes
↓
screen the library
by hybridization to nucleic acid probe or
by immunoreactivity
↓
purify and characterize positive clones

From: *Methods in Molecular Medicine, vol. 30: Vascular Disease: Molecular Biology and Gene Therapy Protocols*
Edited by: A. H. Baker © Humana Press Inc., Totowa, NJ

1.1. Choosing a cDNA Library and Probe

In order to choose the optimal cDNA library for screening, one has to consider the screening strategy, and the frequency of the desired clone. The different type of bacteriophage vectors available for hosting the cDNA libraries exhibit specific characteristics that affect their suitability for different screening strategies *(4)*. For example, cDNA libraries cloned in the λgt 10 vector are suitable for screening with only nucleic acid probes, whereas cDNA libraries generated in λgt 11, also an expression vector, can be screened by both nucleic acid probes as well as by antibody probes. Unfortunately, this added utility of the λgt 11 library is offset by the observation that during amplification of the λgt 11 library some of the recombinants may produce toxic polypeptides which decrease the relative abundance of those recombinants in the library. If the abundance of recombinants are reduced or even lost during amplification, further amplification will not repair the damage.

The frequency of appearance of recombinant clones representing a particular mRNA species in the cDNA library is generally proportional to the abundance of that species in the mRNA population. The expected frequency of the desired RNA among the total mRNA of the cell ranges from 1/1000 to 1/50,000. The amount of the protein in a certain cell type often indicates the abundance of the mRNA. The number of recombinants in the library and the frequency of the expected clone in the library determine the number of bacteriophages that must be screened. In general, one should use the highest density that does not produce confluent lysis. The recommended density of bacteriophages is 20,000–30,000 pfu (plaque forming units)/150 mm plate for first screen.

1.2. Choice of Probe

The type of the probe to be employed might be chosen based on the researcher's goal and the available data, however, the probe must be specific and hybridize only to the desired clones *(5,6)*. There are several methods for generating and labeling the different types of probes. Large DNA pieces might be available for library screening when one seeks to isolate a new isoform of a cloned cDNA or to isolate the analogous cDNA of the same protein in another species, tissue, or cell type. In the latter case, the specific probe can be synthesized by RT-PCR amplification, using oligonucleotide primers based on the known sequence and specific RNA template *(7)*. If short peptide sequences of the protein of interest are accessible, a mixture of synthetic oligonucleotide probes, designed according to the peptide sequence, might be sufficient for library screening *(8)*. The specificity of larger nucleic acid probes is always higher than the specificity of short synthetic oligonucleotide probes. Therefore, as an alternative method, we advise using the synthetic oligonucleotide probes as RT-PCR primers to amplify larger cDNA fragments to serve as more effective probes.

1.2.1. Oligonucleotide Probes

Oligonucleotide probes are used for library screening when only short amino acid sequences are known from the protein of interest. Owing to the degeneracy of the genetic code, degenerate oligonucleotide pools have to be employed. The optimum length of the oligonucleotides in a degenerate pool is approx 17–20 bp. This length is long enough to be specific and short enough not to form mismatched hybrids with cDNAs in the library. We recommend purifying the synthetic oligonucleotides by a spin column before the labeling process and determining the concentration simply by measuring the optical density (OD) at 260 nm. (1 OD unit corresponds to approx 30 μg/mL oligonucleotide concentration). The most commonly used method for labeling is the 5'-hydroxyl end phosphorylation of the oligonucleotide by T4 kinase.

1.2.2. DNA Probes

The most convenient sizes for isolation are 150–1500 bp DNA pieces as they exhibit high specificity with relatively low chance for mismatches. Larger pieces might also be employed; however, the parallel usage of two fragments of a larger piece may give the investigator more information (*see* **Note 1**).

1.3. Expression Libraries

Antibodies recognizing a certain protein are able to identify the desired clones in a recombinant cDNA library *(9,10)*. The DNA inserts are placed in an expression vector and are expressed as fusion proteins. The antibody recognizes the antigenic protein sequence in the fusion protein. However, this recognition does not prove that the DNA insert encodes the protein of interest. Antigenic determinants might be related only at the level of protein structure. Therefore, all positive clones identified by antibody interaction must be verified by an independent method as well.

1.4. Plaque Purification

As it is impossible to pick up a single clone after the first screening step owing to the required high density of bacteriophages, second and third screening steps are necessary. The mixture of bacteriophages, picked from the area where the positive clone was identified, are plated out at lower density—only single plaques should be formed on the plate—and reprobed. If the intensity of the positive signals of the second screening are different, that might indicate the presence of different clones in the first pick. However, this might be the case even when one cannot identify any differences among the signals, indicating it might be beneficial to analyze more than one clone from the second screening.

1.5. Clone Analysis

Different strategies can be employed for the characterization of the positive clones. PCR and/or Southern blot analysis might presort the positive clones of the first screening, especially when dealing with a large number of clones. The purified bacteriophage DNA *(11)* containing the insert of our interest can be sequenced using phage-specific primers. However, the efficiency of the sequencing of the insert in the bacteriophage is low, primarily owing to the relatively small size of the insert compared to the vector. We recommend subcloning the insert into a small plasmid vector before sequencing. It might seem unnecessary to perform this extra step; however, this step will ultimately save a great deal of time when you prepare a large amount of plasmid DNA. The sequencing data may verify the result of screening, particularly if one had previous sequence information. Otherwise the protein of interest, coded by the cloned DNA, has to be expressed and characterized biochemically.

2. Materials

2.1. Library Plating and Transfer

1. LB medium: dissolve 1.0 g of Bacto-tryptone, 0.5 g of Bacto-yeast extract, and 1.0 g of NaCl in 100 mL of water and sterilize by autoclaving.
2. LB Agar: dissolve 1.0 g of Bacto-tryptone, 0.5 g Bacto-yeast extract, 1.0 g of NaCl, and 15 g of Bacto-agar in 100 mL of water and sterilize by autoclaving.
3. Top Agarose: dissolve 1.0 g of Bacto-tryptone, 0.5 g Bacto-yeast extract, 1.0 g of NaCl, and 7.0 g of agarose and dissolve in 1000 mL of water and sterilize by autoclaving.
4. SM buffer: dissolve 2.9 g of NaCl, 1.0 g of $MgSO_4$ and 3.0 g of Tris-HCl in approx 300 mL water, adjust the pH to 7.5 with 2 M HCl, then add 0.05 g of gelatin. Add water up to 500 mL and sterilize by autoclaving.
5. 20X SSPE: dissolve 175.3 g of NaCl, 27.6 g of $NaH_2PO_4.H_2O$, and 7.4 g of EDTA in approx 700 mL of water, adjust the pH to 7.4 with 10 M NaOH. Add water up to 1000 mL and sterilize by autoclaving.
6. 0.5 M NaOH/1.5 M NaCl.
7. 1 M Tris-HCl/1.5 M NaCl.
8. 1 M $MgSO_4$.
9. Maltose.

2.2. Hybridization

1. Rinse buffer: dissolve 6.05 g of Tris-HCl, 0.37 g EDTA (or 1 mL of 0.5 M EDTA, pH 8.0) and 1.0 g of SDS (or 5 mL of 10% SDS) in approx 700 mL water, adjust the pH to 8.0 with 10 M NaOH. Add water up to 1000 mL and sterilize by autoclaving.

2. 50X Denhardt's: dissolve 5.0 g of ficoll (Type 400) and 5.0 g of polyvinylpyrrolidone in water, adjust the volume to 500 mL, then add 5.0 g of gelatin and autoclave.
3. Hybridization buffer: 40 ml of 50X Denhardt's, 60 mL of 20X SSPE, 2 mL of 5% disodium pyrophosphate and 2 mL of 10% SDS in 96 mL of sterile water. Warm in boiling water to dissolve the SDS and filter before use.
4. 20X SSC: dissolve 175.3 g of NaCl and 88.2 g of sodium citrate in approx 700 mL water, adjust the pH to 7.0 with HCl. Add water up to 1000 mL and sterilize by autoclaving.
5. 6X SSC: 300 mL of 20X SSC, 10 mL of 5% disodium pyrophosphate, 10 mL of 10% SDS, and 680 mL of sterile water. Lower X SSC buffers contain the same amount of sodium pyrophosphate and SDS, the amount of 20X SSC decreases appropriately.
6. Herring sperm DNA or yeast torula RNA (Life Technologies, Gaithersburg, MD).

3. Methods

3.1. Plating the cDNA Library (see Note 2)

3.1.1. cDNA Library Stocks

The bacterial host strain depends on the vector, and is provided with the library. Always keep frozen stocks of the host strain (frozen in 15–25% glycerol). For everyday work, prepare a master plate.

1. Streak the bacteria on LB Agar plate (*see* **Note 3**).
2. Incubate overnight at 37°C.
3. Prepare a fresh master plate biweekly and keep at 4°C.

3.1.2. Determination of the Titer of the Library (see Note 4)

Before proceeding with screening, it is critical to check the titer of the library as the titer may drop with storage and the stability varies considerably between libraries and with concentration. In general, the stability of a library is greater when kept at a high titer.

1. Grow the bacterial host culture overnight in 5 mL of LB medium containing 0.2% maltose in a shaker at 37°C. The optical density of the culture should be approx 2.0.
2. Based on the previously determined titer, dilute the library in SM buffer.
3. Add 1 M $MgSO_4$ to the cell culture for a final concentration of 10 mM.
4. Add diluted library to the bacteria as follows:

Tube	Cells	Diluted library
1	300 μL	1 μL
2	300 μL	3 μL
3	300 μL	9 μL

5. Incubate the infected cells at 37°C for 20 min.
6. Add 1 *M* MgSO₄ to 10 mL of top agarose for a final concentration of 10 m*M* (*see* **Note 5**).
7. Add 3 mL of top agarose to each tube of infected cells. Cap the tube and mix by inverting it three times.
8. Pour the mix onto 90-mm LB agar plates (*see* **Note 6**), evenly spread by tilting the plate.
9. Allow the plates to cool at room temperature for 10 min.
10. Invert and incubate the plates at 37°C overnight or 6–8 h depending on the host bacteria.
11. Count the plaques formed and determine the titer using the formula below:

$$\text{pfu/mL} = \text{number of plaques/}\mu\text{L used} \times \text{dilution factor} \times 10^3 \ \mu\text{L/mL}$$

In our experiments, the nonmuscle myosin light chain kinase (MLCK) isoform expressed in human umbilical cord endothelial cells (HUVEC) was cloned from both oligo dT- and random-primed HUVEC cDNA libraries. These libraries were generously provided by David Ginsburg, MD (University of Michigan, Ann Arbor, MI) and were previously utilized to clone human von Willebrand factor (vWF) *(12)*. These libraries were made using the λgt 11 cloning vector and the titer for the libraries at the time of screening was 1–5 × 10⁹ pfu/mL. The bacteria host cell LE392 was utilized to amplify both libraries. This strain of bacteria contains suppressor genes (supE44, supF58), which are especially useful to promote the phage lytic growth when screening the expression libraries. For the most suitable bacteria strain, the investigator is suggested to contact the individual vendors that provides the specific molecular biological products.

3.1.3. Plating the Bacteriophage Library with Transfer to Filter Membranes

The method for plating the library is almost identical to that for library titer determination, with the following differences:

1. Based on the titer of the library and the number of the clones to be screened, determine the volume of the library/150-mm plates × number of the plates. Use approx 30,000 pfu/150-mm plate for first screen.
2. The volume of the top agarose is 12 mL/150-mm plate.
3. As soon as the plaques are formed, place the plates in a plastic bag and refrigerate them (*see* **Note 7**).
4. The transfer of the plaques can be made any time after the plates have cooled down (*see* **Note 8**).

3.1.4. Transfer of the Library to the Membrane

1. Label the nitrocellulose or nylon membranes with a pencil.
2. Cover the bottom of three large dishes with two sheets of Whatman 3M paper.

Wet the 3M papers in the dishes with the buffers as follows:
0.5 *M* NaOH/1.5 *M* NaCl
1 *M* Tris-HCl, pH 8/1.5 *M* NaCl
2X SSPE

3. Place the membrane onto the plate with label facing up for 2 min (*see* **Note 9**). Use forceps or wear gloves. Avoid air bubbles. Mark the orientation of the filter on the plate by stabbing a 20-gauge needle through the filter into the agar close to the edge, at asymmetrical locations.
4. Lift the filter from the plate and place on the 3M papers soaked with NaOH/NaCl for 3 min with the plaque side up.
5. Place the filter on the 3M papers soaked with Tris-HCl/NaCl for 5 min.
6. Place the filter on the 3M papers soaked with 2X SSPE for 5 min.
7. Dry the filters on 3M papers with the plaque side still up.
8. Repeat the whole procedure with the same plate, then with the rest of the plates. It is possible to transfer two plates in parallel.
9. Fix the DNA to the nitrocellulose membrane using an UV crosslinker or by baking at 80°C for 2 h in a vacuum oven. Nylon membranes do not require fixation.
10. Store the membranes at room temperature between filter papers.

For EC MLCK cloning, the oligo dT- and random-primed HUVEC cDNA libraries were plated at a density of 1×10^5 pfu/150-mm plate using a total of 10 plates. Positively charged Nytran membranes (Schleicher Schuell, Keene, NH) were utilized to lift the phage plaques and were subsequently treated according to manufacturer recommendations. These membranes are charged and the phage DNA can be fixed on the membrane under mild alkaline conditions (denaturation step). The membranes consequently were dried overnight at room temperature.

3.2. Probe Hybridization

The hybridization probe is chosen according to the investigator's goal (*see* **Subheading 1.2.**). To avoid nonspecific binding of the probe to the host vector of the library, check the similarity between the sequence of the probe and the vector. Radioactive or nonradioactive labeling of the hybridization probe makes it possible to identify the positive clones in the library (*see* **Notes 10** and **11**).

This step of library screening includes the prehybridization, hybridization, and washing of the filters followed by the detection of the stable hybrids. Prehybridization of the filter membranes with a nonspecific cDNA is required to prevent nonspecific binding of the labeled probe and to decrease the background signal.

3.2.1. Prehybridization

1. Before using the filters, wash them twice in rinse buffer at 42°C for 15 min using a shaker (to remove bacterial cell debris).

2. Prewarm the hybridization buffer. Use approx 25 mL of buffer/10 filters of 13 cm diameter.
3. Boil for 5 min the appropriate amount of sonicated herring sperm DNA or yeast torula RNA to obtain a final concentration of 2 mg/mL or 0.1 mg/mL (respectively), in the hybridization buffer. Then place on ice.
4. Add the appropriate volume of hybridization buffer into one or more Petri dishes (maximum 8–10 filters/dish).
5. Add the herring sperm DNA or the yeast torula RNA and mix.
6. Transfer the wet filters into the dish(es). Be sure that no air remains among the filters.
7. Place the Petri dish into a sealable bag and seal.
8. Prehybridize the filters by placing the bag in a hot-shaker for 2–6 h at 37–42°C (oligonucleotide probe) or 55–65°C (DNA probe).

3.2.2. Hybridization

The hybridization itself is the incubation of the membrane-bound plaques with a solution of the denatured, single-stranded, labeled probe. The probe anneals with its corresponding complementary sequence, resulting in the formation of a hybrid between the labeled probe, and the membrane-bound DNA. However, both related but not homologous and even unrelated interactions may occur. The temperature of the hybridization and the salt concentration of the hybridization solution are two critical variables. During the hybridization step, the salt concentration is always high, indicating low-stringency. The hybridization probe (melting point, degeneracy, and homology of the probe) determines the temperature of hybridization. In general, we want to increase the chance of the formation of the desired hybrid and to minimize the formation of nonspecific hybrids.

1. Prewarm the hybridization buffer.
2. Boil the labeled probe for 5 min and place on ice. Use 1–20 ng DNA probe/mL hybridization buffer, or 0.1–1 ng/each oligonucleotide probe/mL hybridization buffer. The specific activity of ^{32}P-labeled probes have to be >10^7 cpm/mg.
3. Mix the probe and the hybridization buffer in new Petri dish.
4. Transfer the prehybridized filters into the dish containing the probe.
5. Place the dish in a sealable bag and seal.
6. Hybridize the filters overnight in a hot-shaker at 65°C with DNA probe or at a temperature which is 2–5°C below of the melting temperature of the oligonucleotide probe.

3.2.3. Washing

Washing the filters after the hybridization removes the excess probe and probe bound in mismatched hybrids. This reduces the background and the number of the false-positive signals. First, rinse the membranes under low-stringency conditions (low temperature and high salt concentration, e.g., room temperature and 6X SSC, respectively) to remove the excess of the probe, so further hybridization will not occur, then proceed with the higher stringency washes. The positive signals can be detected by autoradiography.

1. Prewarm 6X SSC to the hybridization temperature.
2. Remove the filters from the hybridization solution and rinse them immediately with warm 6X SSC (dispose of the radioactive hybridization buffer properly).
3. Wash the filters twice for 10 min at room temperature in prewarmed 6X SSC with shaking. Use approx 250–300 mL buffer/10 filters of 15 cm diameter.
4. Wash the filters in 6X SSC for 20 min at the hybridization temperature in a hot shaker.
5. Wash the filters in 2X SSC for 20 min at the hybridization temperature in a hot shaker.
6. Check the radioactivity of the filters with a Geiger counter.
7. If the filters show a higher radioactivity than the background, perform an additional wash in 1X SSC for 20 min at the hybridization temperature in a hot shaker (*see* **Note 12**).

3.2.4. Autoradiography

1. Place the wet filters on a used, but blank film and cover with Saran Wrap. Do not allow the filters to dry.
2. Mark the position of the filters by radioactive dye or a fluorescent marker (*see* **Note 13**).
3. Expose the filters to X-ray film at –70°C overnight using intensifying screens.
4. Develop the film. If the background appears too high, perform a wash at higher stringency (use lower salt concentration, 0.2–1X SSC, or higher temperature) and repeat the autoradiography.
5. If the signals are too faint, repeat exposure for 24–72 h.
6. Using the markers align precisely the filters with the autoradiogram, label the points of the needle holes on the filters.
7. Compare the autoradiograms of the duplicate filters. True positive spots must be present on the duplicates in exactly the same place although the intensity of the spots may vary (*see* **Note 14**).

In our experiments to screen the HUVEC cDNA libraries for EC MLCK, we utilized a 3.3 kb cDNA previously subcloned into a pGEM vector which encoded the smooth muscle myosin light chain kinase previously cloned from rabbit *(3)*. This radiolabeled cDNA was utilized as an initial probe to screen the λgt 11 HUVEC cDNA library fixed onto the Nytran membranes. The insert was released from the vector with appropriate restriction enzyme and gel-purified. Approximately 200 ng of DNA representing the purified released insert was random-labeled using a labeling kit (Boehringer Mannheim, IN) with specific activity of 5×10^8 cpm/mg. The prepared Nytran filters were hybridized with the smooth muscle MLCK probe overnight at 65°C in 20–30 mL volume.

3.3. Plaque Purification of the Positive Clones

Since the density of the primary plates does not allow for selecting a single plaque, further (secondary, tertiary) screening steps are necessary. The first screen results generally contain several small libraries, which contain unwanted clones as well as the one (or more) clone that produced the positive signal.

1. Align the autoradiogram with the corresponding plate by the aid of a light box. Cut and remove the area from the plate, which exhibited positive signal using the larger end of a glass Pasteur pipette. The accuracy of the alignment is very important, the positive clones can be lost due to incorrect orientation.
2. Place the "plug" into 1 mL SM buffer containing one drop of chloroform. Let it sit at room temperature for 1 h, vortex every 10–15 min, then keep at 4°C. These are the secondary libraries of the screening. Perform this step even when the first screen provides too many positive clones to investigate at the same time.
3. Determine the titer of the secondary libraries (*see* **Subheading 3.1.2.**).
4. Plate out the secondary libraries at a density of approx 300–600/plate (individual plaques are required), 2–4 plate/library and perform lifting and hybridization as before.
5. Pick the plaque corresponding to the most intense spots on the autoradiogram using a sterile toothpick or the smaller end of a Pasteur pipet, and place into 1 mL of SM buffer containing chloroform.
6. Plate 1 mg of 1-, 10- and 100-fold dilution in SM buffer of this phage stock, carry out lifting and hybridization. Each plaque should hybridize to the probe, other wise this step has to be repeated until the phage is pure (*see* **Note 15**).
7. Make final phage stocks by picking two plaques/clones and store in SM buffer containing chloroform at 4°C.
8. Purify λ-phage using a purification kit (*see* **Note 16**).

3.4. Clone Analysis

The strategy of clone analysis may vary, however, it is recommended to start with a simple restriction analysis utilizing vector-specific enzyme(s) to excise the insert DNA. Separate the digested fragments on an agarose gel and perform Southern blot analysis. Use more than one hybridization probe (from different region of the whole sequence if possible) to gain more information. Based on the size of the cDNA inserts and the result of the Southern blot choose the clones to subclone into a suitable cloning vector for further characterization.

Inserts with similar size and reactivity with the Southern probe(s) may not necessarily be identical. Restriction analysis of the subcloned cDNA helps to recognize identical clones. Use several combinations of restriction enzymes, which do not cut the cloning vector at any site or which cut only at one site. It is very unlikely that two different clones would result in identical restriction maps.

Sequence analysis provides the most definitive feedback of the entire work. Do the analyzed clones contain the sequence which correspond to the known peptide or DNA sequence? Do they span the entire coding region? Do they represent a new isoform? Shall we rescreen the primary library? Probably yes, but based on the result of the first library screening, a more powerful strategy can be employed with a larger variety of probes.

Missing parts of the clone can be amplified by RT-PCR (SuperScript Preamplication System, PCR Reagent System, Life Technology) (*see also* Chapter 15) or RACE-PCR (3' RACE System 5' RACE System, Life Technology, 5'/3' RACE Kit, Boehringer Mannheim) (*see also* Chapter 7). The amplified fragment may serve as an excellent probe to pick the missing clone(s) from the library. Although the validity of the sequence data originated from the lambda phage library is higher, because of the possible mistakes of the PCR amplification, sequencing of the PCR fragments is also safe if high-fidelity enzyme is used. It is always recommended to sequence the DNA fragments in both sense and antisense direction and to compare the sequences of several overlapping clones, whenever it is possible.

In our experiments, positive clones for EC MLCK were identified by identical patterns on duplicate membranes. The plaques corresponding to the signal obtained from the duplicate membranes after the primary screening of the oligo dT-primed HUVEC cDNA library, were individually selected and incubated in the SM buffer overnight. The phage containing the positive EC MLCK inserts were PCR analyzed using a specific primer which was designed from the conserved nucleotide sequences of rabbit, bovine, and chicken smooth muscle MLCK and the λgt 11 vector primers in both reverse and forward orientations. The PCR reactions were run on an agarose gel and the largest positive insert for EC MLCK cDNA was identified. Subsequently, the amplified band was analysed by sequencing and the PCR fragment was subcloned into pBluescript (Ks$^+$ Stratagene LA Jolla, CA) cloning vector. This cycle of continuous screening of the library, sequencing the largest identified clone and designing specific primers for PCR analysis of the positives, was repeated several times using the HUVEC randomly-primed cDNA library until the full length cDNA for EC MLCK was constructed from overlapping fragments.

4. Notes

1. The DNA fragments (PCR product or cut fragment from a plasmid) have to be gel purified before labeling. Load the DNA sample onto a 0.7–1.5% agarose gel and perform electrophoresis. The concentration of the gel depends on the size of the DNA, for the resolution of larger fragments, lower gel concentrations are required. Cut the band of interest from the gel and extract the DNA using a DNA purification kit (Prep-A-Gene, BioRad; Agarose Gel DNA Extraction Kit, Boehringer Mannheim; or Gel Extraction Kit QIAGEN).

2. In most cases, screening an oligo dT-primed cDNA library is sufficient for cloning the desired gene if the transcript size does not exceed 3.0 kb. However, if the transcript size is greater than 3.0 kb as was the case with EC MLCK (8.1 kb), other screening strategies should include randomly-primed cDNA libraries, since these libraries tend to cover more 5' region of the genes than dT-primed libraries.

3. Supplements needed for the bacterial host strain vary with the different strains.

4. The optimum titer for cDNA library is approx 10^9–10^{11} pfu/mL. This is specially important when the abundance of the desired gene is low. Nevertheless, libraries with lower titers can be utilized to clone genes with medium or high abundancy.

5. The top agarose has to be melted completely and kept at 55°C until needed. The top agarose has to be melted completely, but if the top agarose is too warm, this may cause poor bacterial growth.

6. Freshly made plates have to be warmed at 37°C for 20 min. Plates at 4°C need to be incubated at 37°C for 1–2 h to avoid condensation.

7. Since no antibiotics are used and these primary plates will be needed for weeks it is important to take extreme care to avoid contamination.

8. Plaques have to be well formed and the plates cannot be too wet before the transfer to the membrane.

9. Place and lift the membrane with a steady hand and avoid horizontal moving of the membrane in order to produce discrete circles on the autoradiograph, otherwise the identification of the plaques is very difficult.

10. It is essential to purify the probe before labeling, and removing the excess radioactivity, which is not bound in the probe before hybridization is also recommended to minimize the background on the autoradiogram.

11. In general, the chemical principles of the labeling processes are identical, but the detection methods are different. The nonradioactive methods are much safer and several good labeling kits are available. Although they are not less sensitive than the radioactive detection method, the radioactive labeling method more widely utilized as it is cheaper and has proven dependable. Instead of providing one particular recipe for nucleic acid labeling, a brief outline of some commercially available kits are provided (*see* **Table 1**).

12. If the filters still exhibit high radioactivity, repeat the wash in 1X SSC, but increase the temperature by 2–5°C.

13. Fluorescent markers give a sharp signal on the autoradiogram.

14. The amount of radioactive dye to be used has to be optimized in order to get a sharp, strong signal. Precise marking is crucial for the identification of positive plaques.

15. Skipping this step may result the purification of a mixture of phages, confusing restriction analysis, and sequencing data.

16. Efficient and quick lambda DNA purification kits are commercially available (QIAGEN, Stratagene, Promega, etc.).

Table 1
Nucleic Acid Labeling Systems

Labeling kit/company	Application
RTS T4 Kinase Labeling System/Life Technologies	Preparation of radioactive, 5' end-phosphorylated probe.
Random Primers DNA Labeling System/ Life Technologies	Radioactive labeling of DNA. The kit employs Klenow enzyme and random hexamer primers.
PhotoGene System and BioPrime DNA Labeling System/Life Technologies	Generation and detection of biotinylated DNA probes by random priming
DNA 5'-End Labeling Kit/Boehringer Mannheim	Preparation of radioactive, 5' end-phosphorylated probe
Random Primed DNA Labeling Kit/ Boehringer Mannheim	Radioactive labeling of DNA. The kit employs Klenow enzyme and random hexamer primers
DIG/Genius 8 Oligonucleotide 5'-End Labeling Set/Boehringer Mannheim	5'-end labeling of oligonucleotides with digoxigenin
DIG/Genius 1 DNA Labeling and Detection Kit/Boehringer Mannheim	Random primed labeling of DNA with DIG-11-dUTP and detection

References

1. Benton, W. D. and Davis, R. W. (1977) Screening lgt recombinant clones by hybridisation to single plaques in situ. *Science* **196,** 180–182.
2. Huynh, T. V., Young, R. A., and Davis, R. V. (1984) *DNA Cloning: A Practical Approach*, Vol. 1 (D.M. Glover, ed.) pp. 49–78.
3. Garcia, J. G. N., Lazar, V., Gilbert-McClain, L. I., Gallagher, P. J., and Verin, A. D. (1997) Myosin light chain kinase in endothelium: molecular cloning and regulation. *Am. J. Respir. Cell Mol. Biol.* **16,** 489–494.
4. Williams, B. G. and Blasstner, F. R. (1980) Bacteriophage lambda vectors for DNA cloning, in *Genetic Engineering* Vol. 2 (J. K. Setlow and A. Mullander, eds.) p. 201.
5. Denhardt, D. (1966) A membrane filter technique for the detection of complementary DNA. *Biochem. Biophys, Res. Commun.* **23,** 641–646.
6. Southern, E. M. (1975) Detection of specific sequence among DNA fragments separated by gel electrophoresis. *J. Mol. Biol.* **98,** 503–517.
7. Frohman, M. A., Dush, M. K., and Martin, G. R. (1988) Rapid production of full-length cDNAs from rare transcripts: amplification using a single gene-specific oligonucleotide primer. *Proc. Natl. Acad. Sci. USA* **85,** 8998–9002.
8. Lathe, R. (1985) Synthetic oligonucleotide probes deduced from amino acid sequence data. *J. Mol. Biol.* **183,** 1–12.

9. Skalka, A. and Shapire, L. (1976) In situ immunoassays for gene translation produces in phage plaques and bacterial colonies. *Gene* **1,** 65.
10. Young, R. A. and Davis, R. W. (1983) Efficient isolation of genes by using antibody probes. *Proc. Natl. Acad. Sci. USA* **80,** 1194–1198.
11. Benson, S. and Taylor, R. K. (1984) A rapid small-scale procedure for isolation of phage lambda DNA. *Biotechniques* **2,** 126,127.
12. Ginsburg, D., Handin, R. I., Bonthron, D. T., Donlon, T. A., Bruns, G. A., Latt, S. A., and Orkin, S. H. (1985) Human von Willebrand factor (vWF): isolation of complementary DNA (cDNA) clones and chromosomal localisation. *Science* **228,** 1401–1406

7

Cloning Full-Length cDNAs from Vascular Tissues and Cells by Rapid Amplification of cDNA Ends (RACE) and RT-PCR

Rong-Fong Shen

1. Introduction

The isolation of full-length cDNAs remains a frequent task undertaken in many laboratories. A full-length cDNA is often desirable for one of the following purposes: 1) to complete the sequence of a partial cDNA cloned by library screenings or the yeast one- or two-hybrid system; 2) to derive the cDNA sequence encoding a protein, based on peptide sequences; 3) to obtain the sequence of a reported cDNA for functional analysis or expression studies; and 4) to define exon/intron boundaries of a cloned gene or determine transcription start site(s) of a promoter.

Strictly speaking, the term "full-length cDNA" refers to the entire DNA sequence complementary to a mature mRNA, which in most cases consists of a protein coding sequence flanked by the 5' and 3' untranslated regions. Acquiring the end sequences of a cDNA is necessary for such application as those stated in item 4 above. For most other purposes, the isolation of the protein coding sequence with a brief sequence each of the untranslated regions is often sufficient. RACE (rapid amplification of cDNA ends) was introduced 10 years ago by Frohman et al. *(1)* as an efficient way of isolating the ends of a cDNA irrespective of one's prior knowledge of the sequence. Over the years, several modifications have been reported *(2–4)*. RACE takes advantage of the power of polymerase chain reaction (PCR) to amplify trace amounts of the first-strand cDNAs reverse-transcribed from RNA. Because anchored and/or sequence-specific primers are used in nested amplifications, the method is very useful in deriving end sequences of cDNAs of rare transcripts, where alternative methods might be laborious. RACE does not require sophisticated equip-

From: *Methods in Molecular Medicine, vol. 30: Vascular Disease: Molecular Biology and Gene Therapy Protocols*
Edited by: A. H. Baker © Humana Press Inc., Totowa, NJ

ment or expensive reagents. This chapter describes the procedures involved from RNA isolation to the amplification of 5'- or 3'-end of a cDNA by RACE. For the cloning of cDNAs of known sequences, RT-PCR using defined primers is usually the first to be attempted. **Figure 1** briefly outlines steps involved in these approaches.

2. Materials
2.1. RNA Isolation

All buffers need to be sterilized by autoclaving or filtration.

1. DEPC-H_2O: Add 0.2 mL of diethylpyrocarbonate (DEPC) to 100 mL of distilled H_2O and shake rigorously for 2 min. Let the solution stand at room temperature for 1 h before sterilization by autoclaving. Caution: DEPC is a suspected carcinogen and should be handled with care.
2. Denaturing solution: 4 M guanidium thiocyanate, 25 mM citric acid, pH 7.0, 0.5% N-lauryl sarcosine, and 0.1 M 2-mercaptoethanol.
3. DEPC-H_2O-saturated phenol.
4. 3 M NaAc, pH 4.5.
5. RNA Extraction buffer: Combine one volume of denaturing solution, 1 volume of DEPC H_2O-saturated phenol, and 1/15 volume of 3 M sodium acetate, pH 4.5. Mix well by gentle shaking.
6. 2X Binding buffer: 1 M LiCl, 1% SDS, 20 mM Tris-HCl, and 2 mM EDTA, pH 8.0.
7. 1X Binding buffer: Dilute (1:1) 2X binding buffer with DEPC-H_2O.
8. 1X Elution buffer: 0.05% SDS, 10 mM Tris-HCl, and 1 mM EDTA, pH 8.0.
9. Oligo d(T) Column (cat. no. 15939-010, Gibco-BRL, Gaithersburg, MD).
10. Chloroform.
11. Isopropanol.
12. 0.1 N NaOH, 5 mM EDTA, pH 8.0.
13. 5 M NaCl.
14. 100% Ethanol.
15. Polytron homogenizer (Brinkmann).

2.2. cDNA Synthesis, RT-PCR, and RACE

1. 5X Reverse transcription (RT) Buffer: 250 mM Tris-HCl, pH 8.3, 375 mM KCl, 15 mM MgCl$_2$.
2. 10X PCR buffer: 1 M KCl, 200 mM Tris-HCl, pH 9.0, and 20% Triton X-100.
3. Glassmilk (cat. no. 1001-204; BIO 101, CA).
4. 2X Single-strand ligation buffer: 100 mM Tris-HCl, pH 8.0, 20 mM MgCl$_2$, 20 mg/mL BSA, 50% polyethylene glycol (PEG), 2.0 mM hexamine cobalt chloride, 40 mM ATP.
5. Oligo d(T) primer: 17–20mer.
6. 2 mM dNTPs.
7. Moloney murine leukaemia virus reverse transcriptase (MMLV RT).
8. RNAse inhibitor.

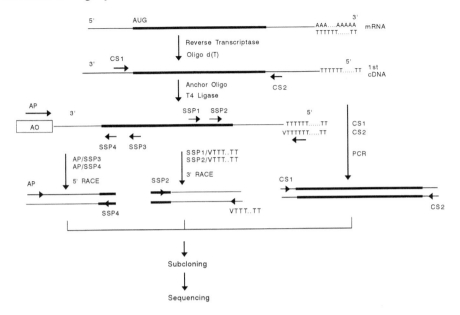

Fig. 1. Outline of Steps Involved in cDNA Amplification by RACE and RT-PCR. mRNA is reverse-transcribed to yield the first-strand cDNA. A single-stranded anchor oligonucleotide, 5' phosphorylated and 3' blocked, is ligated to the first-strand cDNA using T4 ligase. The resulting products are then used as templates in nested PCR reactions (5' or 3' RACE) to obtain end sequences of the cDNAs of rare transcripts. The first-strand cDNA may also be used as the template for direct amplification of the coding sequence using a pair of defined primers. The products are then subcloned and sequenced. The protein coding regions are indicated by thicker lines, while thinner lines are the 5' or 3' flanking sequences. Horizontal arrows indicate primers, pointing from 5' to 3'. CS 1 and 2 are primers for coding sequence amplification. SSP 1-4 are sequence-specific primers. AO, anchor oligonucleotide; AP, anchor primer; V, nucleotide A,G, or C.

9. 50 mM MgCl$_2$.
10. *Taq* DNA polymerase.
11. 4 N NaOH.
12. 4 N acetic acid.
13. 6 N sodium iodide.
14. 80% Ethanol.
15. Glycogen (10 mg/mL).
16. 2 M sodium acetate.
17. T4 RNA ligase.
18. PCR2.1 cloning vector (Invitrogen, CA).
19. T4 DNA ligase.
20. Competent *Escherichia coli* cells (JM109 or equivalent).

21. LB broth: 1% tryptone, 0.5% yeast extract, 1% NaCl (all available from Gibco BRL). Adjust the pH to 7.5 with NaOH. Autoclave and store at room temperature.
22. 10 mM isopropylthio-β-D-galactoside (IPTG).
23. 20 mg/mL 5-bromo-4-chloro-3-indolyl-β-D-galactopyranoside (X-gal) in dimethyl-formamide.
24. LB ampicillin plates: Add 15 g/L agar to 1 L of LB broth, autoclave and allow to cool. Add ampicillin to 50 µg/mL when at 60°C and pour.
25. T7 or M13 sequencing primers.

3. Methods

Both total RNA and poly(A) RNA have been successfully used in RACE and RT-PCR. The RNA isolated by the acid guanidinium thiocyanate procedure *(5)* produces sufficiently high quality RNA for the synthesis of the first-strand cDNA by reverse transcription (RT). For the amplification of sequences from rare transcripts, the use of poly(A) RNA is recommended.

3.1. Total RNA Isolation (see Note 1)

1. Collect vascular cells (2–5 × 10⁷) by centrifugation in a sterile polypropylene tube.
2. Wash the cells once with PBS and lyse with 2 mL of RNA extraction buffer.
3. Homogenize the lysate with a Polytron homogenizer, equipped with a small probe, for three times (10 s each) to shear the chromosomal DNA. (For vascular tissues, use 1 mL of the RNA extraction buffer for each 100 mg of tissue and homogenize directly as in **Subheading 3.1., step 3** [*see* **Note 2**]).
4. Add 1/10 volume of chloroform to the homogenate and vortex vigorously.
5. Centrifuge at approx 2800g for 30 min at 4°C in a table-top centrifuge.
6. Remove the aqueous layer into a new tube and add an equal volume of isopro-panol. Mix and precipitate at room temperature for 10 min.
7. Pellet the RNA by centrifugation at 2800g for 10 min at 4°C.
8. Rinse the pellet once with 70% ethanol and dry in a Speedvac for 5 min (*see* **Note 3**).
9. Resuspend the pellet in DEPC-H$_2$O and determine the concentration. The RNA can be used immediately or stored at –80°C.

3.2. Poly(A)⁺ RNA Purification (6)

1. Prewash an oligo d(T)-cellulose column with 1 ml of 0.1 N NaOH and 5 mM EDTA, pH 8.0 and equilibrate with 1X binding buffer in four 1 mL aliquots.
2. Apply 1 mL of 1X binding buffer to the column and allow 0.5 mL to flow through by gravity.
3. Denature 1–2 mg of RNA from **Subheading 3.1., step 9** at 65°C for 5 min then add an equal volume of 2X binding buffer.
4. Load the sample onto the column and wash the column with 4 mL of 1X binding buffer.
5. Elute the bound poly(A) RNA with 1.5 mL of 1X elution buffer.
6. Precipitate the RNA by adding 3/50 volumes of 5 M NaCl and 2 volumes of ice-cold 100% ethanol. Vortex briefly and store at –20°C for at least 1 h. Recover the RNA as in **Subheading 3.1., step 7**.

3.3. Synthesis of the First Strand cDNA

1. Mix RNA (5 µg of total RNA or 1 µg mRNA) with 0.1 µg of oligo d(T) primer (17–20mer) in an Eppendorf tube.
2. Denature the RNA/primer mix at 75°C for 2 min.
3. Chill on ice and add the rest of components to the tube:
     RNA/primer mix form **step 2**:
     4 µL of 5X RT buffer
     1 µL of 2 mM dNTP
     0.5 µL of RNasin (20 U)
     1 µL of MMLV reverse transcriptase (200 U)
     add H$_2$O to 20 µL (final volume).
4. Incubate the mixture at 42°C for 1 h.
5. Inactivate the reverse transcriptase activity by heating at 94°C for 5 min. Chill on ice for 2 min and flash spin the tube for 10 s in an Eppendorf centrifuge.
6. Store at –80°C until use (this is "first strand cDNA").

3.4. PCR-Amplification of the Coding Sequence (CS) Using Defined Primers of a Reported Sequence

1. Prepare a cocktail solution by mixing the followings:
     5 µL of 10X PCR buffer
     3 µL of 50 mM MgCl$_2$
     10 µL of 2 mM dNTP
     1 µL of *Taq* polymerase (2.5 U)
     1 µL (0.1 µg) of primer CS1 (*see* **Note 4**)
     1 µL (0.1 µg) of primer CS2 (*see* **Note 4**)
     29 µL of water
     50 µL total volume
2. Set up tubes containing the following components for PCR:
     10 µL of the above cocktail solution
     4 µL of the first-strand cDNA from **Subheading 3.3., step 6**
     6 µL of water
     20 µL final volume
3. Carefully overlay with 20 µL of mineral oil on top of each tube.
4. Amplify for 30 cycles under the following conditions (*see* **Note 5**):
     1st cycle:
       Denaturing: 94°C, 3 min
       Annealing: 55°C, 3 min
       Extension: 72°C, 3 min
     Cycles 2–29:
       Denaturing: 94°C, 1 min
       Annealing: 55°C, 1 min
       Extension: 72°C, 1 min
     30th cycle:
       Extension: 72°C, 10 min

5. Take 5 µL of the amplified sample to check for presence of the desired product by agarose gel electrophoresis.
6. Freeze the sample or go on to **Subheading 3.7.** for cloning.

3.5. 3' RACE Using Sequence-specific Primers (SSP) and an V(T)₁₉ Oligomer

1. Prepare a cocktail solution by mixing the followings:
   5 µL of 10X PCR buffer
   3 µL of 50 mM MgCl₂
   10 µL of 2 mM dNTP
   1 µL of *Taq* polymerase (2.5 U)
   1 µL of V(T)₁₉ (*see* **Note 6**) primer (0.1 µg)
   1 µL of primer SSP1 (*see* **Note 6**) (0.1 µg)
   <u>29 µL of water</u>
   50 µL final volume
2. Set up tubes containing the following components for PCR:
   10 µL of the cocktail solution from **Subheading 3.5.**, **step 1**
   4 µL of the first-strand cDNA from **Subheading 3.3.**, **step 6**
   <u>6 µL of water</u>
   20 µL final volume
3. Carry out the PCR reaction, as in the **Subheading 3.4.**, **steps 3** and **4**.
4. Dilute amplified products 100 times with H₂O.
5. Prepare a cocktail as in **Subheading 3.5.**, **step 1**, but substitute SSP1 with SSP2 (*see* **Note 6**).
6. Set up second PCR reaction tube as in **Subheading 3.5.**, **step 2**, but substitute the first strand cDNA with 4 µL the diluted product from **Subheading 3.5.**, **step 4**.
7. Amplify and examine as in **Subheding 3.4.**, **steps 3–5**.
8. Freeze the amplified products at –80°C or continue to **Subheding 3.7.** for subcloning.

3.6. 5' RACE with SSP and an Anchor Primer (AP)

3.6.1. Purification of the Synthesized First-Strand Synthesized cDNAs

1. Synthesize the first-strand cDNA as in **Subheading 3.3.**, but hydrolyze the RNA by the addition of 2 µL of 4 N NaOH. Incubate at 65°C in a water bath for 10 min.
2. Neutralize by the addition of 2 µL of 4 N acetic acid.
3. Bring the volume of the solution up to 30 µL with 6 µL of DEPC-H₂O and flash spin for 10 s in an Eppendorf centrifuge.
4. Add 75 µL of 6 N NaI solution, followed by 5 µL of a 50% glassmilk.
5. Mix by inverting the tube and keep the tube on ice for 10 min.
6. Centrifuge at full speed for 15 s and discard the supernatant.
7. Wash the pellet three times by resuspending it in 500 µL of 80% EtOH.
8. Spin at room temperature for 15 s. Discard the supernatant and air-dry the pellet for 5 min.

9. Resuspend the pellet with 50 µL DEPC-H$_2$O by gentle stirring with a pipet tip. Incubate for 10 min at 65°C.
10. Spin for 2 min and transfer the supernatant containing the cDNA into a new tube.
11. Add 1.5 µL glycogen (10 mg/mL), 5 µL of 2 *M* sodium acetate, and 100 µL EtOH to the tube, briefly vortex, and precipitate at –20°C for 30 min.
12. Centrifuge at 4°C for 20 min. Carefully remove and discard the supernatant.
13. Rinse the pellet with 40 µL of 80% EtOH.
14. Spin the tube at room temperature for 2 min. Remove the supernatant and air-dry the pellet for 5 min.
15. Resuspend the pellet in 6 µL DEPC-H$_2$O.

3.6.2. Ligation of an Anchor Oligo (AO) to the cDNAs (see **Notes 7** and **8**)

1. Set up the following ligation mixture:
   2.5 µL of cDNA from step **Subheading 3.6.1., step 15**
   2.0 µL of AO (4 pmol)
   5.0 µL of 2X single-strand ligation buffer
   0.5 µL of T4 RNA ligase (20U/µL)
   10.0 µL total volume
2. Mix by pipeting up and down several times
3. Incubate at room temperature for 16–22 h. Use immediately or store at –80°C.

3.6.3. Amplification with AP and 3' Sequence Specific Primers, SSP3, and SSP4

1. Set up the following reaction mixture:
   5 µL of 10X PCR buffer
   4 µL of 25 m*M* MgCl$_2$
   1 µL of 10 m*M* dNTP
   1 µL of AO-anchored cDNA from **Subheading 3.6.2., step 3**
   1 µL of SSP3 (*see* **Note 7**) (10 µ*M*)
   1 µL of AP (*see* **Note 7**) (10 µ*M*)
   36 µL H$_2$O
   49 µL final volume
2. Place in a 90°C heat block for 3 min. Remove the tube and cool to room temperature.
3. Add 1 µL (2.5 U) of *Taq* polymerase, mix by gentle stirring with a pipet tip.
4. Amplify as in **Subheading 3.4., steps 3** and **4**.
5. Following amplification, spin the tube at full speed for 30 s.
6. Pipet, from the bottom of the tube, 2 µL of the reaction products into a new tube containing 98 µL H$_2$O. Vortex and take 1 µL into a new PCR tube containing the same components as in **Subheading 3.6.3., step 1** except that the anchored cDNA is omitted and SSP3 is substituted with SSP4 (*see* **Note 7**).
7. Repeat **Subheading 3.6.3., steps 2–5**.
8. Subclone the amplified products following steps in **Subheading 3.7.** (*see below*).

3.7. Subcloning of Amplified cDNAs

1. Set up the following ligation reaction in an Eppendorf tube:
   1 µL amplified cDNAs from **Subheading 3.4., step 6**; **Subheading 3.5., step 8**; or **Subheading 3.6.3., step 7**
   1 µL 10X ligation buffer
   1 µL pCR2.1 vector
   6 µL H_2O
   <u>1 µL DNA ligase (4 U)</u>
   10 µL final volume
2. Incubate at 16°C overnight or at least 4 h.
3. Add 100 µL competent *E. coli* cells to the mixture and incubate on ice for 30 min. Add 1 mL of LB broth and incubate at 37°C for 1 h.
4. While incubating, add 35 µL each of IPTG (10 m*M* in H_2O) and X-gal (20 mg/mL in DMF) on top of LB/ampicillin plates and spread dry.
5. Plate transformed *E. coli* onto the LB agar plates and incubate at 37°C overnight.
6. Select up to 20 white colonies and grow each in 2 mL LB broth overnight.
7. Isolate miniprep plasmid DNA from each culture and digest DNA with appropriate enzymes (e.g., *Eco*RI) to determine the sizes of inserts.
8. Carry out sequencing analysis on at least ten candidate clones using T7 or reverse M13 (both on the pCR2.1 vector) as sequencing primers (*see* **Note 9**).
9. Products from 5' and 3' RACE can be used to assemble a full length cDNA, if primers SSP2 and SSP4 are selected so that the amplified products overlap.

4. Notes

1. All glassware should be baked at least 3 h and gloves worn all the time when handling RNA (*see also* Chapter 4).
2. For a large piece of frozen tissue, grinding under liquid N_2 facilitates homogenization and increases the yield of RNA (*see also* Chapter 4).
3. An over-dried RNA pellet is hard to get back into solution. So, stop drying as long as no apparent liquid is left and the ethanol is completely evaporated
4. CS1 and CS2 are designed according to a published sequence. Oligos of 20-base are usually good enough for this purpose. CS1 should begins at least 10 bases from the translation initiation site so that the Kozak sequence *(7)* for efficient translation is included, while CS2 can be in the 3' UTR or contains at least 10 bases of the 3' UTR. For cDNAs up to 1.5 kb, this simple RT-PCR cloning works efficiently. For those greater than 1.5 kb, a second amplification using nested primers and an aliquot of a diluted product from the first amplification (e.g., 1:20 dilution) increases the chance of specific amplification.
5. The PCR conditions here works well with cDNAs up to 1.5 kb. For those greater than 1.5 kb or rich in G/C content, the conditions may need to be optimized. A 1- to 2- degree increase in denaturing temperature sometimes significantly affects the amplification efficiency.
6. SSP1 and SSP2 are often derived from a partial cDNA sequence. The two oligos may be independent or having up to 10-bases of overlapping in sequence. Oligos

20 bases or longer work well. For subcloning into specific restriction sites, the recognition sequences can be incorporated into the 5' end of SSP2 or $V(T)_{19}$.

7. AO can be a custom-made 35 to 45-base oligomer, which should be 5' phosphorylated and 3' blocked, either by a dideoxynucleotide or an 3'-amino nucleotide. A restriction site can be introduced at the 5' end of AO. AP are designed complementary to the 3' 25–30 bases of AO. A restriction site, if desired, can be added to the 5' end of AP. SSP3 and SSP4 are 20 to 30-base gene specific primers. Best results are obtained when SSP3 and SSP4 are selected so that the amplified products are between 150 and 400 bp. A restriction site, similar to AO or AP, can be incorporated into the 5' end of SSP4 for ease of cloning. Examples of AO and AP, which have been used successfully in our laboratory *(8,9)* are those in the 5' AmpliFinder RACE kit (Clontech, CA).

8. AO-anchored double-stranded cDNAs from several tissues/cell lines ready for amplification with the AP and gene specific primers are available from Clontech.

9. SSP1, SSP3, or the anchor primer can be used as well. This should yield several identical or overlapping clones different only at the 5' sequences. The information will allow determination of the 5' end or ends (due to multiple transcription initiation) of the mRNAs.

References

1. Frohman M.A., Dush, M. K., and Martin, G.R. (1998). Rapid production of full-length cDNAs from rare transcripts: Amplification using a single gene-specific oligonucleotide primers. *Proc. Natl. Acad. Sci. USA* **85,** 8998–9002.

2. Harvey R. J. and Darlison, M. G. (1991) Random-primed cDNA synthesis facilitates the isolation of multiple 5'-cDNA ends by RACE. *Nucleic Acid Res.* **19,** 4002.

3. Frohman M. A. (1993) Rapid amplification of complementary DNA ends for generation of full-length complementary DNAs: thermal RACE. *Meth. Enzymol.* **24,** 340–356.

4. Dumas J. B., Edwards, M., Delort, J., and Mallet J. (1991) Oligodeoxyribonucleotide ligation to single-stranded cDNAs: a new tool for cloning 5' ends of mRNAs and for constructing cDNA libraries by in vitro amplification. *Nucleic Acid Res.* **19,** 5227–5232.

5. Chomczynski, P. and Sacchi, N. (1987) Single-step method of RNA isolation by acid guanidinium thiocyanate-phenol-chloroform extraction. *Anal. Biochem.* **162,** 156–159.

6. Aviv, H. and Leder, P. (1972) Purification of biologically active globin messenger RNA by chromatography on oligothymidylic acid-cellulose. *Proc. Natl. Acad. Sci. USA* **69,** 1408–1412.

7. Kozak M. (1991) Structural features in eukaryotic mRNAs that modulate the initiation of translation. *J. Biol. Chem.* **266,** 19,867–19,870.

8. Lee, K.-D., Baek, S. J., and Shen, R.-F. (1994) Cloning and characterization of human thromboxane synthase gene promoter. *Biochem. Biophys. Res. Comm.* **201,** 379–387.

9. Zhang, L., Xiao, H., Schultz, R. A. and Shen, R.-F. (1997) Genomic organization, chromosomal localization and expression of the murine thromboxane synthase gene (*Tbxas1*). *Genomics* **45,** 519–528.

8

Use of cDNA Representational Difference Analysis to Identify Disease-Specific Genes in Human Atherosclerotic Plaques

Kerry Tyson and Catherine Shanahan

1. Introduction

Changes in gene expression underlie many biological phenomena, including cellular differentiation and activation, embryonic development, and pathological processes. In recent years, much attention has been focused on the identification of genes that are differentially expressed between normal and disease states: the isolation of disease-specific genes is not only essential for our understanding of the molecular basis of pathological conditions, but may potentially highlight novel therapeutic targets.

Our work has focused on the isolation of disease-specific genes from human atherosclerotic plaques, using RNA extracted from aortic tissue samples. A major constraint on the design of our experiments was the limited amount of human tissue available to us, and the quantity and quality of the RNA that we were able to extract from such pathological samples. Delays in obtaining and processing the tissue samples inevitably lead to a partial degradation of the RNA by cellular ribonucleases, affecting both the quality and yield of RNA. Indeed, the yield of RNA from aortic tissue is relatively low, even in the absence of apparent degradation. Thus, the selection of an experimental strategy that would allow efficient use of the material in hand was necessary. Here we describe cDNA representational difference analysis (cDNA RDA) *(1)*, a polymerase chain reaction (PCR)-based technique, that has allowed us to isolate several disease-specific clones using only microgram quantities of RNA *(2)*.

From: *Methods in Molecular Medicine, vol. 30: Vascular Disease: Molecular Biology and Gene Therapy Protocols*
Edited by: A. H. Baker © Humana Press Inc., Totowa, NJ

1.1. Approaches to Isolating Differentially Expressed Genes

Initial approaches to the cloning of differentially expressed mRNAs relied on the construction of cDNA libraries coupled to techniques such as differential hybridization *(3–5)*. However, these techniques are both time consuming and labor intensive, and furthermore require the isolation of large amounts of high-quality polyA$^+$ RNA for the construction of representative libraries. More recently, the development of several PCR-based techniques, such as differential display RT-PCR (DDRT-PCR) *(6)*, serial analysis of gene expression (SAGE) *(7)* and cDNA RDA, have obviated the need for substantial amounts of starting material, making the isolation of differentially expressed genes from limited sources of mRNA possible.

Of the three PCR-based techniques listed above, the most widely used in the current literature is DDRT-PCR *(6)* (*see* Chapter 9), which relies on the direct visual comparison of randomly amplified fragments from the two cDNA populations of interest: differences in the banding pattern generated by a particular pair of primers from the two cDNA samples is indicative of differential gene expression. Whereas DDRT-PCR has been used successfully to identify differentially expressed genes in some pathological conditions *(8–12)*, it presents some important technical problems. These include the isolation of false-positive clones, which on further investigation prove not to be differentially expressed, and the requirement for multiple PCRs with different primer combinations to obtain the full spectrum of differentially expressed genes. In addition, the use of an oligo-dT primer for PCR amplification generates fragments from the 3' ends of transcripts, which may consequently hinder the identification and characterization of the PCR product. Furthermore, the success of DDRT-PCR relies on the reproducibility of banding patterns generated by a particular primer pair from similar samples. However, we found that identical PCRs, using cDNAs derived from different tissue pieces of the same pathological state, gave very different results, making it impossible to identify true differences when comparing healthy and diseased samples. This is most probably due to variation between the individual samples, reflecting the complex nature of the atherogenic process, and demonstrates that precise classification of pathological specimens is essential when using DDRT-PCR.

SAGE *(7)* is a technique that allows the rapid analysis of thousands of genes by amplifying and sequencing small expressed sequence tags (ESTs). This technique requires only small amounts of total RNA (5 µg) as the starting material, and can both identify the genes expressed by a particular cell type and provide information on the relative abundance of transcripts within the mRNA population. However, the sequence tags generated are small and located at the 3' end of transcripts, and so provide little sequence information of novel genes that are amplified. Unlike DDRT-PCR, there are few examples in the literature of this technique being used to identify differentially expressed genes *(13–15)*.

In contrast to DDRT-PCR and SAGE, cDNA RDA *(1)* is a positive selection technique that couples subtractive hybridization to PCR amplification, an approach that has several advantages over DDRT-PCR and SAGE. First, only sequences that are differentially expressed are amplified, avoiding the need for comparison of PCR fragments and reducing the isolation of false-positive clones. Second, the subtractive hybridization steps generate a difference product representing all of the differentially expressed genes that are amplified in a single reaction. In addition, unwanted difference products can be eliminated during the hybridization step *(1,16)*. Furthermore, the fragments generated by RDA are more likely to include sequences derived from the open reading frame of the cDNA, facilitating the identification of clones and providing useful information for novel cDNAs. Finally, cDNA RDA allows the isolation of clones representing rarely expressed mRNAs *(17)*, and has been used to clone differentially expressed genes from a variety of systems *(16,18–21)*.

1.2. Overview of cDNA RDA

We have used cDNA RDA to isolate differentially expressed genes from human atherosclerotic plaques, using only minimal amounts of total cytoplasmic RNA. Although on first reading this technique may appear complicated, in reality it involves only PCR, restriction digests, and ligations, which are techniques commonly used in most laboratories.

It is worth noting that in our experiments using total RNA, some fragments derived from 18S and 12S rRNAs and ribosomal protein S4 RNA were cloned from the final difference product. As expected, these sequences were not differentially expressed between our two RNA samples, and thus represent false-positive clones. However, we have been able to identify several plaque-specific genes, some of which represent rarely expressed mRNAs, demonstrating that cDNA RDA is an efficient means of detecting differentially expressed genes when only small amounts of total RNA are available.

cDNA RDA can be divided into three steps:

1. the generation of "representative amplicons" (the starting material for subtractive hybridization),
2. hybridization and selective amplification of differentially expressed sequences, and
3. cloning, sequencing, and identification of "difference products."

The first two steps are illustrated schematically in **Fig. 1** and are described in **Subheading 1.2.1.**

A

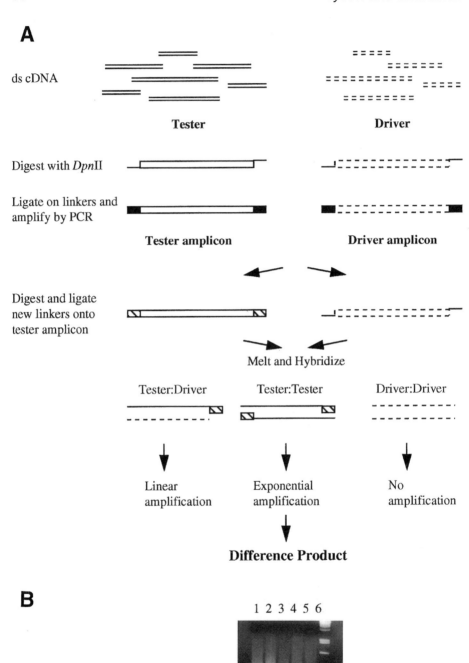

ds cDNA

Tester   **Driver**

Digest with *Dpn*II

Ligate on linkers and
amplify by PCR

Tester amplicon   **Driver amplicon**

Digest and ligate
new linkers onto
tester amplicon

Melt and Hybridize

Tester:Driver   Tester:Tester   Driver:Driver

Linear   Exponential   No
amplification   amplification   amplification

Difference Product

B

1 2 3 4 5 6

1.2.1. Generation of Representative Amplicons

In this step, double-stranded cDNA is synthesized from the two mRNA populations of interest: the sample containing the target genes is referred to as the tester, whilst the sample containing sequences common to both populations is referred to as the driver. Only small amounts of RNA are required as the cDNA is amplified by PCR to generate sufficient material for the subsequent hybridization step. To achieve this, the ds cDNA is digested with a four-cutter restriction enzyme (*Dpn*II), ligated to adaptors containing binding sites for PCR primers and amplified to produce the tester and driver "amplicons." The frequency of restriction sites for a four-cutter enzyme (approx every 256bp), ensures that the majority of cDNAs will contain at least one *Dpn*II fragment and thus be "represented" in the final amplicon. In addition, digesting the ds cDNAs decreases the size of the fragments to be amplified. This is important for achieving efficient amplification of all the sequences in an amplicon. PCR is most efficient at amplifying short sequences, and thus large cDNAs tend to be under-represented when amplifying full-length cDNAs. Digesting the cDNA to liberate small fragments ensures that even large cDNAs are represented in the tester and driver amplicons.

1.2.2. Hybridization and Amplification

Selective amplification of sequences unique to the tester amplicon is achieved by ligating new adaptors, with different PCR primer binding sites, onto the tester amplicon fragments prior to hybridization with an excess of driver. Sequences that are common to the two amplicons form tester:driver hybrids and are amplified linearly in the subsequent PCR step: these single-stranded molecules are eliminated by treating the PCR mixture with mung bean

---

Fig. 1. (**A**) Schematic representation of cDNA RDA. Tester and driver cDNAs are represented by solid and dashed lines, respectively. Following digestion with *Dpn*II, R-oligonucleotides (black boxes) are ligated onto both samples and the fragments are amplified by PCR to generate the representative amplicons. The hatched boxes represent the J- (or N-) oligonucleotides that are ligated onto the tester amplicon, allowing selective amplification of tester sequences following hybridization with an excess of driver. The technique is illustrated up to the generation of the first difference product. To generate second and third difference products, the product is reintroduced at the hybridization stage, increasing the ratio of driver:tester as described in the method. (**B**) Agarose/EtBr gel illustrating the different steps of cDNA RDA. Lanes 1 and 2 contain PCR-amplified *Dpn*II fragments derived from healthy (driver) and diseased (tester) aortic tissue RNA samples, respectively. Lanes 3–5 contain the difference products obtained after each of three successive rounds of subtractive-hybridization and amplification, using tester: driver ratios of 1:100, 1:800 and 1:400,000, respectively. The difference products in lane 5 were subsequently cloned and sequenced (*2*). Lane 6 contains a DNA size marker.

nuclease. Only those sequences that are unique to the tester, and therefore of interest, are amplified exponentially. Thus, the reaction is enriched for sequences unique to the tester amplicon. Further enrichment is achieved by repeating the hybridization and amplification steps a further two times, increasing the ratio of driver:tester in each hybridization.

Figure 1B shows the results of an experiment to identify genes expressed in human atheromatous plaques. Tester and driver amplicons were generated using cDNA derived from diseased and healthy aortic tissue samples, respectively. The complexity of the tester amplicon decreased with each successive round of subtraction and amplification, resulting in a final difference product containing discrete bands. Twenty-eight different fragments were cloned from the final difference product, and included fragments from genes expressed by macrophages, T cells, and vascular smooth muscle cells (VSMC) *(2)*. Thus, we were able to isolate markers from the different cell types found in human atheromatous plaques. Several fragments representing unknown genes were also isolated and are currently under investigation.

2. Materials

2.1. RNA

If sufficient material is available, polyA$^+$ RNA should be used as the template for cDNA synthesis. However, for our experiments we used total cytoplasmic RNA extracted from diseased and healthy aortic tissue samples, with only minor modifications to the basic technique. The tissue pieces were digested with collagenase and elastase, prior to RNA extraction (*see* Chapter 4).

2.2. Oligonucleotides

1. The following oligonucleotides are required:
   R-Bgl- 12: 5'-GATCTGCGGTGA-3'
   R-Bgl-24: 5'-AGCACTCTCCAGCCTCTCACCGCA-3'
   J-Bgl- 12: 5'-GATCTGTTCATG-3'
   J-Bgl-24: 5'-ACCGACGTCGACTATCCATGAACA-3'
   N-Bgl- 12: 5'-GATCTTCCCTCG-3'
   N-Bgl-24: 5'-AGGCAACTGTGCTATCCGAGGGAA-3'

The oligonucleotides should be desalted and resuspended in water at a stock concentration of 5 µg/µL (*see* **Note 1**).

2.3. Enzymes

1. *Dpn*II (10 U/µL), New England Biolabs Inc., Beverly, MA.
2. Mung Bean Nuclease (10 U/µL), New England Biolabs Inc.
3. T4 DNA ligase (3 U/µL), Promega Corp., Madison, WI.
4. *Taq* DNA polymerase (5 U/µL), Promega Corp.

5. MMLV reverse transcriptase (200U/μL), Promega Corp.
6. RNAse H (0.5 U/μL), Promega Corp.
7. DNA polymerase I (5 U/μL), Promega Corp.

2.4. Buffers and Reagents

All solutions, glassware, and pipet tips for the synthesis of cDNA should be free from RNAse. Solutions should be made with Diethyl pyrocarbonate (DEPC)-treated water *(22)*. All buffers and reagents should be stored at room temperature unless otherwise stated.

1. Oligo-dT (12-18) primer (1 μg/μL).
2. 5 mM dNTPs, store at –20°C.
3. 0.1 M Dithiothreitol (DTT), store at –20°C.
4. 0. 1 M ATP, store at –20°C.
5. 10X first strand buffer: 0.5 M Tris-HCl, pH 7.6, 0.7 M KC1, 0.1 M MgCl$_2$, store at –20°C.
6. 5X second strand buffer: 35 mM MgCl$_2$, 0.5 M Tris-HCl, pH 7.4, 75 mM (NH$_4$)$_2$SO$_4$, store at –20°C.
7. EE × 3 buffer: 30 mM EPPS (N-[2-hydroxyethyl]-piperazine-N'-3-propane-sulfonic acid), pH 8.0 at 20°C, 3 mM ethylenediaminetetra-acetic acid disodium salt (EDTA).
8. TE buffer: 10 mM Tris-HCl, pH 8.0 at 20°C, 1 mM EDTA.
9. 10X PCR buffer: 500 mM KC1, 100 mM Tris-HCl, pH 9.0 at 25°C, 1.0% Triton-X-100, 15 mM MgCl$_2$.
10. 10 M Ammonium acetate.
11. 3 M Sodium acetate, pH 5.3.
12. 5 M NaCl.
13. 50 mM Tris-HCl, pH 8.9.
14. Phenol/chloroform/isoamyl acohol (IAA) (25:24:1), store at 4°C.
15. Chloroform/isoamyl alcohol (IAA) (24: 1), store at 4°C.
16. 100% and 70% (v/v) ethanol.
17. Isopropanol.
18. 4 mM dNTPs, store at –20°C.
19. Yeast tRNA (5 μg/μL in TE), store at –20°C.
20. Glycogen (1 μg/μL in water), store at –20°C.
21. 1.2% Agarose in 1X TBE/EtBr prep-gel (*see* **Note 2**).
22. 10X loading buffer: 0.25% bromophenol blue, 0.25% xylene cyanol FF, 15% Ficoll type 400.
23. Sterile distilled water.

3. Methods

3.1. Synthesis of Double-Stranded cDNA

Double stranded cDNA should be prepared using an oligo-dT primer using 5 μg polyA$^+$ RNA from both tester and driver samples (*see* **Note 3**). Care should be taken to ensure that the cDNA is of a good size (*see* **Note 3**). 2 µg of ds cDNA from both tester and driver are required (*see* **Note 4**). The method for generating ds cDNA described below is modified from the procedure of Gubler and Hoffman *(22,23)*. An oligo-dT primer is used to prime synthesis of the first cDNA strand to generate a cDNA:RNA hybrid. Nicks are introduced into the RNA strand of the hybrid molecules by RNAse H, generating initiation sites for nick translation by DNA polymerase I. The fragments of the second strand are then ligated together to generate double stranded cDNAs.

3.1.1. First Strand Synthesis

1. Mix together in an Eppendorf, 5 µg polyA$^+$ RNA and sufficient DEPC-treated water to bring the volume to 21 µL.
2. Heat to 65°C for 10 min and then place immediately on ice.
3. Briefly spin the tube to collect any condensate.
4. To the denatured RNA, add: 5 µL 10X first-strand buffer; 10 µL oligo-dT (12–18) (1 µg/µL); 10 µL 5 m*M* dNTPs; 2 µL 0.1 *M* DTT; 2 µL MMLV reverse transcriptase. Mix by gently pipeting and incubate at 37°C for 1 h.

3.1.2 Second-Strand Synthesis

1. To the first strand reaction, add the following: 20 µL 5X second-strand buffer, 2 µL RNAse H, 10 µL DNA polymerase I, and 68 µL water. Mix by gently pipeting and incubate at 16°C for 4 h.
2. To the second-strand reaction, add: 1.5 µL 0.1 *M* ATP and 3 µL T4 DNA ligase. Mix by pipeting and incubate at room temperature for 30 min.
3. Extract the sample with an equal volume of phenol/chloroform/IAA.
4. Precipitate the ds cDNA by adding 1/10 volume of 3 *M* NaAc, pH 5.3 and 2.5 volumes of 100% ethanol.
5. Mix and incubate at –20°C for 20 min.
6. Centrifuge the sample at 14,000 *g* and at 4°C for 15 min.
7. Wash the pellet with 70% ethanol, dry, and resuspend in 20–50 µL of TE buffer.

3.2. Generation of Representative Amplicons

Perform the following digestion, ligation and amplification on both tester and driver cDNA samples.

3.2.1. Digestion of Double-Stranded cDNA with DpnII

1. Mix together: 2 µg cDNA, 10 µL 10X *Dpn*II buffer, and 5 µL *Dpn*II and add sterile water to make the volume up to 100 µL.
2. Incubate at 37°C for 2–4 h.
3. Extract each sample twice with an equal volume of phenol/chloroform/IAA, and once with an equal volume of chloroform/IAA.
4. Precipitate the cDNA fragments by adding 2 µL of glycogen (1 µg/µL), 50 µL of 10 *M* NH$_4$OAc and 650 µL of 100% ethanol. Mix and incubate on ice for 20 min, then spin in a minifuge for 15 min at 14,000 *g* and at 4°C.

5. Wash the pellet with 500 µL of 70% ethanol. Air dry the pellet until the residual ethanol has evaporated and then resuspend the DNA in 20 µL of TE.

3.2.2. Ligation of Adaptors

Using the digested cDNA samples from the previous step:

1. Mix together: 12 µL *Dpn*II digested cDNA (approx 1.2 µg), 4 µL R-Bgl-24 oligo (2 µg/µL), 4 µL R-Bgl-12 oligo (1 µg/µL), 6 µL 10X ligase buffer, and 31 µL water.
2. Anneal the oligos by heating the reaction in a PCR machine to 50°C for 1 min, then cool to 10°C over 1 h (*see* **Note 5**).
3. Add 3 µL of T4 DNA ligase and incubate at 15°C overnight.

3.2.3. Amplification (see **Notes 6** and **7**)

1. Dilute the tester and driver ligations from **Subheading 3.2.2.** by adding 140 µL of TE. Prepare 20–30 reactions (200 µL each) for both tester and driver. This should generate approx 0.5 mg of each representative amplicon.
2. For each reaction, mix together in a 0.5-mL Eppendorf: 158 µL water, 20 µL 10x PCR buffer, 17 µL 4 m*M* dNTPs, 2 µL R-Bgl-24 oligo (1 µg/µL), and 2 µL diluted ligation.
3. Overlay the reactions with mineral oil, place the tubes in a PCR machine and run the following program: Dissociate the 12-mer by heating to 72°C for 3 min. Add 1 µL *Taq* DNA polymerase and incubate at 72°C for 5 min to fill in the ends. Then 20 cycles of: 1 min at 95°C and 3 min at 72°C. Followed by 10 min at 72°C.
4. Combine each set of reactions separately (four reactions per 1.5-mL Eppendorf) and extract twice with 700 µL of phenol/chloroform/IAA, and once with 700 µL of chloroform/IAA.
5. Precipitate the DNA by adding 75 µL of 3 *M* NaOAc, pH 5.3 and 800 µL of isopropanol, mix and incubate on ice for 20 min.
6. Spin for 15 min at 14,000*g* at 4°C. Wash the pellet with 500 µL of 70% ethanol, air dry and resuspend at 0.5 µg/µL (*see* **Notes 8** and **9**).

3.3. Digestion of Representations

This step removes the adaptors ligated onto the tester and driver amplicons in **Subheading 3.2.2.**, and should be performed on both amplicons.

1. Mix together: 600 µL representative DNA (approx 300 µg), 140 µL 10X *Dpn*II buffer, 100 µL *Dpn*II, and 560 µL water.
2. Incubate at 37°C for 4 h.
3. Divide the digest into 2X 700 µL aliquots and extract twice with 700 µL of phenol/chloroform/IAA, and once with 700 µL of chloroform/IAA. Precipitate the DNA by adding 70 µL of 3 M NaOAc, pH 5.3 and 700 µL of isopropanol. Mix and incubate on ice for 20 min, then spin at 14,000*g* and 4°C for 15 min. Wash the pellet with 500 µL of 70% ethanol. Air dry the pellet and resuspend in water at a concentration of 0.5 mg/mL.

The DRIVER is now ready for hybridization. The TESTER amplicon requires purification and the addition of new adaptors.

3.4. Preparation of TESTER Amplicon for Hybridization

In this step the tester amplicon is purified on an agarose prep-gel to remove the digested adaptors. The tester fragments are then ligated to new adaptors, containing different PCR primer binding sites, that will allow selective amplification of tester sequences following the subtractive hybridization.

1. Mix 40 μL (approx 20 μg) of the digested tester representation with 50 μL of TE and 10 μL of 10× loading buffer, and load onto a 1.2% agarose/TBE/EtBr prep-gel. Electrophorese the sample until the bromophenol blue has migrated about 2 cm. The digested adaptors, which migrate at approx 25 bp, should be clearly separated from the amplicon.
2. Excise the gel slice containing the amplicon, leaving behind the digested adaptors. Purify the amplicon from the agarose gel slice, using either electroelution or a commercially available purification kit (*see* **Note 10**).
3. Precipitate or elute the DNA and adjust the final volume to 120 μL with TE. Estimate the concentration by running a small sample on a 1.3% agarose/EtBr gel (*see* **Note 11**).
4. Mix together: 2 μg gel purified tester DNA, 6 μL 10× ligase buffer, 4 μL J-Bgl-24 (2 μg/μL), 4 μL J-Bgl-12 (1 μg/μL), and add water to make the volume up to 57 μL.
5. Anneal the oligos by heating the reaction in a PCR machine to 50°C for 1 min, then cool to 10°C over 1 h (*see* **Note 5**).
6. Add 3 μL of T4 DNA ligase and incubate at 15°C overnight.
7. Dilute the J-ligated TESTER by adding 120 μL of TE, to give an approximate concentration of 10 ng/μL.

3.5. Subtractive Hybridization

1. Mix 80 μL (40 μg) of digested DRIVER from **Subheading 3.3.**, with 40 μL of diluted, J-ligated TESTER (0.4 μg) from **Subheading 3.4.** Extract once with an equal volume of phenol/chloroform/IAA, and once with an equal volume of chloroform/IAA.
2. Add 30 μL of 10 M NH_4OAc, 380 μL of 100% ethanol, mix, and precipitate at −70°C for 20 min. Spin at 14,000g and at 4°C for 15 min. Wash the pellet twice with 500 μL of 70% ethanol, spinning between each wash, and air dry the pellet.
3. Resuspend the pellet thoroughly in 4 μL of EE × 3 buffer by pipeting for 2 min, followed by incubation at 37°C for 5 min. Vortex the mixture, spin to the bottom of the tube and transfer to a 0.5-mL Eppendorf. Overlay the sample with mineral oil.
4. Place the tube in a PCR machine and denature by heating to 98°C for 5 min. Cool the sample to 67°C, in the PCR machine, and then immediately add 1 μL of 5 *M* NaCl directly to the DNA. Hybridize at 67°C for at least 20 h.

3.6. Generation of First Difference Product

In this step sequences unique to the tester sample are selectively amplified in two stages. The hybridization mix is diluted and subjected to a few rounds of amplification. The PCR mixture is then treated with mung bean nuclease to remove single-stranded DNA molecules, as these represent the amplification products of sequences common to both tester and driver. The remaining ds DNA molecules are then further amplified to generate the first difference product.

1. Remove the annealed DNA from under the mineral oil and dilute by adding 8 µL of TE containing 5 µg/µL of yeast RNA. Mix well by pipeting. Add 25 µL of TE, mix by pipeting, and finally add 362 µL of TE to bring the final volume to 400 µL. Vortex to mix.

2. Set up four PCRs as follows: 20 µL diluted hybridization mix (from above), 20 µL 10× PCR buffer, 17 µL 4 mM dNTPs, and 140 µL water. Overlay the sample with mineral oil, place in a PCR machine and run the following program: Dissociate the 12-mer by incubating at 72°C for 3 min. Add 1 µL of *Taq* DNA polymerase and incubate at 72°C for 5 min to fill in the ends. Add 2 µL J-Bgl-24 (1 µg/µL). Then 10 cycles of: 1 minute at 95°C and 3 min at 70°C. Followed by 10 min at 72°C.

3. Combine the four reactions and extract twice with 700 µL of phenol/chloroform/IAA, and once with 700 µL of chloroform/IAA. Precipitate the DNA by adding 2 µL of glycogen (1 µg/µL), 75 µL of 3 M NaOAc, pH 5.3, 800 µL of Isopropanol and incubating on ice for 20 min. Spin at 14,000 g and at 4°C for 15 min. Wash the pellet with 500 µL of 70% ethanol. Air dry the pellet and resuspend in 40 µL of 0.2X TE. This sample is now treated with mung bean nuclease.

4. Mix together: 20 µL DNA, from above, 14 µL water, 4 µL 10 × mung bean nuclease buffer, and 2 µL mung bean nuclease. Incubate at 30°C for 35 min, then terminate the reaction by adding 160 µL of 50 mM Tris-HC1, pH 8.9 and incubating at 98°C for 5 min to denature the enzyme. Place the tube on ice.

5. Set up four PCRs as follows: 20 µL mung bean nuclease treated DNA, from above, 140 µL water, 20 µL 10× PCR buffer, 17 µL 4 mM dNTPs, and 2 µL J-Bgl-24 (1 µg/µL). Overlay the sample with mineral oil, place in a PCR machine and run the following program: 1 min at 95°C to denature the DNA, then cool to 80°C and add 1 µL *Taq* DNA poymerase. Then 18 cycles of: 1 min at 95°C and 3 min at 70°C. Followed by 10 min at 72°C.

6. Combine the four reactions and extract twice with 700 µL of phenol/chloroform/IAA, and once with 700 µL of chloroforom/IAA. Precipitate the DNA by adding 75 µL of 3 M NaOAc, pH 5.3, 800 µL of Isopropanol and incubating on ice for 20 min. Spin at 14,000g and at 4°C for 15 min. Wash the pellet with 500 µL of 70% ethanol, air dry, and resuspend in 50 µL of TE. Adjust the concentration to 0.5 mg/mL.

This is the *first difference product.*

3.7. Changing Adaptors on a Difference Product

1. Mix together: 40 µL (20 µg) of first difference product, 215 µL water, 30 µL 10 × *Dpn*II buffer, 15 µL *Dpn*II, and incubate at 37°C for 2–4 h.
2. Extract twice with 300 µL of phenol/chloroform/IAA, and once with 300 µL of chloroform/IAA. Precipitate by adding 33 µL of 3 *M* NaOAc, pH 5.3 and 800 µL of 100% ethanol. Mix and incubate at –20°C for 20 min. Spin at 14,000*g* at 4°C for 15 min, then wash the pellet with 500 µL of 70% ethanol. Air dry the pellet and resuspend in TE to a concentration of 0.5 µg/µL.
3. Dilute 1 µL of the digested first difference product DNA to 50 ng/µL by adding 9 µL of TE. Mix together: 4 µL diluted DNA (200 ng), from above, 39 µL water, 6 µL 10× ligase buffer, 4 µL N-Bgl-24 (2 µg/µL), and 4 µL N-Bgl-12 (1 µg/µL).
4. Place in a PCR machine and anneal the oligos by heating to 50°C for 1 min, and then cooling to 10°C over 1 h (*see* **Note 5**).
5. Add 3 µL of T4 DNA ligase and incubate at 15°C overnight.
6. Dilute the N-ligated DNA by adding 100 µL of TE, to give a concentration of 1.25 ng/µL.

3.8. Generation of Second Difference Product

1. Mix together: 40 µL (50 ng) of diluted N-ligated DNA, from **Subheading 3.7.**, 80 µL (40 µg) of DRIVER, from **Subheading 3.3.**, and repeat the subtraction and amplification steps in **Subheadings 3.5.** and **3.6.**

3.9. Generation of Third Difference Product

1. Digest 20 µg of the second difference product with *Dpn*II as described in **Subheading 3.7.** Repeat the ligation step, using J-oligos.
2. Dilute the J-ligated second difference product to 1 ng/µL by adding 140 µL of TE. Then dilute 10 µL of this with 990 µL of TE containing 30 µg of yeast RNA, to give a final DNA concentration of 10 pg/µL.
3. Mix together: 10 µL (100 pg) of diluted J-ligated DNA, from above, and 80 µL (40 µg) of DRIVER, from **Subheading 3.3.** and repeat the subtraction and amplification steps in **Subheadings 3.5.** and **3.6.** above, increasing the final number of PCR cycles from 18 to 22.

3.10. Cloning and Identificiation of Final Difference Products

The final difference product may contain several bands, which can be agarose gel-purified or shotgun cloned into a T/A cloning vector. Alternatively, the DNA fragments may be digested with *Dpn*II prior to purification and cloned into a compatible site (e.g., *Bam*HI, *Bgl*II, *Bcl*I) in a suitable vector (*see* **Note 12**).

Confirmation of differential expression may be obtained in several ways (*see* **Notes 13–17**).

4. Notes

1. O'Neill and Sinclair *(17)* report that HPLC purification of the adaptor oligonucleotides, to remove truncated molecules, reduces the isolation of false-positive clones.
2. A 1.2% agarose prep-gel in 1 × TBE is required for purification of the tester amplicon from the adaptor oligonucleotides. The wells should be able to accommodate a 100 µL sample volume.
3. There are several commercially available kits for the synthesis of double stranded cDNA. We used the Pharmacia cDNA synthesis kit (Pharmacia Biotech Inc., Uppsala, Sweden), and monitored cDNA synthesis by incorporation of $[\alpha\text{-}^{32}P]dCTP$ into the first strand, followed by alkaline agarose gel electrophoresis *(22)*. Undegraded polyA+ RNA should yield firststrand cDNA molecules in the size range of 700–8,000 nucleotides. The yield of ds cDNA can be calculated by diluting 1 µL of the cDNA sample in 100 µL of water, and measuring the absorbance at 260 nm (an absorbance of 1.0 is equivalent to a concentration of 50 µg/mL).
4. For our experiments, we synthesized ds cDNA from total cytoplasmic RNA extracted from healthy and diseased aortae. 5 µg of total RNA was used as the template for cDNA synthesis. The entire sample was used in the generation of representative amplicons.
5. The adaptor oligonucleotides are allowed to anneal by denaturing at 50°C and then slowly cooling to 10°C over 1 h. This is best achieved by incubating the annealing reaction in a PCR machine that is programmed to cool from 50–10°C incrementally, i.e., cooling by 0.6°C/min. Alternatively, the annealing reaction can be left on the bench to cool to room temperature and then placed on ice.
6. The amount of material generated by the amplification of representations is usually sufficient to serve as both tester and driver in reciprocal subtractions.
7. When using total RNA as the starting material, it may be necessary to increase the number of cycles of amplification to obtain 0.5 mg DNA. Increase the number of cycles to 20–21 cycles. If this does not generate sufficient material, consider using more RNA in the cDNA synthesis reaction.
8. We recommend measuring the concentration of samples at all stages to ensure that the correct amount of material is used for each step. Dilute 1 µL of the DNA sample in 100 µL of water and measure the absorbance at 260 nm (an absorbance of 1 is equivalent to 50 µg/mL for ds DNA). As phenol extraction and precipitation of DNA samples results in a loss of material, the volume of water/TE required to resuspend pellets to a given concentration may need adjusting. As a rough guide, assume 50% loss of DNA when resuspending pellets, and adjust the volume after measuring the concentration.
9. At most stages in the protocol an excess of amplified material is generated. It is advisable to store any unused samples at –20°C, as these provide a backup should any of the subsequent steps fail.
10. The tester DNA can be purified from the agarose gel slice using a commercially available kit such as QIAEX II (Qiagen, Chatsworth, CA) or Wizard PCR Preps (Promega Corp., Madison, WI). Alternatively, the DNA may be

electroeluted from the gel slice *(22)*, phenol/chloroform/IAA extracted and ethanol precipitated.

11. Estimating the concentration of the gel-purified tester amplicon is easily achieved by running a small aliquot of the tester alongside a known volume of the driver from **Subheading 3.3.** (i.e., 2 µL of driver = 1 µg DNA), and comparing the intensity of the ethidium bromide staining.

12. The final difference product often contains multiple bands which may be cloned in several ways. We found that in addition to a few bands that were clearly visible on an agarose/EtBr gel (*see* **Fig. 1B**), the final difference product also contained a number of minor species. To clone these fragments we digested the final difference product with *Dpn*II and randomly ligated the fragments into the *Bam*HI site of pBluescript KS(+) (Stratagene, La Jolla, CA). We were then able to sequence the cloned fragments using the T3 and T7 primers.

13. The cloned fragments may be used to probe a Southern blot of the Tester and Driver amplicons. We found that this was a useful way of confirming differential expression for most of the cloned difference products prior to sequencing. However, some of the cloned fragments could not be detected by this technique, presumably because they were present at a very low level in the tester and driver amplicons.

14. If sufficient material is available, differential expression may be demonstrated by Northern analysis. This provides more accurate information about the relative levels of expression than probing the tester and driver amplicons. As an alternative to Northern analysis, we also probed virtual Northern blots to analyze expression of our difference products (*see* **Note 15**).

15. We have used virtual Northern analysis to confirm the differential expression of some of our disease-specific clones. To do this we used Clontech's SMART PCR cDNA synthesis kit (Clontech Laboratories Inc., Palo Alto, CA) to generate and amplify cDNA from the two RNA samples used in our experiments. The cDNAs were Southern blotted and probed using the cloned difference products.

16. The ability of cDNA RDA to detect rarely expressed mRNAs can present difficulties when trying to confirm differential expression by Northern analysis. In such cases we have usually been able to confirm differential expression by RT-PCR. However, this requires sequencing of the cloned fragments before differential expression can be verified.

17. The next logical step is to sequence the cloned difference products: the identity of the differentially expressed genes can then be determined by searching available databases. If novel genes are identified, the cloned fragments can be used as probes to screen cDNA libraries to try and obtain a full length cDNA clone. Alternatively, additional sequence information may be obtained by RACE experiments (*see* Chapter 7).

References

1. Hubank, M. and Schatz, D. (1994) Identifying differences in mRNA expression by representational difference analysis of cDNA. *Nucl. Acids. Res.*, **22**, 5640–5648.

2. Tyson, K. L., Weissberg, P. L., and Shanahan, C. M. Unpublished observations.
3. Duguid, J. R., Rohwer, R. G., and Seed, B. (1988) Isolation of cDNAs of scrapie-modulated RNAs by subtractive hybridization of a cDNA library. *Proc. Natl. Acad. Sci.,* **85,** 5738–5742.
4. Duguid, J. R. and Dinauer, M. C. (1990) Library subtraction of cDNA libraries to identify differentially expressed genes in scrapie infection. *Nucl. Acids Res.,* **18,** 2789–2792.
5. Shanahan, C. M., Weissberg, P. L., and Metcalfe, J. C. (1993) Isolation of gene markers of differentiated and proliferating vascular smooth-muscle cells. *Circ. Res.,* **73,** 193–204.
6. Liang, P. and Pardee, A. B. (1992) Differential display of eukaryotic messenger RNA by means of the polymerase chain reaction. *Science,* **257,** 967–971.
7. Velculescu, V. E., Zhang, L., Vogelstein, B., and Kinzler, K. W. (1995) Serial analysis of gene expression. *Science,* **270,** 484–487.
8. Utans, U., Liang, P., Wyner, L. R., Kamovsky, M. J., and Russell, M. E. (1994) Chronic cardiac rejection: identification of five upregulated genes in transplanted hearts by differential mRNA display. *Proc. Natl. Acad. Sci.,* **91,** 6463–6467.
9. Hu, E., Liang, P., and Spiegelman, B. M. (1996) AdipoQ is a novel adipose-specific gene dysregulated in obesity. *J. Biol. Chem.,* **271,** 10,697–10,703.
10. Lee, I. J., Soh, Y. J., and Song, B.J . (1997) Molecular characterization of fetal alcohol syndrome using mRNA differential display. *Biochem. Biophys. Res. Comm.,* **240,** 309–313.
11. Li, Y. L. and Youssoufian, H. (1997) MxA overexpression reveals a common genetic link in four Fanconi anemia complementation groups. *J. Clin. Invest.* **100,** 2873–2880.
12. Patel, I. R., Attur, M. G., Patel, R. N., Stuchin, S. A., Abagyan, R. A., Abramson, S. B., and Amin, A. R. (1998) TNFα convertase enzyme from human arthritis-affected cartilage: Isolation of cDNA by differential display, expression of the active enzyme and regulation of TNFα. *J. Immunol.,* **160,** 4570–4579.
13. Velculescu, V. E., Zhang, L., Zhou, W., Vogelstein, J., Basrai, M. A., Bassett, D. E., Hieter, P., Vogelstein, B., and Kinzler, W. (1997) Characterization of the yeast transcriptome. *Cell,* **88,** 243-251.
14. Madden, S. L., Galella, E .A., Zhu, J. S., Bertelsen, A. H., and Beaudry, G. A. (1997) SAGE transcript profiles for p53-dependent growth regulation. *Oncogene,* **15,** 1079–1085.
15. Gonzalez-Zulueta, M., Ensz, L. M., Mukhina, G., Lebovitz, R. M., Zwacka, R. M., Engelhardt, J.F., Oberley, L. W., Dawson., V. L., and Dawson, T. M. (1998) Manganese superoxide dismutase protects nNOS neurons from NMDA and nitric oxide-mediated neurotoxicity. *J. Neurosci.,* **18,** 2040–2055.
16. Wada, J., Kumar, A., Ota, K., Wallner, E. I., Batlle, D. C., and Kanwar, Y. S. (1997) Representational difference analysis of cDNA of genes expressed in embryonic kidney. *Kidney Int.,* **51,** 1629–1638.
17. O'Neill, M. J. and Sinclair, A.H. (1997) Isolation of rare transcripts by representational difference analysis. *Nucl. Acids Res.* **25,** 2681,2682.

18. Don, M. and Manuelidis, L. (1996) Visualization of viral candidate cDNAs in infectious brain fractions from Creutzfeldt-Jakob disease by representational difference analysis. *J. Neurovirol.* **2,** 240–248.
19. Niwa, H., Harrison, L. C., DeAizpurua, H., and Cram, D. S. (1997) Identification of pancreatic beta cell-related genes by representational difference analysis. *Endocrinology* **138,** 1419–1426.
20. Gress, T. M., Wallrapp, C., Frohme, M., MullerPillasch, F., Lacher, U., Friess, H., Buchler, M., Adler, G., and Hoheisel, J. D. (1997) Identification of genes with specific expression in pancreatic cancer by cDNA representational difference analysis. *Genes Chromosomes and Cancer* **19,** 97–103.
21. Tajima, Y., Tashiro, K., and Camerini, D. (1997) Cloning of human chromosome 17-specific cDNAs using representational difference analysis and human-mouse hybrid cells. *Genomics* **42,** 353–355.
22. Sambrook, J., Fritsch, E. F., and Maniatis, T. (1989) *Molecular Cloning: A Laboratory Manual.* 2nd ed., Cold Spring Harbor Laboratory Press, New York.
23. Gubler, U. and Hoffman, B. J. (1983) A simple and very efficient method for generating cDNA libraries. *Gene* **25,** 263.

9

The Use of Differential mRNA Display (DDRT-PCR) to Identify Genes Differentially Expressed in Normal and Diseased Vascular Cells

Paul J. Adam

1. Introduction

In 1992 a new approach for identifying differentially expressed genes was described by Liang and Pardee *(1)*. Their method allowed the simultaneous differential display of mRNA from two or more cell types by means of the polymerase chain reaction (PCR). In a subsequent study demonstrating the technique Bauer, et al. *(2)* named it differential display reverse transcription PCR (DDRTPCR) in accordance with the series of steps required to identify differences in gene expression. Differential mRNA display offered a number of advantages over existing cDNA library hybridization based methods used to identify differentially expressed genes. Firstly, screening is fast, reproducible, and technically easier than existing protocols, especially since cDNA libraries do not need to be constructed. Secondly, PCR amplification not only detects low abundance mRNA species, but also allows the comparison of gene expression from very small amounts of starting material such as vascular biopsies.

The basic principles underlying DDRTPCR are illustrated in **Fig. 1**. Small amounts of total RNA are required from each of the cell or tissue samples being compared. The RNA is reverse transcribed using specific oligo(dT) anchored primers, each of which only allows a fraction of the total mRNA to be converted to cDNA. Each set of cDNAs are subdivided further by forty PCR cycles using the original oligo(dT) anchored primer in combination with an arbitrary decamer and an annealing temperature of 42°C. The manageable number (50–100/reaction) of radiolabeled cDNAs generated by this PCR step can then be "displayed" on a standard 6% acrylamide DNA sequencing gel. Each primer combination provides a unique banding pattern, or fingerprint,

From: *Methods in Molecular Medicine, vol. 30: Vascular Disease: Molecular Biology and Gene Therapy Protocols*
Edited by: A. H. Baker © Humana Press Inc., Totowa, NJ

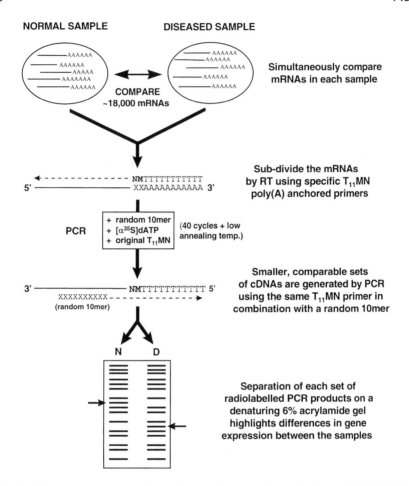

Fig. 1. Schematic representation of the basic principles underlying DDRTPCR. The two sets of mRNA transcripts being compared are initially divided into 12 sets of cDNAs by reverse transcription using each of 12 T$_{11}$MN 3' anchored primers. These are subdivided further by PCR amplification using the same T$_{11}$MN primer, an arbitrary decamer primer, and a low annealing temperature. The PCR products from these reactions can then be resolved by 6% acrylamide gel electrophoresis to "display" a distinct banding pattern; differences in banding between the samples being compared highlights differences in gene expression.

which can be independently analyzed for every sample being compared. Differentially displayed bands can be isolated from the gel, re-amplified with the original primer combination, then used as probes for Northern blots to confirm differential expression (refer to Chapter 16) and sequenced. Further characterization of differentially displayed PCR products can include; isolating the full-length transcript by either screening a cDNA library (*see* Chapters 5 and 6) or by RACE (*see* Chapter 7); using *in situ* hybridisation to localise the expression of the differentially expressed gene in normal and diseased vascular tissue (*see* Chapter 17).

To date, there are a number of studies which have successfully applied differential mRNA display to the identification of genes differentially expressed in normal and diseased vascular tissue *(3–5)*. The following protocol has been used to isolate differentially expressed vascular smooth muscle cell (VSMC) genes. However, modifications to the method described do exist and where relevant have been outlined in **Subheading 4.**

2. Materials

2.1. Isolation and Preparation of RNA Samples

1. Diethylpyrocarbonate (DEPC). DEPC is an inhibitor of RNase's and is commonly used for the treatment of solutions and equipment which are to be used for RNA work. DEPC-treated H_2O is prepared by adding 1 ml DEPC to 500 mL distilled H_2O, shake vigorously and let stand at room temperature for 1 h. Autoclave the solution to inactivate the remaining DEPC. This compound is highly toxic.
2. DNase digestion buffer: 10 mM Tris-HCl, pH 7.8, 50 mM KCl, 1.5 mM MgCl$_2$. Store at 4°C.
3. Recombinant ribonuclease inhibitor (RNasin), 20 units/µl (Promega). Store at –20°C.
4. RNase-free DNase 1, 1 unit/µl (Promega). Store at –20°C.
5. 1:1 phenol/chloroform, pH 7.8, RNase free. Store at 4°C. This mixture is toxic.
6. 3 M sodium acetate, pH 4.8, RNase free.
7. 100% and 70% ethanol.
8. A spectrophotometer or equivalent, suitable for measuring the optical density at 260 nm (OD$_{260}$) of RNA solutions.

2.2. Reverse Transcription (RT)

1. M-MLV reverse transcriptase, 200 U/µL (Gibco BRL). Store at –20°C.
2. 5× reverse transcription buffer (supplied with M-MLV RT enzyme): 250 mM Tris-HCl, pH 8.3, 375 mM KCl, 15 mM MgCl$_2$, 100 mM DTT. Store at –20°C.
3. 0.1 M DTT. Store at –20°C.
4. Pre-mixed deoxynucleotide triphosphates (dNTPs) (200 µM each of dATP, dTTP, dCTP, dGTP). 100 mM stocks of each dNTP can be obtained from Pharmacia Biotech.
5. 50 µM oligo(dT) anchored primers (*see* **Note 1**). A set of 12 nondegenerate $T_{11}MN$ primers (where M = A, C, or G, and N = A, C, G, or T) can be synthesised. Alternatively, a set of 4 degenerate $T_{12}VA$ primers (where V is threefold degenerate for G, C, or A) can be used (GenHunter Corp.). Store at –20°C.

2.3. Polymerase Chain Reaction (PCR)

1. 0.5 mL thick-walled PCR reaction tubes (GeneAmp, Perkin Elmer).
2. A programable PCR thermal cycler. Use in a fume-hood when thermal cycling reactions containing (α-^{35}S)dATP (*see* **Note 2**).
3. 200 μM premixed dNTPs (as used in **Subheading 2.2.**).
4. *Taq* DNA polymerase (5–10 U/μL). Store at –20°C.
5. 10× PCR buffer (MgCl$_2$-free): 500 mM KCl, 100 mM Tris-HCl , pH 9.0, 1.0% Triton X-100. This is often supplied with *Taq* enzyme (Promega).
6. 20 mM MgCl$_2$.
7. (α-^{35}S)dATP isotope (800 Ci/mmol, 10–12.5 mCi/mL) (Amersham or DuPont NEN, Boston, MA) (*see* **Note 2**).
8. 50 μM T$_{11}$MN anchored primers (as used in **Subheading 2.2.**).
9. Set of random 10mer oligonucleotide primers (10 μM each) (*see* **Note 3**).
10. Mineral oil (molecular biology grade) (Sigma).

2.4. Resolution of PCR Products

1. Formamide loading buffer: 95% formamide, 20 mM EDTA, 0.05% bromophenol blue, 0.05% xylene cyanol FF.
2. 96-well microsample plates (Pharmacia LKB Biotechnology).
3. DNA sequencing grade glass plates with 0.5-mm thick spacers and comb. Siliconize the surface of one plate (Repelcote VS, BDH) to allow easy separation of this plate from the gel, and thoroughly clean both plates with 95% ethanol.
4. Denaturing 6% acrylamide gels *(6)*. Mix 75 mL 40% acrylamide/bis (19:1), 25 mL 10X TBE, 230 g urea (ultrapure), make up to 500 mL with dH$_2$O, filter through scintered glass, and store at 4°C for no longer than 1 mo. Each gel will require approx 50 mL of this mix.
5. 1X TBE, pH 7.4: 89 mM Tris base, 89 mM boric acid, 2 mM EDTA, pH 7.4.
6. Sequencing gel apparatus and a power unit capable of supplying 34 W (1750 V).
7. X-ray film (35 × 43 cm) (Kodak X-OMAT AR or Fuji RX) and film cassette.

2.5. Isolation and Reamplification
of Differentially Displayed PCR Bands

Additional materials to those already required for previous procedures are;

1. Luminescent autorad markers (Glogos II, Stratagene).
2. TE buffer, pH 7.4: 10 mM Tris-HCl, pH 7.4, 1 mM EDTA, pH 8.0.
3. 85% Ethanol.
4. 10 mg/mL glycogen (molecular biology grade).
5. Dry ice.

3. Methods
3.1. Isolation and Preparation of RNA Samples

The quality of RNA samples is critical to the successful application of differential mRNA display. Many problems associated with the generation of a clear and reproducible differential mRNA display can be attributed to the isolation of poor quality RNA. Any protocol for total RNA isolation can be used, such as guanidinium/cesium chloride ultracentrifugation *(6)*, alternatively, an NP-40 lysis method was used for the isolation of cultured VSMC RNA *(7)* (also *see* Chapter 4). The isolation of good quality RNA from cardiovascular tissue biopsies is often technically challenging, particularly if the samples are small, and is dependent on the processing of fresh sample to minimize RNase degradation of the RNA. There are, however, commercially available kits for high yield total RNA isolation from tissue samples (RNAqueous, Ambion).

Another common problem associated with differential mRNA display is the PCR amplification of "false positive" bands, which do not represent differentially expressed genes. This is often a result of DNA contamination of the RNA samples. To minimise DNA contamination, each RNA sample must be treated with DNase 1 in the presence of an RNase inhibitor. The procedure described below is suitable for the DNase 1 treatment of up to 50 µg of total RNA.

1. Make each RNA sample to a volume of 50 µL with DEPC-treated H_2O in a sterile (RNase-free) 1.5-mL Eppendorf tube.
2. Add (in the following order): 50 µL of DNase digestion buffer, 10 U (0.5 µL) of RNase inhibitor and 10 U (10 µL) of DNase 1.
3. Mix by gently pipeting up and down, spin briefly (5 s) at 14,000g, then incubate at 37°C for 30 min to allow DNA digestion.
4. To extract the enzymes add 100 µL 1:1 phenol/chloroform (pH 7.8), vortex for 20 s, then spin at 14,000g for 2.5 minutes (*see* **Note 5**).
5. Carefully remove the upper aqueous phase to a fresh 1.5-mL Eppendorf tube and precipitate the RNA by adding 1/10 volume (10 µL) 3 M sodium acetate (pH 4.8) and 2.5 volumes (250 µL) of 100% ethanol.
6. Vortex briefly, then chill at –70°C for 2 h.
7. Recover the precipitate by centrifugation at 14,000g for 15 min. Carefully remove and discard the supernatant then gently rinse the pellet with 200 µL 70% ethanol.
8. Air dry the pellet at room temperature for 1 h then resuspend in 25 µL of DEPC-treated H_2O.
9. Determine the concentration of the DNA-free RNA spectraphotomerically by diluting 2 µL in 200 µL of DEPC-treated H_2O, mix and measure its absorbance (A) at 260 nm. The concentration can be calculated as follows;

$$\text{Concentration } (\mu g/mL) = [(A_{260})(\text{dilution } (100)](40 \ \mu g/mL)$$

10. Dilute the RNA samples to a concentration of 0.2 µg/µL in DEPC-treated H_2O.
11. Check the quality of each RNA sample by electrophoretically analyzing 2 µL on a 1.5% agarose gel containing 0.5 µg/mL ethidium bromide (*see* **Note 6**).

3.2. Reverse Transcription (RT)

Subdivision of each set of RNA transcripts is initially achieved by independently reverse transcribing 0.2 μg using specific 3' anchored primers. To help minimise false positive bands later in the procedure perform the reactions outlined below using at least two independent RNA isolates from each sample being compared (*see* **Note 7**).

1. Set up 20 μL RT reactions on ice containing the following:

	Final concentration	Volume (μL)
0.2 μg total RNA	0.01 μg/mL	1
5X RT buffer	1X	4
0.1 M DTT	10 mM	2
Premixed dNTPs (200 μM each)	40 μM	4
50 μM anchored T$_{11}$MN primer	2.5 μM	1
DEPC-treated H$_2$O	–	7

2. Denature the RNA by heating at 65°C for 5 min, spin the tubes briefly at 14,000g to collect any condensation.
3. Add 1 μL (200 U) M-MLV reverse transcriptase, mix briefly by stirring with the pipet tip, and incubate at 37°C for 1 hr.
4. Stop the reaction by denaturing the reverse transcriptase at 95°C for 5 min. Spin the tubes briefly at 14,000g and either store at –20°C or place on ice for the PCR step.

3.3. Polymerase Chain Reaction (PCR)

Each T$_{11}$MN-primed set of cDNAs is subdivided further by PCR amplification using random 10mer oligonucleotide primers (*see* **Note 3**).

1. Using 0.5-mL thick-walled PCR tubes set up each 20 μL PCR reaction on ice containing the following:

	Final concentration	Volume (μL)
Specific RT products	—	1
10X PCR buffer (MgCl$_2$-free)	1X	2
20 mM MgCl$_2$	1 mM	1
Premixed dNTPs (200 μM each)	10 μM	1
(α-^{35}S)dATP (10-12.5 μCi/μL)	—	1
50 μM anchored T$_{11}$MN primer	2.5 μM	1
(the same one used for the initial RT)		
10 μM random 10mer primer	0.5 μM	1
Distilled H$_2$O	—	12

2. Add 0.5 μL (2.5–5 U) *Taq* DNA polymerase and mix the components of the reaction thoroughly with the pipet tip.
3. Overlay each PCR reaction with two drops of mineral oil and amplify in a thermal cycler using the following parameters; 30-s denaturation at 94°C, 60-s annealing at 42°C, 30-s extension at 72°C, for 40 cycles, followed by a final 5-min extension at 72°C.

3.4. Resolution of PCR Products

The products of each PCR reaction are displayed and compared after electrophoresis on denaturing 6% acrylamide gels.

1. Remove 8 µL of the products from each PCR reaction (taking care not to pipet any mineral oil) and mix with 4 µL formamide loading buffer in the well of a microsample plate (these eliminate using many tubes and decrease handling times).
2. Prepare a 0.5-mm thick denaturing 6% acrylamide gel using large glass sequencing plates.
3. Denature the samples at 80°C for 4 min and load 6 µL of each onto the gel. When loading be careful not to let samples spill over into adjacent wells.
4. Run the gel at 34 W for between 4–5 h (*see* **Note 8**).
5. Carefully transfer and dry the gel onto Whatman card.
6. Expose the gel to X-ray film for 24–72 h (depending on the intensity of the signal) and analyse for differentially displayed bands. A typical example of the banding pattern obtained is shown in **Fig. 2**.

3.5. Isolation and Reamplification of Differentially Displayed PCR Bands

When differentially displayed bands are identified the cDNA can be recovered from the gel and reamplified using the original primer combination.

1. Using luminescent autorad markers for accurate orientation, carefully align and tape (to prevent slipping) the film on top of the gel. Using a fresh scalpel blade for each differentially displayed band, carefully excise the small portion of the gel containing the DNA of interest by cutting through the film into the gel. Try to recover the smallest piece of gel possible to minimize the risk of isolating and reamplifying adjacent "false positive" bands.
2. Soak each dried gel fragment in 100 µL TE for 10 min, boil for 15 min, then spin at 14,000g for 2 min to pellet the gel and paper debris.
3. Transfer the supernatant to a fresh microfuge tube and add 10 µL 3 M sodium acetate (pH 4.8), 5 µL glycogen (10 mg/mL), and 450 µL 100% ethanol.
4. Precipitate the DNA at –80°C on dry ice for 1 h, then spin for 15 min at 14,000g to pellet the DNA.
5. Remove the supernatant, wash the pellet with 200 µL 85% ethanol, then leave to dry at room temperature for 1 h.
6. Resuspend the DNA in 10 µL dH$_2$O and use 5 µL of this for PCR reamplification using the same primer combination which identified the band. The PCR conditions are the same as those used originally (*see* **Subheading 3.3.**) except that no isotope is added and the final dNTP concentration is 100 µM.
7. Resolve the amplified band on a 1% agarose gel and confirm that it is approximately the same size as the band on the differential mRNA display gel (*see* **Notes 9** and **10**).

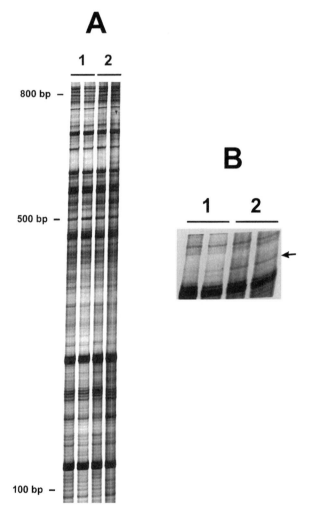

Fig. 2. (**A**) A typical "RNA fingerprint" generated by differential mRNA display. DNA-free RNA was obtained from control (1) and growth factor stimulated (2) vascular smooth muscle cells. Gene expression was compared in duplicate samples by DDRTPCR using a $T_{11}MN$ and random 10mer primer combination. (**B**) A detailed example of a differentially displayed band (arrowed). The band shown was excised from the gel, reamplified, and using Northern blot analysis, was found to represent a gene whose expression was upregulated 20-fold by growth factor treatment.

4. Notes

1. Subdivision of mRNA at the reverse transcription step was originally described using a set of non-degenerate $T_{11}MN$ primers *(1)*, where the two 3' nucleotides (MN) hybridise to the 5' end of the poly(A) region. Since N = A, C, T, or G and

M = C, G, or A, all possible combinations of these two nucleotides mean that 12 primers, therefore 12 reverse transcription reactions, are required. $T_{12}VA$ primers, where V is threefold degenerate for G, C, or A, have also been used for DDRTPCR. These four primers cut down the number of RT reactions and much of the redundancy often associated with the 12 nondegenerate primers (8). However, degenerate primers tend to under-represent certain populations of mRNAs. More recently, one-base anchored oligo(dT) primers have been used in combination with longer arbitrary primers (9) (*see* **Note 3**), these also reduce the number of RT reactions required but overcome the limitations of degenerate primers (10).

2. $(\alpha\text{-}^{35}S)$dATP has been widely used for differential mRNA display because of its ability to produce very high resolution bands (1) (*see* **Fig. 2**). However, $(\alpha\text{-}^{32}P)$dATP can be used (11,12), or more favorably $(\alpha\text{-}^{33}P)$dATP which combines the sensitivity of $(\alpha\text{-}^{32}P)$dATP with the resolution of $(\alpha\text{-}^{35}S)$dATP (2,12). When using $(\alpha\text{-}^{35}S)$dATP for differential mRNA display it is important to note that this isotope can decompose during thermal cycling resulting in the escape of a volatile vapour through the top of the PCR tube (12). Therefore, perform all thermal cycling in a fume hood and monitor the cycler and tubes for contamination afterwards.

3. The length of the random oligonucleotide primers used for differential mRNA display determines the approximate number of bands displayed. It was found that 10 nucleotides gave an ideal number of bands (between 50–100) when used in combination with a nondegenerate $T_{11}MN$ anchored primer (1). Baur, et al. (2) described a selection of 26 arbitrary 10mers which, in theory, would allow the detection of every expressed gene in a cell when used in combination with each of the 12 $T_{11}MN$ primers. Longer arbitrary primers have been used for differential mRNA display, but only in combination with one-base anchored oligo(dT) primers (9).

4. Any source of *Taq* polymerase can be used. However, It has been demonstrated that different sources of PCR reaction tubes (13) and *Taq* polymerase (14) can produce different banding patterns when all other DDRTPCR conditions are identical. Thus, to obtain reproducible results and minimize false positives it is important that identical reagents are used throughout the procedure.

5. The DNase 1 treatment of RNA samples and subsequent phenol/chloroform extraction and ethanol precipitation steps may result in the loss of approx 10–30% of the sample. This is particularly important when comparing gene expression in small vascular biopsies where the initial yield of RNA is low.

6. After DNase 1 treatment always analyze a small aliquot (approx 0.2 µg) of each RNA sample on a 1.5% agarose gel. This not only allows the quality of the RNA to be assessed, but also confirms the spectrophotomeric analysis of its concentration. Good quality RNA should show tight 28S, 18S, and 5S ribosomal RNA bands and no obvious signs of degradation.

7. A common problem associated with the differential mRNA display technique is the isolation of differentially displayed bands which do not represent differentially expressed genes. In some cases these artifacts may be due to infidelity of

the *Taq* polymerase during the PCR step. To minimize the risk of isolating these "false positives," it is important that at least duplicates of each DDRTPCR reaction, preferably using independent RNA preparations, be compared alongside each other such that only bands which are differentially displayed in each identical reaction are characterised further.

8. This allows small PCR products (< 80 bp) to run off the gel and allows greater resolution of the larger, more informative bands.

9. In most cases differentially displayed bands are successfully reamplified after the DNA has been extracted from the gel. If no product is generated by one round of PCR take 5 μL of this reaction and use it as template for a second round. However, this second reamplification often generates multiple PCR products where each may have to be screened by Northern blot analysis to identify, which represents the differentially expressed gene.

10. Further analysis of each differentially displayed band can be carried out after firstly cloning the amplified DNA into a T:A cloning vector. Northern blot analysis can be used to confirm differential expression (*see* Chapter 16). The identity of the gene which each band represents can be determined by a combination of DNA sequencing, screening a cDNA library to isolate full-length cDNAs (*see* Chapters 5 and 6), or RACE analysis (*see* Chapter 7).

References

1. Liang, P. and Pardee, A. B. (1992) Differential display of eukaryotic messenger RNA by means of the polymerase chain reaction. *Science* **257,** 967–971.

2. Bauer, D., Muller, H., Reich, J., Riedel, H., Ahrenkiel, V., Warthoe, P., and Strauss, M. (1993) Identification of differentially expressed mRNA species by an improved display technique (DDRT-PCR). *Nucl. Acids Res.* **21,** 4272–4280.

3. Hsieh, C-M., Yoshizumi, M., Endege, W. O., Kho, C-J., Jain, M. K., Kashiki, S., Santos, R., Lee, W-S., Perrella, M. A., and Lee, M-E. (1996) APEG-1, a novel gene preferentially expressed in aortic smooth muscle cells, is down-regulated by vascular injury. *J. Biol. Chem.* **271,** 17,354–17,359.

4. Sibinga, N. E. S., Foster, L. C., Hsieh, C-M., Perrella, M. A., Lee, W-S., Endege, W. O., Sage, E. H., Lee, M-E., and Haber, E. (1997) Collagen VIII is expressed by vascular smooth muscle cells in response to vascular injury. *Circ. Res.* **80,** 532–541.

5. Nishio, Y., Aiello, L. P., and King, G. L. (1994) Glucose induced genes in bovine aortic smooth muscle cells identified by mRNA differential display. *FASEB J.* **8,** 103–106.

6. Sambrook, J., Fritsch, E. F., and Miniatis, T. (1989) *Molecular Cloning: A Laboratory Manual*, 2nd ed., Cold Spring Harbor Laboratory, Plainview, NY.

7. Adam, P. J., Weissberg, P. L., Cary, N. R. B., and Shanahan, C. M. (1997) Polyubiquitin is a new phenotypic marker of contractile vascular smooth muscle cells. *Cardiovasc. Res.* **33,** 416–421.

8. Liang, P., Averboukh, L., and Pardee, A. B. (1993) Distribution and cloning of eukaryotic mRNAs by means of differential display: refinements and optimization. *Nucl. Acids Res.* **21,** 3269–275.

9. Liang, P., Zhu, W., Zhang, X., Guo, Z., O'Connell, R. P., Averboukh, L., Wang, F., and Pardee, A. B. (1994) Differential display using one-base anchored oligo-dT primers. *Nucl. Acids Res.* **22,** 5763–5764.

10. Liang, P. and Pardee, A. B. (1995) Recent advances in differential display. *Curr. Opin. Immunol.* **7,** 274–280.

11. Welsh, J., Chada, K., Dalal, S. S., Cheng, R., Ralph, D., and McClelland, M. (1992) Arbitrary primed PCR fingerprinting of RNA. *Nucl. Acids Res.* **20,** 4965–4970.

12. Trentmann, S. M., Van der Knaap, E., and Kende, H. (1995) Alternatives to ^{35}S as a label for the differential display of eukaryotic messenger RNA (letter; comment). *Science* **267,** 1186–1187.

13. Chen, Z., Swisshelm, K., and Sager, R. (1994) A cautionary note on reaction tubes for differential display and cDNA amplification in thermal cycling. *Biotechniques* **16,** 1003–1005.

14. Haag, E. and Raman, V. (1994) Effects of primer choice and source of *Taq* DNA polymerase on the banding patterns of differential display RT-PCR. *Biotechniques* **17,** 226–228.

10

Identification of Novel Protein Kinases in Vascular Cells

Ian Zachary, Spiros Servos, and Barbara Herren

1. Introduction

Protein kinases play pivotal roles in almost all signal transduction pathways in eukaryotic cells *(1–4)* and are implicated in most major human diseases, including atherosclerosis and associated vasculoproliferative disorders of arteries such as restenosis and graft stenosis *(5)*. Several hundred distinct kinases have already been molecularly cloned, and it is likely that as a result of new information generated through large-scale genome sequencing projects this number will increase. Despite this flood of information, and with several important exceptions, there is a relative lack of knowledge regarding the identity of kinases specifically expressed in vascular tissues or cells and more particularly, it remains unclear how the expression of kinases alters in cardiovascular disease states. The first step in approaching this question is to identify the repertoire of kinases present in vascular tissues and cells. The protein tyrosine kinase (PTK) receptors for several polypeptide growth factors, including platelet-derived growth factor (PDGF), insulin-like growth factor-I (IGF-I) and basic fibroblast growth factor (bFGF) have been implicated in neo-intimal and atherosclerotic disease *(5)*. Apart from these and a few other exceptions, surprisingly little is known regarding the patterns of expression of specific PTKs or other kinases in neo-intima formation. The use of anti-phosphotyrosine antibodies, selective tyrosine kinase inhibitors and kinase-specific antibodies is limited. Antibody detection using anti-phosphotyrosine antibodies does not distinguish tyrosine kinases from their targets, not all tyrosine kinases are easily detected by antiphosphotyrosine antibodies, the use of PTK-specific antibodies is restricted to a candidate kinase approach and PTK-specific inhibitors are still not widely available.

From: *Methods in Molecular Medicine, vol. 30: Vascular Disease: Molecular Biology and Gene Therapy Protocols*
Edited by: A. H. Baker © Humana Press Inc., Totowa, NJ

An alternative approach is to take advantage of the homologies which exist between all kinases. All kinases share the enzymatic activity essential to their role in signal transduction, namely the transfer of phosphate from the gamma phosphoryl moiety of ATP to an acceptor protein, either on serine/threonine residues, tyrosine residues, or both in the case of some dual-specificity kinases such as the mitogen-activated protein kinase kinases. The corollary is that all kinases share motifs in their amino acid sequences and corresponding DNA protein coding sequences which encode highly conserved regions in their catalytic domains necessary for binding ATP and the enzymatic transfer of the phosphate group. The high degree of conservation of these motifs between diverse kinases and across species has made it possible to adopt an homology-based approach using polymerase chain reaction (PCR) methodology and oligonucleotide primers with built-in degeneracy *(6–8)*. In this chapter a strategy for identification and molecular cloning of PTKs in vascular cells is described.

2. Materials

All solutions and buffers unless provided with kits should be autoclaved prior to use and H_2O should always be double-distilled, deionised and autoclaved. Special precautions apply to use of reagents and buffers when preparing or working with RNA (*see* **Subheading 2.1.**).

2.1. mRNA Preparation

1. Glassware: should be made RNase-free by cleaning with detergent, rinsing thoroughly and baking at >210°C for at least 3 h. If facilities for baking are not available, an alternative is to treat glassware with DEPC-treated water and then autoclave.
2. Plasticware: Eppendorf tubes and tips should be autoclaved. All materials and reagents should be handled with latex gloves and adopt microbiological aseptic techniques during all procedures involving RNA.
3. Refrigerated microcentrifuge (Eppendorf, Sigma, or Heraeus).
4. Water bath.
5. Rotary shaker.
6. Phosphate-buffered saline: 137 mM NaCl, 2.7 mM KCl, 10 mM Na_2HPO_4, 1.8 mM KH_2PO_4, pH 7.4. Store at room temperature.
7. Micro-Fast Track™ mRNA kit (Invitrogen cat. no. k1520-02) (store +4°C).
8. Electrophoresis apparatus.

2.2. RT-PCR

1. Oligonucleotide primers: primers should be made by custom oligonucleotide synthesis (e.g., Gibco/BRL). The method described utilizes degenerate oligonucleotides previously described *(4,5)*. The primers correspond to highly conserved motifs in subdomains VI and IX of PTK catalytic regions, primer I correspond-

ing to the IHRDL motif and primer II to the DVWSFG motif (*see* **Fig. 1** and *see* **Note 1**). In the original oligonucleotide design *Bam* HI and *Eco*RI restriction sites were added to the primers to facilitate ligation. If custom-made kits for subcloning PCR fragments are used, these restriction sites should **not** be incorporated into the oligonucleotide design (*see* **Note 2**).

2. Thermocycler: a PerkinElmer Cetus DNA Thermal Cycler widely available in and before 1990 was used by the author, but others are suitable and may have improved performance. The PTC-100™ Programmable Thermal Controller (MJ Research Inc.) is recommended.
3. Water bath or heating block (Techne).
4. Gene Amp RNA PCR Core kit (Perkin Elmer, cat. no. N808-0143). Store -20°C.

2.3. PCR Amplification of PTKs

1. *Taq* polymerase and buffer. Store –20°C.
2. Oligonucleotide primers (GibcoBRL). Store –20°C.

2.4. Subcloning of PCR Products

1. *E. coli* Gene Pulser and cuvettes (Bio-Rad).
2. Cooling water bath (–20–100°C; Grant L6 DTG; optional).
3. GENECLEAN® kit (BIO 101). Store room temperature.
4. TAQench PCR cloning enhancer (Gibco BRL). Store at –20°C.
5. pBluescript II KS(+/–) vector or other standard subcloning vectors (Stratagene). Store –20°C).
6. T4 DNA ligase and buffer (GibcoBRL). Store both at –20°C. Aliquot buffer before storage.
7. Restriction endonucleases: *Bam*HI, *Eco*RI, and others (GibcoBRL). Store at –20°C.
8. Calf intestinal alkaline phosphatase (GibcoBRL). Store at +4°C.
9. LB-agar plates with 100 µg/mL ampicillin: 0.5 mM IPTG and 40 µg/mL Bluogal (or X-gal) (All components from GibcoBRL). Autoclave LB-agar, then while LB-agar is still in liquid equilibrate at 50°C. Add ampicillin, Bluo-gal and IPTG to desired final concentrations. Pour the plates and leave on the bench for 2–3 h and store upside down at +4°C.
10. pGEM-T Easy vector system I (Promega) required for subcloning PCR fragments. Store –20°C.
11. *E. coli* XL-1 blue (or other suitable strain, e.g., DH5α). Store –70°C.

2.5. DNA Sequencing

1. DNA sequencing apparatus (Bio-Rad or ABI) or automated sequencer if available.
2. Gel Dryer (Bio-Rad).
3. Plasmid DNA: prepare using QIAprep Spin minipep kit (Qiagen; Cat.No.27104). Store at +4°C.
4. Automated sequencing: ABI Prism dRhodamine Dye terminator cycle sequencing ready reaction kit with Amplitaq DNA polymerase FS (cat. no. P/N 402080). Store at –20°C. Which fluorophore (i.e., Rhodamine or another) is used may

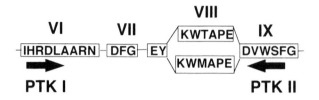

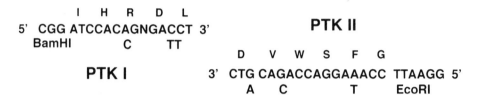

Fig. 1. Design of degenerate oligonucleotides for homology-based amplification of a ~210 bp region of PTK catalytic domains. The top of the figure shows the domain structure of part of the catalytic domains of PTKs, with the consensus amino acid sequences (amino acid residues are denoted using the single letter code) characteristic of each subdomain according to the system of Hanks, Hunter and Quinn *(3,4)*. The bottom of the figure shows the degenerate oligonucleotides, PTK I and II, corresponding to subdomains VI and IX respectively, used for amplification of this region. N denotes the use of all four bases at that position and use of alternative bases is indicated below the oligonucleotide sequence. The corresponding amino acid consensus is indicated above the nucleotide sequence. The consensus PTK II coding sequence was reversed and complemented before oligonucleotide synthesis and *Bam*HI and *Eco*RI restriction endonuclease sites were added with an additional CG and G in the case of *Bam*HI and *Eco*RI, respectively, to ensure efficient digestion close to the ends of oligonucleotides.

depend on the available settings of the automated sequencer.

Manual sequencing: T7 Sequenase version 2.0 DNA sequencing kit (Amersham; store –20°C) and [α-^{35}S]dATP. Store at –20°C and remove from freezer 1–2 h to allow to thaw prior to use.

5. 10X TBE stock buffer: dissolve 108 g Tris/Base and 55 g Boric acid in 800 mL H$_2$O, add 40 mL 0.5 *M* EDTA, pH 8.0, and make up to 1000 mL final volume with H$_2$O. Dilute to working concentration as required. Store room temperature.

6. 12% methanol/10% acetic acid.

7. Denaturing solution: 1 *M* NaOH, 1 m*M* EDTA.

8. 2.5 *M* sodium acetate, pH 5.2.

9. Ultrapure urea.

10. Acrylamide and bis-acrylamide.

11. TEMED.

12. Ammonium persulphate (APS).

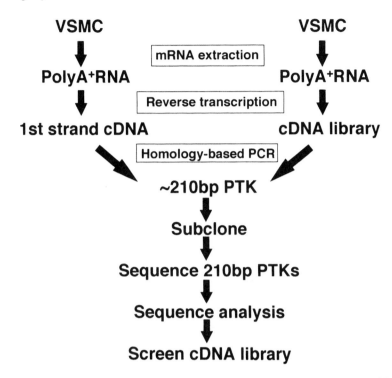

Fig. 2. Flow diagram showing the key stages in the identification of PTKs by homology-based PCR amplification using either a cDNA library or single-stranded cDNA as template.

2.6. Library Screening (see also Chapters 5 and 6)

1. cDNA libraries can be purchased from Clontech, Stratagene, Gibco BRL, or other companies. Libraries cloned into λZap II are recommended.

3. Methods
3.1. mRNA Preparation

Either a complementary DNA library or single-stranded cDNA synthesised by reverse-transcriptase(RT)-PCR are suitable templates for PCR amplification of PTKs (**Fig. 2**). We have used a rat VSMC cDNA library *(9)* and rabbit VSMC cDNA synthesised by RT-PCR from either polyA$^+$RNA or total RNA. In either case the starting material is good-quality RNA. Though either polyA$^+$ or total RNA can be used for RT-PCR, polyA$^+$RNA is strongly recommended. We have obtained good yields of high-quality polyA$^+$ RNA using the Micro-FastTrack™ mRNA isolation kit (*see* **Note 3**). Typically, 2.5–3.5 µg of polyA$^+$RNA are obtained from 2–5×10^6 cells. Use 2–5×10^6 vascular smooth muscle cells (VSMC) or cell type of choice for each isolation. Arterial or other vascular tissue may also be used (*see* **Note 4**).

1. Wash cells in phosphate-buffered saline (PBS) at 4°C and detach the cells by mild trypsinisation.
2. Collect the cell pellet by centrifugation and wash the pellet with PBS at 4°C.
3. Transfer to a 1.5-µL microcentrifuge tube at room temperature and add 1 µL of lysis buffer to the pellet.
4. Resuspend cells by carefully passing through a sterile plastic syringe fitted with an 18–21-gage needle 3–5 times in order to avoid foaming.
5. Incubate the suspension at 45°C for 15–20 min in a water bath. Slow shaking is desirable, but if a shaking water bath is not available, shake the suspension by hand every 2–3 min.
6. Remove any insoluble material by centrifugation at 4000g for 5 min at room temperature.
7. Adjust the NaCl concentration to 0.5 M by addition of 63 µL of 5 M NaCl to every 1 mL of lysate.
8. Mix and then shear the DNA by passing the lysate through a sterile plastic syringe fitted with an 18–21-gauge needle 3–5 times.
9. Add one oligo (dT) cellulose tablet to the lysate and allow to disperse by gently agitating the tube by hand. Rock tube gently on a rotary shaker at room temperature for 20 min.
10. Pellet the oligo (dT) cellulose at room temperature in a microcentrifuge at 4000g for 8 min.
11. Carefully aspirate the supernatant and suspend the oligo (dT) cellulose in 1.3 mL of binding buffer.
12. Pellet as before and repeat washing with binding buffer (1.3 mL) until buffer is no longer cloudy (3–5 times).
13. After the final wash, resuspend the oligo (dT) cellulose pellet in 0.3 mL of binding buffer.
14. Transfer some of the sample to a spin column in a microcentrifuge tube and spin for 10 s at 5000g. Repeat until the whole sample is transferred to the spin column. Discard the liquid inside the microcentrifuge tube.
15. Return the spin column to the tube and wash by adding binding buffer and centrifuging as in **step 14** above. Repeat 3-5 times until the OD of the flow through is < 0.05.
16. Wash off non-polyA$^+$RNA by adding 200 µL of low salt wash buffer and gently mixing it into the cellulose bed in the spin column using a pipet tip. Centrifuge as in step 14 and repeat wash.
17. Transfer the spin column to a fresh microcentrifuge tube and add 100 µL of elution buffer to the spin column and mix it into the cellulose as in **step 16**. Centrifuge as in **step 14** and repeat process using 100 µL of fresh elution buffer. If less than 200 µL of the polyA$^+$ RNA eluate is collected in the bottom of the tube, spin in a microcentrifuge again for 1 min.

18. Quantitate the polyA$^+$ RNA by measuring the OD_{260}/OD_{280} ratio. This should be between 1.8 and 2.1 (*see* **Note 5**).
19. Precipitate the RNA by adding to each 200 μL of polyA$^+$ RNA, 10 μL of a 2 mg/μL solution of glycogen, 30 μL 2 *M* sodium acetate, pH 5.2 and 600 μL 100% ethanol and placing on dry ice until the solution has solidified. Keep at –70°C for up to 6 mo.
20. Recover the RNA by spinning in a microcentrifuge at +4°C at maximum speed for 15 min.
21. Aspirate the ethanol supernatant, spin again briefly (1 min), aspirate residual ethanol, and resuspend RNA in 1–10 μL of elution buffer (10 m*M* Tris, pH 7.5).

3.2. cDNA Synthesis

Perform first-strand cDNA synthesis by reverse transcription using approximately 100–500 ng of polyA$^+$RNA or 1 μg total RNA, the Murine Leukaemia Virus Reverse Transcriptase (MuLV), either Oligo d(T)16 or random hexamer primers and the GeneAmp RNA PCR kit (Perkin Elmer).

1. Heat the RNA to 65–70°C for 10 min immediately prior to reverse transcription in order to disrupt RNA secondary structure.
2. Place the RNA to ice and then add the following components in a 0.5-mL microcentrifuge tube:

Component	Volume	Final concentration
25 m*M* MgCl$_2$	4 μL	5 m*M*
10X PCR buffer	2 μL	1X
dGTP	2 μL	1 m*M*
dATP	2 μL	1 m*M*
dTTP	2 μL	1 m*M*
dCTP	2 μL	1 m*M*
RNase inhibitor	1 μL	1 U/μL
MuLV Reverse transcriptase	1 μL	2.5 U/μL
Random hexamers	1 μL	2.5 m*M*
(or Oligo d(T)16, if preferred)		
polyA$^+$RNA or total RNA	1 μL	100–500 ng of polyA$^+$RNA
		1 μg of total RNA
DEPC-treated water		add to make final volume 20 μL

3. Overlay the reaction mix with ~50 μL of mineral oil, and incubate at room temperature for 10 min to allow extension of primers by reverse transcriptase.
4. Incubate at 42°C for 15 min (reverse transcription), 96°C for 5 min (*see* **Note 6**) and 5°C for 5 min.

3.3. PCR

3.3.1. PCR Using the First-Strand cDNA as a Template

1. For PCR with degenerate oligonucleotides and first-strand cDNA as template, add the following components in a 0.5-mL microcentrifuge tube:

Primer I	1 μL (50 pmol)
Primer II	1 μL (50 pmol)
10x PCR reaction buffer	5 μL
25 mM MgCl$_2$	2 μL
Taq polymerase	0.5 μL (2.5 U)
First-strand cDNA mix (from **Subheading 3.3.**, step 3)	20 μL
H$_2$O	20.5 μL
Final volume	50 μL

2. Overlay with ~ 50 μL (i.e., 1 volume) of heavy mineral oil.
3. Mix vigorously by flicking the tube sharply several times.
4. Spin in a microcentrifuge for 30 s at top-speed.
5. Amplify using the following cycle for 35 cycles: 1.5 min at 95°C (denaturation), 2 min at 37°C (annealing), and 3 min at 63°C (elongation). The cycle parameters should be optimised according to the particular thermocycler and type of tubes (*see* **Note 7**).

3.3.2. PCR Using a cDNA Library as the Template

1. If using a cDNA library as the template, mix the following components in a 0.5-mL microcentrifuge tube, omitting the *Taq* polymerase and dNTPs:

Primer I	1 μL (50 pmol)
Primer II	1 μL (50 pmol)
10X PCR reaction buffer	5 μL
25m*M* MgCl$_2$	2 μL
cDNA library	2 μL (should be equivalent to ~ 10^7 cDNA clones)
H$_2$O	37.5 μL

Briefly agitate the cDNA library before addition to the PCR mix.
2. Heat the reaction mix to boiling for 7 min. A boiling water bath is recommended for this purpose. Remember to seal the tube tightly to prevent evaporation during boiling.
3. Cool the reaction mix rapidly by placing on ice for ~ 2 min.
4. Spin in a microcentrifuge for 10 s at maximum speed and then keep on ice.
5. Add to the mix, 1 μL of 20 m*M* of each dNTPs (i.e., dGTP, dATP, dTTP, and dCTP), and 0.5 μL (2.5 U) of *Taq* polymerase (Boehringer-Mannheim or enzyme supplied by a kit). The final volume should be 50 μL.
6. Overlay with ~ 50 μL of heavy mineral oil and mix vigorously.
7. Spin in a microcentrifuge (10 s, maximum speed) and perform PCR as in **Subheading 3.3.1.**, step 5 (*see* **Note 7**).

3.3.3. Analysis of PCR Reactions

1. Place the reactions on ice after amplification. The mineral oil can be removed by extraction with chloroform/isoamyl alcohol by transferring the tube to –20°C where the PCR reaction freezes but the oil does not and removing the oil.
2. Analyze the PCR products by running a small aliquot of the PCR product (2–5 μL should be sufficient) on a 2% agarose gel.

3. Stain the gel with ethidium bromide. The predicted PCR product obtained with these degenerate primers should be ~210 bp (*see* **Notes 8** and **9**).

3.4. Subcloning PCR Fragments

1. Purify the remainder of the PCR fragment by preparative agarose gel electrophoresis on a 2% agarose gel (*see* **Notes 10** and **11**). Isolate sufficient DNA for several ligations. It is important at this step that the purest grade agarose (molecular biology grade, Gibco/BRL) is used because small impurities carried over from the gel purification step is a common cause of the failure of ligations.
2. Locate the ~210 bp band under ultraviolet light and excise using a clean sterile scalpel (CAUTION: use gloves, cover other exposed parts of the body and use an appropriate face shield while using a UV light source).
3. Place the band in a preweighed microfuge tube and calculate the weight of the agarose band.
4. Purify the DNA using a GENECLEAN® kit by adding the sodium iodide solution provided at 3 times the volume of the gel (0.1 g, ~0.1 mL).
5. Melt the agarose by heating to 55°C for 5–10 min and gently mixing the contents every 2 min.
6. Add the glassmilk according to the manufacturer's instructions and allow DNA to bind for at least 10 min.
7. Pellet, wash and elute DNA according to the protocol provided.
8. Digest the purified fragment with *Eco*RI and *Bam*HI for 4 h at 37°C and purify the digested ~210 bp fragment from solution using the GENECLEAN® kit by adding 3 volumes of the NaI solution provided to the restriction digest and mixing by gentle inversion (do not vortex). Perform the remainder of the purification according to the kit protocol but using only gentle mixing and without vortexing (*see* **Note 12**).
9. In parallel with the previous step, digest the vector (pBluescript/SK-) with *Eco*RI/*Bam*HI, dephosphorylate by addition of 1 μL calf intestinal alkaline phosphatase (GibcoBRL) during the final 30 min of the digestion, and then purify using the GENECLEAN® kit as in **step 8**.
10. Estimate the concentrations of both vector and PCR fragments by gel electrophoresis of aliquots against molecular weight markers.
11. Ligate the PCR fragment to ~50 ng vector using an excess (two- to 10-fold) molar concentration of the PCR fragment.
12. Mix the PCR product and vector in the appropriate molar ratio with 1 μL 10x ligation buffer (*see* **Notes 13** and **14**) but excluding *E. coli* DNA ligase and ATP.
13. Heat to 60°C in a water bath for 20 min.
14. Allow to cool slowly to room temperature by leaving in the water bath without heat. This allows annealing to occur between complementary ends of the vector and T4 DNA ligase.
15. Add 1 μL of *E. coli* DNA ligase, 1 μL of ATP (to give a final concentration of 1 mM) and make up to a total volume of 10 μL with H_2O.
16. Incubate the ligations overnight at 15°C using a cooling water bath (see **Note 15**).

17. Prior to electro-transformation, reduce the ionic strength, and concentrate the DNA as follows *(10)*. Denature *E. coli* DNA ligase at 65°C for 10 min.
18. Add H_2O to 50 µL (30–40 µL, depending on the volume of the ligation).
19. Add 500 µL n-butanol and vortex mix tube for 30 s.
20. Centrifuge at maximum speed in a microcentrifuge for 10 min. Discard the supernatant and dry the pellet either using a DNA concentrator (Speed-Vac) or by air-drying.
21. Resuspend the pellet in 3 µL of H_2O and electroporate 100 µL of electrocompetent (see **Note 16**) *E. coli* XL-1 blue (or another suitable *E. coli* strain) using a GenePulser (Bio-Rad) according to the manufacturer's instructions (see **Note 17**).
22. Spread transformed cells onto LB-agar plates containing 100 µg/mL ampicilin, Bluo-gal or X-gal (Bluo-gal gives a darker blue colour than the more commonly used X-gal) and isopropylthio-β-galactoside (IPTG) and incubate at 37°C overnight. Typical yields of colonies vary from 2–5 X 10^3 per ligation, of which at least 30–60% should be white colonies.
23. Pick white colonies using sterile sticks.
24. Prepare DNA minipreparations and digest a small aliquot with suitable restriction enzymes (e.g., *Bam*HI and *Eco*RI). Use minipreps which have an insert of ~210 bp for sequencing. Up to 200 colonies with inserts of the predicted size should be sequenced initially (see **Note 18**).

3.5. Sequencing of DNA Minipreparations

3.5.1. Preparation of Sequencing Gels

The quality of gel electrophoresis is essential for obtaining clear sequencing information. Many investigators may choose to use automated sequencing facilities either provided through commercial outlets or provided as a service in their institution. For those for whom these options are not available, good quality sequence information can be readily obtained by 'manual' sequencing.

1. Clean the gel plates thoroughly by wiping both sides alternately with water and 70% ethanol using tissue wipes (KimWipes are ideal for this purpose). This should be repeated three times ensuring that any residual acrylamide gel or crystallized urea left from prior use is removed. It is also recommended that the gel side of one glass plate is siliconized to facilitate separation of the gel from the siliconized glass plate after electrophoresis (see **Note 19**).
2. Prepare gel solution by mixing in a beaker: urea, 34.5 g; 38% acrylamide, 2% bis-acrylamide, 11 mL; 10X TBE, 7.5 mL; water, 50 mL
3. Stir until urea is completely dissolved (1–2 h should be sufficient) and make up to a final total volume of 75 mL with water (see **Note 20**).
4. Filter the gel solution.
5. While the urea is dissolving, assemble the gel apparatus and seal the bottom of gel using strong electrical tap. (see **Note 21**).
6. Pour the sequencing gel. To the remainder of the gel solution, add while stirring, 90 µL of TEMED and 300 µL of 10%APS. Immediately pour the gel using a

25-mL pipet. It is essential that bubbles are not introduced, while pouring the gel. This is best achieved by holding the gel assembly at a steep angle and pipetting the solution slowly and evenly down one side, and gradually lowering the angle of the plates as they fill up. Fill the plates up to the top, and insert a flat-edged comb into the top to a depth of ~4 mm. Allow the gel to set at a slight angle by placing a falcon tube under the top end of the gel.

7. After the gel has completely set (allow 1–2 h), remove the comb and sealing tape from bottom if necessary. Remove any excess crystallized urea and acrylamide by rinsing the outside of assembled gel thoroughly using water and paper towels. Using a 50-mL syringe filled with 1X TBE and fitted with a needle, rinse the top of the gel. Place gel in the electrophoresis chamber and fill chamber with 1X TBE.

8. Insert the comb. Clean the comb with 1X TBE, and after 1X TBE has been added to upper chamber of electrophoresis chamber, insert the comb teeth downwards carefully and evenly into the top of the gel, ensuring that the comb is not inserted too far. Test for leaks by adding running buffer on the upper tank only. If there is a leak, seal with 2% agarose. N.B. *See* **Note 22** for simple methods of maximizing sequence information

3.5.2. Manual Sequencing

Sequence ~210 bp PCR products obtained from isolated colonies by the dideoxyribonucleoside triphosphate chain termination method *(11)*. Sequencing gels (*see* **Subheading 3.5.1.**) should be prepared prior to performing sequencing reactions.

1. Denature the DNA by addition of 3 µL of denaturing solution (1 *M* NaOH, 1 m*M* EDTA) to 12 µL of DNA (~2–5 µg) and incubate at 60 °C for 30 min (*see* **Note 23**).
2. Precipitate the DNA by addition of 2 µL 2.5 *M* Sodium acetate, pH 5.2 and 60 µL of 100% ethanol and incubate at –20°C for at least 15–30 min. DNA precipitation can also be performed overnight at –20°C if this is more convenient.
3. Spin in a microcentrifuge at maximum speed for 20 min at 4°C and wash pellet once with 70% ethanol preincubated at –20°C. Allow the pellet to dry and resuspend in 7 µL of water.
4. Anneal the template to the primer by mixing 7 µL of DNA, 1 µL of primer (10 pmol) and 2 µL of reaction buffer (primer and buffer both supplied with Sequenase® kit).
5. Heat to 65°C in a water bath for 3 min and allow to cool slowly to below 30°C over at least 30 min by allowing the water bath to cool at room temperature to anneal primer to DNA.
6. For the labeling reaction, add the following on ice: annealed DNA/primer, 10 µL; labeling mix (dGTP,dCTP,dTTP, diluted 1:5 in H_2O), 2 µL; [α-^{35}S]dATP (see **Note 24**), 1 µL (10 µCi); sequenase (diluted 1:8 in dilution buffer, *see* **Note 25**), 2 µL.

7. Mix carefully (and without introducing bubbles) by pipeting up and down a few times.
8. Incubate at room temperature for up to 5 min.
9. For termination reactions, add 2.5 μL of each dideoxyNTP (ddNTP) to wells in a microtitre plate on ice (for each labelling reaction you will need 4 wells).
10. Prewarm the plate (with the lid on to minimize evaporation) to 37°C by placing on a preheated hot block with the smooth surface uppermost for ~ 1 min.
11. Add 3.5 μL of labeling mix to each well containing a different ddNTP and mix by briefly pipetting up and down.
12. Incubate the plate with its lid attached on a hot block at 37°C for 3–10 min.
13. Add 4 μL of stop solution and keep samples on ice. If necessary store samples at –20°C.
14. Immediately prior to loading the samples onto the gel, heat the samples to 80°C for 3 min by placing microtitre plate on a preheated hot block.
15. Return the plate to ice and load 1.5–3 μL of each termination reaction on a sequencing gel.

3.5.3. Electrophoresis of Sequencing Gels

1. Prerun the gel at 60 W until the temperature of the mounted gel assembly is 55°C (approx 30 min). The temperature can be gauged conveniently using a stick-on temperature indicator.
2. After the prerun, and before loading samples, flush wells thoroughly using 50-mL syringe filled with 1x TBE and fitted with angled needle (simply bend a needle for this purpose).
3. Load samples in the order GATC (see **Note 26**). Load 8–12 samples and run into the gel (at 60 W) until the two dyes just separate.
4. Load another 8–12 samples and repeat until all the samples are loaded.
5. Run the gel at 60 W for shorter runs (2.5–3.5 h) or 55W for longer runs (6–7 h) (see **Note 27**).
6. After the gel has run, switch off the power supply and leave for a few minutes.
7. Dismantle the gel apparatus and very carefully separate the gel plates. The gel should remain on the nonsiliconized plate!
8. Remove the urea by rinsing the gel thoroughly and carefully with 12% methanol/10% acetic acid. This is most conveniently done at the sink, by laying the gel flat and pipetting the 12% methanol/10% acetic acid slowly over the gel. Repeat until 500 mL has been used. Rinse the gel once with H_2O (*see* **Note 28**).
9. Transfer the gel to 3MM Whatman chromatography paper as follows. Make sure the gel is flat. Lay the dry unwetted paper onto the gel on the glass plate, beginning at one end, and carefully smoothing the paper onto the gel. After the paper has been added, remove the paper carefully from the plate. The gel should stick firmly to the paper (*see* **Note 29**).
10. Cover the gel with cling film and smooth out any wrinkles. Dry under vacuum at 80°C (1–2 h).
11. Remove cling film from the dried gel and expose to film at room temperature without screens.

3.6. Analysis of Results

It should be possible to sequence an entire ~210 bp fragment in one sequencing run even using manual sequencing (*see* **Note 30**). Sequences should be analysed and homologies with known PTKs determined using BLAST. BLAST is located on the internet at http://www.ncbi.nlm. nih.gov/BLAST.

3.7. The Next Steps

1. Full-length cDNA clones for PTKs of interest can be obtained by hybridizing the corresponding ~210 bp fragment labeled with [α-^{32}P]dCTP to a cDNA library of choice and using standard cloning techniques *(12)* (**Fig. 2**; *see* Chapters 5 and 6). This approach has been successfully used previously (**refs. *7,8,13,14*** and I. Zachary, unpublished results). Ideally the cDNA library should be made from RNA prepared from the same cells used for the initial identification. If such a cDNA library is not available, the same ~210 bp fragment should be used to probe RNAs prepared from various tissues, and a commercially available cDNA library corresponding to a tissue giving strong expression used for cloning the full-length cDNA.
2. Once positive clones have been confirmed by taking them through three successive rounds of plaque purification and hybridisation, it is useful to perform a preliminary analysis in the gel plugs of plaques containing bacteriophage particles using PCR amplification with non-degenerate primers specific to the PTK of interest. Amplification of a ~210 bp band will confirm the presence of the corresponding sequence used for screening the cDNA library.
3. Once the relatively straightforward aim of obtaining the full-length cDNA for a PTK has been achieved, the more difficult one of defining its function can be embarked upon. Analysis of mRNA expression by Northern blot should be performed in tissue and cell-derived mRNAs (*see* Chapter 16). For functional as well as expression studies of PTKs, the generation of good antibodies is essential. From the point of view of cardiovascular disease, studies of mRNA and protein expression in atherosclerotic lesions or other neointimal lesions derived from animal or other models are clearly important goals.

3.8. Limitations of the Homology-Based Strategy

The homology-based PCR methodology has been very successful in identifying novel members of the PTK family *(6–8,13)* and it is ideal for identifying the PTKs expressed in a particular tissue or cell type. Some important PTKs may be resistant to amplification using the homology-based approach. For example, focal adhesion kinase (FAK) was not amplified using three different cell-derived mRNAs even though this PTK is expressed at the protein level in all of the cells used (I. Zachary, unpublished results). FAK has a large noncatalytic region at its COOH end, and it may be that cDNAs containing its catalytic domains are more rarely represented in cDNA libraries. The FAK-related PTK, Cell adhesion kinase β, was however successfully cloned using the homology-based approach and a rat brain cDNA library *(13)*.

Another important limitation of the protocol described is the nonquantitative nature of the data produced. The number of independent colonies obtained expressing a particular PTK PCR product should **not** be used as a good guide to the level of expression of that PTK. Quantitative expression data is ideally obtained by Northern analysis of mRNA or quantitative PCR.

3.9. Other Applications of the Homology-Based Strategy

The degenerate oligonucleotides used in this protocol are specifically designed to amplify a region in PTK catalytic domains. It is possible to refine the technique to selectively amplify particular subsets of PTKs such as receptor PTKs *(8, see* **Note 1**). Due to the high degree of sequence homology within this region between the catalytic domains of all protein kinases, this method may also occasionally amplify serine/threonine protein kinases. Cloning of at least one novel serine/threonine protein kinase has been achieved as a result *(14,15)*. For the identification of serine/threonine protein kinases, degenerate oligonucleotides can be designed specifically tailored to their catalytic domains as described *(15)*. In theory the homology-based approach can be used to identify the members of any family of proteins in which certain sequence motifs are highly conserved. Such an approach has been successfully used to identify novel phosphatases *(16)* and to identify members of the metalloproteinase-like, disintegrin-like cysteine-rich protein (MDC) family in endothelial cells *(17)*.

4. Notes

1. The homology-based approach can be refined to tailor the investigation to a particular subset of PTKs. For example, most receptor-like PTKs have a consensus motif KWMAPE in subdomain VIII of the catalytic domain. In contrast, most non-receptor PTKs do not possess a methionine in the third position and typically have the motif KWTAPE or FWYAPE. Some important exceptions are the EPH family of receptor PTKs which all possess a threonine in place of a methionine *(18)* and the nonreceptor PTK focal adhesion kinase which has the motif, KWMAPE *(19)*. Receptor PTKs also almost all have the sequence DLAARN in subdomain VI. Thus by using receptor PTK-specific degenerate primers corresponding to DLAARN and WMAPE motifs, members of this subset will be selectively amplified *(8)*.

2. Efficient subcloning of PCR fragments can now be achieved by taking advantage of the ability of *Taq* polymerase to add a single deoxyadenosine in a template-independent fashion to the 3'-ends of amplified fragments. The resulting A-tailed products can then be subcloned into purpose-designed vectors such as pGEM-5Zf(+) (Promega) with 3'-T overhangs *(20)*. The A-tailing activity of *Taq* is shared by some other thermostable polymerases (e.g., *Tfl* and *Tth*), but Vent (*Tli*) and *Pfu* produce blunt-ended products.

3. All of the buffers and solutions referred to in **steps 1–22** are provided with the kit.

4. For extraction of mRNA from contractile VSMC use fresh aortic tissue *(see* Chapter 4). Remove medial strips from the aorta (rabbit or rat) after denuding the endothelium by gentle abrasion as described *(21,22)*. Cut the medial strips into small pieces (1 mm^2 or smaller) using a McIlwain tissue chopper. Place the pieces onto plastic film, cover and grind the tissue using a mortar and pestle into a fine powder on dry ice or liquid N$_2$. Then collect the tissue into a 1.5-mL microcentrifuge tube, wash with PBS and extract with lysis buffer as described in **Subheading 3.1.**

5. To minimize wastage of polyA$^+$RNA, it is recommended that ODs are measured using microvolume cells which require samples up to 50 μL. It is also recommended that the integrity of the polyA$^+$ RNA is checked by running an aliquot on a denaturing gel. Total RNA should have prominent 28S and 18S ribosomal RNA bands with no smearing, while polyA$^+$RNA typically has weaker 28S and 18S ribosomal RNA bands with a smear between, above and below these bands.

6. This step inactivates the reverse transcriptase, which can inhibit subsequent PCR reactions if not inactivated.

7. The cycle that is most suitable will be affected both by the rate of thermal increase, thermal homogeneity and other specifications of the particular thermocycler used and by the types of tubes. The protocol described here has been used with an older model PerkinElmer Cetus DNA Thermal Cycler and 0.5-mL microcentrifuge tubes. This model has now been superceded by more recent and improved thermocyclers. Thin-walled 0.5-mL tubes designed specifically for PCR are now also widely available. Investigators are **strongly advised** to optimise the cycle parameters for use in their particular thermocycler and/or if using thin-walled tubes. The effect of these modifications is likely to be to reduce the denaturation temperature (to 92 or 93°C), and decrease the cycle times for all three steps. Compare for example the cycle used with a different homology-based PCR approach in the PTC-100™ Programmable Thermal Controller (B. Herren, personal communication and **ref. *17***).

8. Despite the low stringency annealing conditions used during the amplification step, we have not uncommonly obtained a single ~210 bp product with little product of other sizes. It is not unlikely that other products will be obtained, however, and the presence of other bands should not necessarily be taken as an indication that the PCR has been unsuccessful. *See* **Note 9**, however.

9. If the major PCR products are not of the predicted size, check for contamination of RNA with genomic DNA by performing a control RT-PCR reaction without reverse transcriptase. If PCR products are obtained in the absence of reverse transcriptase, pretreat the RNA sample with RNase-free DNase I.

10. Purification of PCR products can be performed before and after restriction endonuclease digestion. Alternatively, the first DNA purification step (i.e., **steps 1** and **2**) can be avoided by carrying out the restriction endonuclease digestion in the PCR reaction as follows. Add 1 μL Taquench per 50 μL of PCR reaction. Taquench PCR Cloning Enhancer is a proprietary inhibitor that has been designed

for use in restriction endonuclease cloning of PCR products where 3' recessed ends or blunt ends are generated. Then adjust the solution to make it compatible with the appropriate enzyme buffers. It is also advisable to allow the digestion to proceed for a longer time to ensure complete digestion.

11. The ligation of the PCR product to vector can also be conveniently and efficiently performed by in-gel ligation. If this method is preferred use the following protocol and go directly to **step 22** (except for digestion and purification of the vector). Prepare a 2% gel using low melting point agarose (NuSieve, FMC BioProducts) in TAE buffer. It is important to use a thin gel and to load as much of the PCR product in one well as possible. After running the gel, estimate the amount of DNA from gel using a known amount of molecular weight marker as a guide. Excise the band under long wave UV and transfer to a 1.5-mL microcentrifuge tube. Melt the gel slice at 69°C. Measure the volume with pipet after 2 min, calculate volume needed to have insert in desired molar excess over vector. In a second tube, prepare ligation mix with 1 μL 10x ligation buffer, 1 μL digested dephosphorylated and purified vector, 1 μL T4 DNA ligase and water to a final volume of 10 μL. Add required volume of melted gel to the ligation mix and quickly mix by pipetting up and down. Incubate 15°C overnight. For transformation of electrocompetent *E. coli* (*see* **Note 16** for preparation of electrocompetent cells), melt the ligation mix at 69°C for 5 min, add 40 μL water to dilute the agarose and vortex. Spin in a microcentrifuge for 10 s at maximum speed. Use 1–2 μL for electroporation of 100 μL competent cells.

12. After the restriction enzyme digestion, it is important to minimize damage to cohesive ends. DNA purification of the digested PCR fragment and vector should be performed in solution, that is in the restriction digest without prior gel isolation, and should be performed gently without vortexing or vigorous mixing.

13. It is strongly advised that several ligation reactions are set up using a fixed amount of vector and varying amounts of insert. Ligation of insert to vector will be favoured by using a molar excess of insert, and insert:vector molar ratios from 2:1 up to 10:1 are recommended. If a suitable water bath is not available ligations can also be conveniently and effectively performed over a weekend in the door of a fridge.

14. Polyethylene glycol is an important constituent of most ligation buffers because it excludes water and increases the effective molar concentrations of complementary cohesive ends.

15. If ligations are performed with PCR products and vectors containing single-base overhangs (*see* **Note 2**), low temperature ligations (<15°C) are required as higher temperatures will tend to favour blunt-end ligations of non-tailed vector.

16. Electrocompetent cells for transformation can be purchased or cells can be made competent according to the following simple protocol. Add 1 mL of an overnight *E. coli* XL-1 blue culture to 100 mL LB-broth and shake at 37°C for 2.5 h (incubations for much longer for this are not desirable). Transfer to a mixture of ice and water. Spin at 4°C to collect cells and resuspend pellet by addition of 2 mL H_2O and gently pipeting up and down. Add a further 13 mL of H_2O. Spin and resuspend the cell pellet in 25 mL of ice-cold 10% glycerol (in H_2O). Spin and

resuspend the cell pellet in 2 mL of 10% glycerol. The final cell density should be 5×10^{10} to 10^{11} cells per mL. Aliquot 100 μL into separate microcentrifuge tubes and store at –70°C for up to 2 yr or more. Use 100 μL of ice-cold cells for each electroporation.

17. Electroporation produces a transformation efficiency 100–1000 times greater than that obtained using $CaCl_2$/heat shock transformation procedures. This is particularly desirable for transformation with ligated DNA which produces a much lower efficiency of transformation. If an electroporater is not available, the $CaCl_2$ and heatshock method can be used as described in standard textbooks *(12)*.

18. It is important to sequence a large number of subcloned amplified fragments because many of the most abundantly represented species are more likely to be already known.

19. Siliconize in a fume-cabinet by pouring a small amount of silicone onto the gel surface of one plate and spreading over the plate using a paper tissue. Leave for several hours and rinse well with H_2O.

20. When making up the sequencing gel solution, it is important to remember that as the urea dissolves the volume of the solution will increase substantially. Allow for this increase by adding a smaller amount of water initially than would be necessary to make up to the final desired volume. It is better to underestimate the amount of water at this stage. If some urea is left undissolved, determine the volume and add some more water until the final volume is reached.

21. Alternatively, the bottom can be sealed with a small amount of polymerized gel as follows. Impregnate two strips of 3MM Whatman filter paper with a small volume of gel solution (~10 mL) to which has been added a high concentration of temed and ammonium persulfate (90 μL TEMED and 300 μL 10% ammonium persulfate) to ensure rapid polymerization. Immediately place the bottom of the gel on to the impregnated filter paper and hold in place very firmly until the gel has polymerized. Inspect the bottom of the gel to ensure that the solution has polymerized across the whole width of the gel assembly.

22. Two ways to maximise the sequence information from a particular piece of DNA in a single run are described here. The first method is to load the same sample twice on the same gel, but load the two aliquots 2–3 h apart. Another simple method is to use electrolyte gradient DNA sequencing gels as follows. Make and mount the sequencing gel as usual, fill the upper chamber with 0.5 x TBE. For the buffer in the lower chamber add 0.5 volume of 3 *M* sodium acetate (made by simply dissolving sodium acetate salt in H_2O; not necessary to pH) to 1x TBE to give a final concentration of 1 *M* sodium acetate (it does not matter that the TBE will be less than 1 x). Add buffer to the lower chamber. Run gel as usual. Electrophoresis will take approx 75% longer than with usual buffer system *(23)*. These methods should not be necessary for sequencing the ~210 bp PTK fragments but they will be useful for sequencing the cDNAs obtained at later stages of the project.

23. 37°C may be sufficient, but the higher temperature is desirable for sequences rich in GC base pairs and is preferable overall.

24. Specific activity of [α-^{35}S]dATP should be 1000-1500 Ci/mmol.
25. Dilute sequenase immediately prior to use in the sequencing reaction and only dilute into the dilution buffer.
26. The order GATC is used because most sequence problems involve the reading of G and C bases. Separating G and C helps to facilitate reading the sequence.
27. For sequencing the ~210 bp PTK PCR products runs of 2.5–3.5 h should be sufficient.
28. It is possible to dry the gel without first washing with methanol/acetic acid. Nonremoval of the urea may affect the resolution of the bands, however.
29. If the gel is proving difficult to transfer to paper and is becoming distorted or is in danger of being damaged, transfer the glass plate with gel to a large tray and smooth out distortions in the gel and repair tears by wetting with liberal amounts of 1X TBE. Prewet paper with 1X TBE and place onto the gel. Remove most of the excess TBE. Hold the bottom of the glass plate and the top of the filter firmly between flattened hands and quickly invert the gel. With the paper on the bottom, ease the plate away from the paper using 1X TBE to encourage separation.
30. If a sequence is particularly GC-rich and problems are being encountered with G/C compressions, reactions in which dITP is substituted for dGTP should be performed and run on the same gel as parallel reactions with dGTP. If using dITP keep labeling and termination reactions to 5 min or less.

References

1. Vandenberger, P., Hunter, T., and Lindberg, R. A. (1994) Receptor protein-tyrosine kinases and their signal transduction pathways. *Annu. Rev. Cell Biol.* **10,** 251–337.
2. Hanks, S. K. and Hunter, T. (1995) Protein kinases, the eukaryotic protein kinase superfamily - kinase (catalytic) domain structure and classification. *FASEB J.* **9,** 576–596.
3. Hanks, S. K., Quinn, A. M., and Hunter, T. (1988) The protein kinase family: conserved features and deduced phylogeny of the catalytic domain. *Science,* **241,** 42–52.
4. Hanks, S. K. and Quinn, A. M. (1991) Protein kinase catalytic domain sequence database: identification of conserved features of primary structure and classification of family members. *Methods Enzymol.* **200,** 38–61.
5. Ross, R. (1993) The Pathogenesis of atherosclerosis: a perspective for the 1990s. *Nature* **362,** 801–809.
6. Wilks, A. F. (1989) Two putative protein-tyrosine kinases identified by application of the polymerase chain reaction. *Proc. Natl. Acad. Sci. USA,* **86,** 1603–1607.
7. Wilks, A. F. (1991) Cloning members of the protein-tyrosine kinase family using polymerase chain reaction. *Methods Enzymol.* **200,** 533–545.
8. Hovens, C. M., Stacker, S. A., Andres, A-C., Harpur, A. G., Ziemiecki, A., and Wilks, A. F. (1992) RYK, a receptor tyrosine kinase-related molecule with unusual kinase domain motifs. *Proc. Natl. Acad. Sci. USA,* **89,** 11,818–11,822.

9. Shanahan, C. M., Weissberg, P. L., and Metcalfe, J. C. (1993) Isolation of gene markers of differentiated and proliferating vascular smooth muscle cells. *Circ. Res.* **73,** 193–204.

10. Thomas M. R. (1994) Simple, effective cleanup of DNA ligation reactions prior to electro-transformation of E. coli. *Biotechniques* **16,** 988–990.

11. Sanger, F., Nicklen, S., and Coulson, A. R. (1977) DNA sequencing with chain-terminating inhibitors. *Proc. Natl. Acad. Sci. USA* **74,** 5463–5467.

12. Sambrook, J., Fritsch, E. F., and Maniatis, T. (1989) *Molecular Cloning: A Laboratory Manual.* Cold Spring Harbor Laboratory Press.

13. Sasaki, H., Nagura, K., Ishino, M., Tobioka, H., Kotani, K., and Sasaki, T. (1995) Cloning and characterisation of cell adhesion kinase β, a novel protein-tyrosine kinase of the focal adhesion kinase subfamily. *J. Biol. Chem.* **271,** 21,206–21,219.

14. Valverde, A. M., Sinnett-Smith, J., Van Lint, J., and Rozengurt, E. (1994) Molecular cloning and characterization of protein kinase D: a target for diacylglycerol and phorbol esters with a distinctive catalytic domain. *Proc. Natl. Acad. Sci. USA* **91,** 8572–8576.

15. Johannes, F-J., Prestle, J., Eis, S., Oberhagemann, P., and Pfizenmaier, K. (1994) PKCμ is a novel, atypical member of the protein kinase C family. *J. Biol. Chem.* **269,** 6140–6148.

16. Sun, H., Charles, C. H., Lau, L. F., and Tonks, N. K. (1993) MKP-1 (3CH134), an immediate early gene product, is a dual specificity phosphatase that dephosphorylates MAP kinase in vivo. *Cell* **75,** 487–493.

17. Herren, B., Raines, E. W., and Ross, R. (1997) Expression of a disintegrin-like protein in cultured human vascular cells and in vivo. *FASEB J.* **11,** 173–180.

18. Lhotak, V., Greer, P., Letwin, K., and Pawson, T. (1991) Characterisation of ELK, a brain-specific receptor protein tyrosine kinase. *Mol. Cell. Biol.* **11,** 2496–2502.

19. Schaller, M. D., Borgman, C. A., Cobb, B. S., Vines, R. R., Reynolds, A. B., and Parsons, J. T. (1992) pp125[FAK], a structurally distinctive protein-tyrosine kinase associated with focal adhesions. *Proc. Natl. Acad. Sci. USA* **89,** 5192–5196.

20. Mead, D. A., Pey, N. K., Herrnstadt, C., Marcil, R. A., and Smith, L. M. (1991) A universal method for the direct cloning of polymerase chain reaction-amplified nucleic acid. *Bio-Technology* **9,** 657.

21. McMurray, H., Parrott, D. P., and Bowyer, D. E. (1991) A standardised method of culturing aoric explants suitable for the study of factors affecting the phenotypic modulation, migration and proliferation of aortic smooth muscle cells. *Atherosclerosis* **86,** 227–237.

22. Southgate, K. M., Davies, M., Booth, R. F. G., and Newby, A. C. (1992) Involvement of extracellular matrix-degrading metalloproteinases in rabbit smooth muscle cell proliferation. *Biochem. J.,* **288,** 93–99.

23. Sheen, J-Y. and Seeds, B. (1988) Electrolyte gradient gels for DNA sequencing. *BioTechniques* **6,** 942–944.

III

Methods for Mapping Transcriptional Start Sites and Measurement of Promoter Activity in Vascular Cells

11

Primer Extension Analysis
to Map Transcription Start Sites of Vascular Genes

Yutaka Kitami and Kunio Hiwada

1. Introduction

The principle of the technique presented in this chapter is illustrated in **Fig. 1**. As with S1 mapping or riboprobe mapping, this technique can be used to determine precisely the start site of transcription of a mRNA sequence *(1–3)*. Since this technique is relatively easier than other techniques, it is readily used for the primary determination of the transcription start site of a target gene. A radiolabeled probe derived entirely from within the gene is hybridized to mRNA complementary to the probe and extended using reverse transcriptase (RT). The cloned probe is normally derived from a region near the 5' end (cap site) of the gene and the extension reaction terminates at the extreme 5' end of the mRNA. Since only a small fragment of DNA probe is required as a primer, synthetic oligonucleotides are now almost exclusively used (although it is possible to use double-stranded DNA fragments or single-stranded primers generated by restriction enzyme digestion and gel electrophoresis) *(4)*.

Previously we have reported the transcription start sites of several vascular genes including platelet-derived growth factor (PDGF) receptors *(5,6)* and CCAAT/ enhancer-binding protein (C/EBP)-δ *(7)*. Shown in **Fig. 2** are typical results obtained when the primer extension technique is used to analyze the reverse transcripts of the C/EBP-δ gene. In this experiment a synthetic oligonucleotide was hybridized to poly(A)+ mRNA prepared from cultured vascular smooth muscle cells (VSMC) and extended using avian myeloblastosis virus (AMV) RT.

From: *Methods in Molecular Medicine, Vascular Disease: Molecular Biology and Gene Therapy Protocols*
Edited by: A. H. Baker © Humana Press Inc., Totowa, NJ

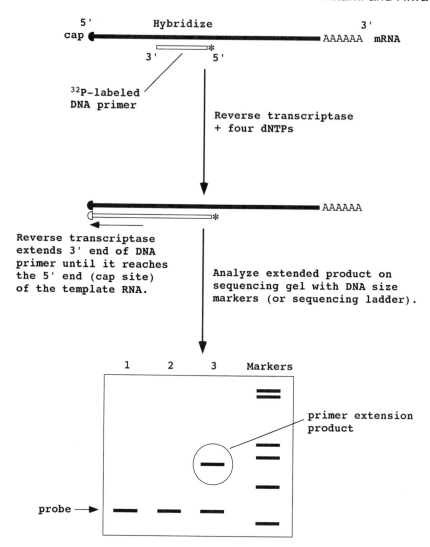

Fig. 1. The principle of primer extension analysis using a 5' end-labeled probe. The diagram illustrates how the 5' terminus of a poly(A)⁺ mRNA might be determined using a 5' end-labeled single-stranded DNA probe (or synthetic oligonucleotide). Usually the probe would be a fragment derived from a cloned copy of the gene by cleavage with appropriate restriction enzymes or an oligonucleotide synthesized from the known cDNA sequence. The schematic representation of the autoradiogram demonstrates the results expected from a typical experiment. **Lane 1**, untreated probe; **lanes 2** and **3**, probe incubated under annealing conditions in the absence or presence of mRNA complementary to the probe, respectively, and then incubated with RT in the presence of unlabeled four deoxynucleoside trisphosfates (dNTPs). Only when complementary mRNA is present to form a hybrid with the primer, a primer extension product is synthesized as shown in lane 3.

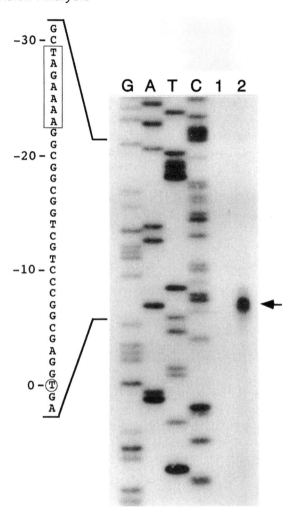

Fig. 2. The identification of the transcription start site of a vascular gene by primer extension analysis. In this experiment a 26-mer synthetic oligonucleotide primer specific for the rat CCAAT/enhancer-binding protein (C/EBP)-δ gene was hybridized to poly(A)⁺ mRNA obtained from rat cultured VSMC (7). The probe was end-labeled with T4 polynucleotide kinase and hybridized to 2 μg yeast tRNA (**lane 1**) or 2 μg vascular poly(A)⁺ mRNA (**lane 2**) for 1 h at 58°C. Primer extension was carried out with 5 U AMV RT for 1 h at 42°C and primer extension products were resolved on a 6% polyacrylamide/7 *M* urea gel. The single transcription start site of the rat C/EBP-δ gene was identified by a single reverse transcript (marked arrow) corresponding to the thymine base (T) of the sequencing ladder (marked open circle). A sequence "TAGAAAA" (marked open box) is one of TATA box-like sequences found at 23–29 bp upstream of the transcription start site. Most promoters have a sequence called TATA box, "TATAAAA," usually located within 30 bp upstream of the transcription start site.

2. Materials

2.1. End-Labeling of Synthetic Oligonucleotides

1. Synthetic oligonucleotides to be labeled (10 pmol) (*see* **Table 1**), and appropriate DNA size markers (e.g., dephosphorylated φX174 Hinf I markers available from Promega, Madison, WI) (*see* **Note 1**).
2. 1 *M* Dithiothreitol (DTT): Dissolve 3.09 g DTT in 20 mL 0.01 *M* sodium acetate, pH 5.2, and sterilize by filtration. Dispense into 1-mL aliquots and store at –20°C.
3. 10 X forward reaction buffer: 500 m*M* Tris-HCl, pH 7.5, 100 m*M* MgCl$_2$, 50 m*M* DTT (*see* **Note 2**), 1 m*M* spermidine (*see* **Note 3**). Stored at –20°C.
4. [γ-^{32}P]ATP (6,000 Ci/mmol, 10 mCi/mL).
5. T4 polynucleotide kinase (8–10 U/μL) (*see* **Note 4**). Add fresh from frozen aliquots.
6. Sephadex G-25 spun column equilibrated with TE buffer (10 m*M* Tris-HCl, pH 7.6, and 1 m*M* EDTA, pH 8.0) (e.g., MicroSpin G-25 Column; Pharmacia, Uppsala, Sweden). Stored at 4°C.
7. Whatman DE81 circular filter (2.3 cm diameter).

2.2. Hybridization and Primer Extension Reactions

1. Radiolabeled oligonucleotide probes (*see* **Subheading 2.1.**).
2. RNA samples (*see* **Note 5**).
3. 10 mg/mL yeast tRNA solution (*see* **Note 6**).
4. AMV RT (5 U/μL) (*see* **Note 7**). Add fresh from frozen aliquots.
5. 100 m*M* dNTPs: Dissolve each dNTP (dATP, dCTP, dGTP, or dTTP) in nuclease-free water at an approx concentration of 100 m*M*. Using a micropipet, adjust the pH of each of the solutions to 7.0 with 0.05 *M* Tris base (use pH paper to check the pH) and dilute the solutions with nuclease-free water to a final concentration of 50 m*M* dNTP. Store each separately in small aliquots at –70°C.
6. 2X hybridization/extension (H/E) buffer: 100 m*M* Tris-HCl, pH 8.3 at 42°C, 100 m*M* KCl, 20 m*M* MgCl$_2$, 20 m*M* DTT, 1 mM spermidine, and 2 m*M* each dNTP (*see* **Note 8**).
7. 5 mg/mL actinomycin D solution (*see* **Note 9**).
8. 40 mM sodium pyrophosphate (*see* **Note 10**). Store at –20°C.
9. 10 mg/mL deoxyribonuclease-free ribonuclease A (DNase-free RNase A) solution in 10 m*M* Tris-HCl, pH 8.0 containing 50% glycerol (e.g., Sigma, St. Louis, MO, cat. no. R 4642). Add fresh from frozen aliquots.
10. Phenol/chloroform/isoamylalcohol (25:24:1): in buffer 10 m*M* Tris-HCl, pH 8.0 containing 1 m*M* EDTA. Store at 4°C.
11. 3 *M* sodium acetate, pH 5.5.
12. Loading dye: 98% formamide (*see* **Note 11**), 10 m*M* EDTA, 0.1% xylene cyanol, and 0.1% bromophenol blue. Store at –20°C in small aliquots.

2.3. Preparation of Denaturing Polyacrylamide Gels

1. Sequencing gel electrophoresis apparatus: vertical electrophoresis tank, glass plate (40–60 cm long), 0.4-mm spacers, and shark's tooth comb.

Table 1
Amount of Primer Needed to Equal 10 pmol

Primer length	Nanograms of primer equal to 10 pmol
15-mer	50
16-mer	53
17-mer	56
18-mer	59
19-mer	63
20-mer	66
24-mer	80

2. 5X Tris-borate electrophoresis (TBE) stock buffer: 1X TBE (90 mM Tris-borate and 2 mM EDTA) is prepared as a concentrated stock solution (5X TBE) (to prepare 5X TBE stock, mix 54 g Tris base, 27.5 g boric acid, and 20 mL 500 mM EDTA, pH 8.0, and add distilled water to 1 L final volume). Keep in a plastic bottle and store at room temperature.

3. Urea, ultra pure (e.g., Sigma, cat. no. U 5378).

4. 40% acrylamide stock solution (19:1, acrylamide:bisacrylamide): Mix 38 g acrylamide, 2 g N,N'-methylene bisacrylamide, and water to 100 mL final volume. Dissolve the chemicals by heating the solution to 37°C with constant stirring. Filter the solution through a 2-μm membrane filter and store it at 4°C in a foil-wrapped bottle. Stock solution is stable for several weeks (*see* **Note 12**).

5. 10% (w/v) ammonium persulfate. Store at -20°C in small aliquots.

6. N,N,N',N'-tetramethyl ethylenediamine (TEMED). Store at 4°C.

7. Whatman 3MM paper and plastic wrap.

8. Vacuum-type gel dryer (e.g., Model 585 gel dryer; Bio-Rad, Hercules, CA).

3. Methods

3.1. 5'-End-Labeling of Synthetic Oligonucleotides by Phosphorylation

1. Mix the following reagents in a nuclease-free microcentrifuge tube: 10 pmol of oligonucleotide primer (*see* **Table 1**), 2 μL; 10 X forward reaction buffer, 1 μL; [γ-^{32}P]ATP (6,000 Ci/mmol, 10 mCi/mL), 3 μL; nuclease-free water, 3 μL to 9 μL final volume. DNA markers used for size determination can also be prepared by the end-labeling method (*see* **Subheading 3.2.**).

2. Add 1 μL of T4 polynucleotide kinase (8–10 U/μL) and mix gently. Incubate for 15 min at 37°C.

3. Heat for 2 min at 90°C to inactivate the T4 polynucleotide kinase, spin briefly in a microcentrifuge tube and add 40 μL nuclease-free water to 50 μL final volume. To determine the percent incorporation, spot 1 μL of mixture onto Whatman circular filter (F1) and keep it until counting.

4. Centrifuge the reaction mixture through a Sephadex G-25 spun column. Spot 1 μL of excluded probe onto another Whatman DE81 filter (F2). Dry the filters and measure the radioactivity of each filter using Cerenkov counting. The percentage incorporation is calculated by the average cpm for F1 and F2 filters:

$$\text{Percent incorporation } (\%) = (\text{cpm F2/ cpm F1}) \times 100$$

5. Bring the final concentration of the end-labeled specific primer to 100 fmol/μL by adding more nuclease-free water. The specific activity should be more than 10^6 dpm/pmol of primer.

3.2. 5′-End-Labeling of DNA Size Markers by Phosphorylation

1. Mix the following reagents in a nuclease-free microcentrifuge tube: Dephosphorylated φX174 Hinf I DNA markers (50 ng/μL), 5 μL; 10 X forward reaction buffer, 1 μL; [γ-^{32}P]ATP (6,000 Ci/mmol, 10 mCi/mL), 3 μL; T4 polynucleotide kinase (8–10 U/μL), 1 μL to 10 μL final volume.
2. Incubate for 15 min at 37°C.
3. Heat for 2 min at 90°C to inactivate the T4 polynucleotide kinase, spin briefly in a microcentrifuge tube and add 190 μL of nuclease-free water to 200 μL final volume. Store at –20°C. Typically loading 1 μL of the diluted markers onto a gel will provide dark bands on an autoradiogram following an overnight exposure (*see* **Note 13**).

3.3. Procedures for Hybridization and Primer Extension

1. RNA sample [poly(A)$^+$ mRNA or total RNA]: Typically use 100 fmol of probe at a specific activity of 10^6 dpm/pmol with five- to 10-fold excess of DNA over RNA complementary to the DNA probe. Therefore adjust the volume to 5 μL in nuclease-free water containing 10–20 fmol complementary RNA (i.e., 4–8 ng of a 1 kb mRNA) (*see* **Note 14**). In addition, prepare a "no complementary RNA" control tube by adding the diluted yeast tRNA solution (e.g., 5 μg yeast tRNA in 5 μL nuclease-free water) for each primer.
2. In a nuclease-free microcentrifuge tube, mix the following reagents gently: RNA sample, 5 μL; ^{32}P-labeled primer (100 fmol/μL) ,1 μL; 2 X H/E buffer, 5 μL to 11 μL final volume.
3. Heat the tubes for 2 min at 90°C, transfer the tubes into prewarmed water bath at an appropriate temperature, e.g., 58°C (*see* **Note 15**), and anneal the primer with complementary RNA by incubating for 2 h (*see* **Note 16**).
4. Place the tubes at room temperature to cool for 10 min, spin briefly, and combine the components for a "master" reverse transcriptase mixture (RT mix). For example, to ensure sufficient mix for five reactions, prepare a master RT mix for six tubes. Add the AMV RT last and mix gently.

	1 reaction	6 reactions
2X H/E buffer	5 μL	30 μL
40 m*M* sodium pyrophosphate	1.4 μL	8.4 μL
5 mg/mL actinomycin D	0.2 μL	1.2 μL

Nuclease-free water	1.4 μL	8.4 μL
AMV reverse transcriptase (5 U/μL)	1 μL	6 μL
	to a final volume	to a final volume
	of 9 μL	of 54 μL

5. Add 9 μL of master RT mix to each tube and incubate for 1 h at 42°C.
6. Add 1 μL of DNase-free RNase A solution (10 mg/mL) and incubate for 30 min at 37°C. (This step is optional. However, performing this step usually generates clear bands of autoradiographic images).
7. Bring a final volume to 100 μL by adding nuclease-free water, extract twice with phenol/chloroform/isoamylalcohol and once with chloroform. Then collect the DNA following precipitation with 0.1 vol of 3 *M* sodium acetate, pH 5.5 and 2.5 vol of ethanol.
8. Incubate the tubes for 30 min at –70°C and centrifuge at 10,000*g* for 15 min at 4°C.
9. Rinse the DNA pellet with 75% ethanol. Then leave it open to dry at room temperature.
10. Dissolve directly the dried pellet in 10 μL of loading dye. Typically 2–4 μL of the 10 μL volume are used to load onto a denaturing polyacrylamide gel. Store the remainder of the samples at –20°C.

3.4. Denaturing Polyacrylamide Gel Analysis

1. Prepare the denaturing polyacrylamide/7 M urea gel. Choose an appropriate gel concentration for 50 mL gels (*see* **Table 2**).
2. Preelectrophorese the gel at constant power (40–45 W) for at least 30 min in 1X TBE running buffer.
3. Heat the sample tubes at 90°C for 10 min and then load the samples (2–4 μL) immediately onto the preelectrophoresed gel alongside radiolabeled DNA size markers or sequencing ladder.
5. Continue electrophoresis at the same constant power in 1X TBE running buffer until the bromophenol blue dye is 1–2 cm from bottom of the gel.
6. Stop the electrophoresis and dismantle the apparatus leaving the gel adhering to one plate.
7. Place a piece of Whatman 3MM paper on top of the gel, and apply gently pressure so that the paper becomes firmly attached to the rough surface of the paper. Quickly flip the plate over, and lay the gel on a dry piece of protective paper.
8. Cover the gel with a plastic wrap and dry it for 1 h under vacuum on a commercially available gel dryer set at 80°C.
9. Establish an autoradiography by exposing the gel to X-ray film at –70°C with an intensifying screen. An RNA constituting only 0.1% of the population can easily be detected in an overnight exposure of the gel.

4. Notes

1. Sequencing ladder can be also used to determine precisely the transcription start site of the target gene.
2. Do not autoclave DTT or solutions containing DTT.

Table 2
Preparation of Denaturing Polyacrylamide/7 *M* Urea Gel

	Polyacrlymode gel concentration (%)			
	5	6	7	8
40% acrylamide stock (mL)	6.25	7.5	8.75	10.0
5X TBE stock buffer (mL)	10.0	10.0	10.0	10.0
Urea (g)	21	21	21	21
Water (mL)	16.25	15.0	13.75	12.5
10% ammonium persulfate (mL)	0.25	0.25	0.25	0.25
TEMED (µL)	30	30	30	30

3. Spermidine stimulates incorporation of $[\gamma\text{-}^{32}P]$ATP and inhibits a nuclease present in some preparations of bacteriophage T4 polynucleotide kinase.
4. Ammonium ions are strong inhibitors of bacteriophage T4 polynucleotide kinase. Therefore DNA should not be dissolved in, or precipitated from, buffers containing ammonium salts prior to treatment with T4 polynucleotide kinase.
5. The primer extension reaction is more sensitive and yields cleaner results using poly(A)$^+$ mRNA rather than total RNA. When using total RNA, primer extension yields a relatively large number of prematurely terminated transcripts. This is presumably caused by cellular inhibitors of RT, which are removed by oligo(dT)-cellulose chromatography. [Commercially available kits (i.e., oligo(dT)-latex; Qiagen, Chatsworth, CA) are convenient for multiple preparations of poly(A)$^+$ mRNA.] However, with a DNA probe derived from near the 5' end of the mRNA (within 100–200 nucleotides), reasonable results can be obtained even if using total RNA.
6. This solution can be prepared by dissolving commercially available yeast tRNA at a concentration of 10 mg/mL in sterile TE, pH 7.6, containing 0.1 *M* NaCl. The solution is extracted twice with phenol (equilibrated in Tris-HCl, pH 7.6) and once with chloroform, and the RNA is precipitated with 2.5 vol of ethanol at room temperature. The RNA is recovered by centrifugation at 5000*g* for 15 min at 4°C, redissolved at a concentration of 10 mg/mL in nuclease-free TE, pH 7.6, divided into small aliquots, and stored at –20 °C.
7. Reverse transcriptase obtained from different manufacturers varies greatly in activity per unit. The figure of 5 units is based on the enzyme obtained from Gibco-BRL (Grand Isalnd, NY).
8. Stock solutions of 100 m*M* of each dNTP are commercially available (e.g., Pharmacia) if you do not want to prepare your own. Use the four stock solutions to make a single working solution containing each of the four dNTPs at a concentration of 2 m*M* dNTP. Store the mixture in small aliquots at –70°C.
9. Actinomycin D inhibits synthesis of double-stranded DNA by RT without significantly affecting the yield of first-strand DNA. It therefore prevents the synthesis of "hairpin" molecules that are formed when the first strand of DNA serves

as a primer/template. Usually stock solutions of actinomycin D are prepared in ethanol at a concentration of 5 mg/mL, stored at –20°C in the dark, and dilute it into the reaction mixture immediately before use. Caution: Actinomycin D is a teratogen and a carcinogen. Stock solutions should be prepared while wearing gloves and a mask and in a chemical hood, not on an open bench.

10. Sodium pyrophosphate may precipitate in solutions that are cooler than room temperature. Therefore, prewarm the 40 mM sodium pyrophosfate, nuclease-free water and 2X H/E buffer to 37°C to maximize solubility.

11. Many batches of reagent-grade formamide are sufficiently pure to be used without further treatment. However, if any yellow color is present, the formamide should be deionized by adding mixed-bed resin (e.g., Bio-Rad AG 501-X8), stirring on a magnetic stirrer for 1 h and filtering twice through Whatman No. 1 paper. Deionized formamide should be stored in small aliquots under nitrogen at –70°C.

12. Caution: Acrylamide is a neurotoxin.

13. For accurate sizing of single-stranded denatured DNA, it is important that the DNA markers should be denatured before loading them on the gel. Add the markers directly to 1–2 μL loading dye, heat at 90°C for 10 min and then immediately load them onto the denaturing gel (*see* **Subheading 3.4.**).

14. It is necessary to exercise care in optimizing the conditions under which the probe is hybridized to the RNA. The hybridization reaction should be performed under conditions of moderate excess of the primer over the target RNA. However, a massive excess of primer should not be used because this will lead to nonspecific priming during the extension reaction. Therefore, it is better to perform the reaction using different proportions of the primer/RNA around the expected optimum.

15. Optimum temperature for the hybridization mainly depends on the GC-content or length of the primer. Using a primer (e.g., 50% GC-content and 20–30 mer-length), the optimum temperature will normally be between 50 and 60°C. However, it is best to perform hybridization reactions in parallel at different temperatures (e.g., from 10°C below to 10°C above, in 5°C steps). This will also aid interpretation of the data obtained.

16. Incubation time for the hybridization also depends on the primer to be used. When incubate for a longer time (e.g., 4 h to overnight), it should be necessary to prevent from evaporation during the incubation (e.g., lay small aliquots of mineral oil onto each reaction mixture).

References

1. Sambrook, J. and Fritsch, E. F., and Maniatis, T. (1989) *Molecular Cloning: A Laboratory Manual.* 2nd ed. Cold Spring Harbor Laboratory Press, Cold Spring Harbor, NY.

2. Ausbel, F. M., Brent, R., Kingston, R. E., Moore, D. D., Seidman, J. G., Smith, J. A., and Struhl, K. (1989) *Current Protocol in Molecular Biology.* Greene Publishing Associate, NY.

3. Hames, B. D. and Higgins, S. J. (1989) *Gene Transcription: A Practical Approach.* IRL Press, New York, NY.

4. Hames, B. D. and Higgins S. J. (1989) *Nucleic Acid Hybridization: A Practical Approach*. IRL Press, New York, NY.
5. Kitami, Y., Inui, H., Uno, S., and Inagami, T. (1995) Molecular structure and transcriptional regulation of the gene for the platelet-derived growth factor α receptor in cultured vascular smooth muscle cells. *J. Clin. Invest.* **96**, 558–567.
6. Kitami, Y., Fukuoka, T., Okura, T., Takata, Y., Maguchi, M., Igase, M., Kohara, K., and Hiwada, K. (1998) Molecular structure and function of rat platelet-derived growth factor β-receptor gene promoter. *J. Hypertens.* **16**, 437–445.
7. Fukuoka, T., Kitami, Y., Kohara, K., and Hiwada, K. (1997) Molecular structure and function of rat CCAAT-enhancer binding protein-delta gene promoter. *Biochem. Biophys. Res. Commun.* **231**, 30–36.

12

Use of Liposome-Mediated DNA Transfection to Determine Promoter Activity in Smooth Muscle Cells

Rosalind P. Fabunmi

1. Introduction

The transfer and expression of DNA plasmids containing promoter fragments of heterologous genes linked to reporter cDNAs in mammalian cells has become an invaluable technique for studying the regulation of gene expression. Several reporter genes such as luciferase, β-galactosidase, chloramphenicol acetyl transferase, and green flourescent protein are ideal to study promoter activities as their gene products are not endogenous to smooth muscle cells (SMC) and their expression can be readily detected using convenient assays (1). Among these genes, a popular choice is the firefly luciferase, as its expression can be easily detected in cells using a highly sensitive chemiluminescent assay (2). The firefly luciferase catalyses a rapid, ATP-dependent oxidation of the substrate, luciferin, which then emits light. Reactions catalyzed by firefly luciferase are:

$$\text{luciferase} + \text{luciferin} + \text{ATP} \rightarrow \text{luciferase. luciferyl-AMP} + PP_i$$

$$\text{luciferase.luciferyl-AMP} + O_2 \rightarrow \text{luciferase} + \text{oxyluciferin} + \text{AMP} + CO_2 + \text{light}$$

Total light output is measured which is maximal at 562 nm and is proportional to the amount of luciferase present (3). Luciferase activity is linear up to 200 μg protein in cell extracts.

An important consideration in reporter assays for the analysis of gene promoter regulation is to correct for differences in transfection efficiency. This may be achieved by cotransfection of a second reporter gene such as β-galactosidase (β-gal) under the control of a strong constitutive promoter (4). The

From: *Methods in Molecular Medicine, Vascular Disease: Molecular Biology and Gene Therapy Protocols*
Edited by: A. H. Baker © Humana Press Inc., Totowa, NJ

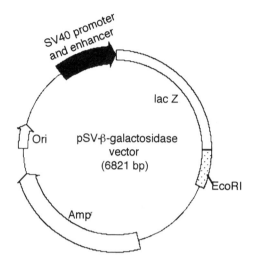

Fig. 1. pSV-β-gal vector for monitoring transfection efficiencies in SMC. The SV40 early promoter and enhancer drive expression of the bacterial *lac* Z gene which, in turn, is translated into the β-gal enzyme. Additional features of the plasmid include an ampicillin resistance gene (Amp^r) conferring ampicillin resistance in *Escherichia coli* and an origin of plasmid replication in *E. coli* (ori). The arrow within *lac* Z indicates the direction of transcription of the *lac* Z gene.

Simian virus (SV40) early promoter, rous sarcoma virus (RSV), and the cytomegalovirus (CMV) promoters are commonly used for this purpose (**Fig. 1**). β-gal activity in cell extracts can be readily assayed using a simple spectrophotometric assay in which β-gal catalyses the conversion of *o*-nitrophenol-β-D-galactoside (ONPG), a galactoside derivative, to galactose and the chromophore, *o*-nitrophenol, which is detected by measuring absorbance at 420 nm (*5*). However, this assay has limitations owing to its poor sensitivity with a detection limit of 100 pg. An improved chemiluminescent reporter assay has been developed with greater sensitivity and a detection limit of 2 fg (*6*). In this assay, β-gal cleaves a chemiluminescent 1,2-dioxetane substrate and the reaction is terminated by the addition of a luminescence accelerator reagent that accelerates light emission, which can be measured in a luminometer. β-gal is not ideal as a reporter gene in several cell types including macrophages as its expression is endogenous to the cell, though this may be partially overcome by heat inactivation (*7*).

Several methods for transfecting cells are available, which include the use of electroporation, calcium phosphate, and liposomes. Of these methods, liposome-mediated DNA transfection is considered to be effective in transfecting most cell types. Liposome-mediated DNA transfection employs the use of cationic lipids as vehicles for DNA transfer *(8)* (*see also* Chapters 24, 25, and 31). Many different preparations of liposomes are available commercially and differ in their lipid components. The prototype of cationic liposomes is composed of a positively charged lipid, N[1-(2,3-dioleyloxy)propyl]-N,N, N-trimethylammonium (DOTMA), and a neutral lipid, dioleoyl phosphatidylethanolamine (DOPE) and is commercially available as Lipofectin. An improved polycationic lipid formulation has been developed called Lipofectamine, which has been reported to achieve up to 30-fold higher activity than monocationic liposome reagents such as Lipofectin *(9)*. The cationic lipid vesicles introduce DNA into the cell by interacting with the negatively charged phosphate groups on the DNA resulting in the formation of a liposome/polynucleotide complex. Endocytosis is thought to be the major cellular uptake pathway for the DNA/lipid complex. The DNA/lipid complex is released from endosomes before reaching the lysosomes, where the majority of the complex is degraded. The remainder of the DNA/lipid complex is delivered to the cytosol followed by translocation to the nucleus where the DNA is retained, mainly extrachromosomally and expressed *(8)*. Liposome-mediated transfection is quick and easy to perform. It does not require the use of specialized equipment, and, when suitably optimized, can lead to relatively high transfection efficiency and low toxicity in vascular cells.

This chapter describes the use of liposome-mediated DNA transfection to introduce promoter-luciferase reporter gene constructs in to primary rabbit aortic SMC in vitro.

2. Materials

2.1. Cell Culture and Transfection

1. Primary rabbit aortic smooth muscle cells (*see* **Note 1**).
2. Complete media: Dulbecco's modification of Eagles medium (DMEM) supplemented with 15% fetal calf serum, 8 mM L-glutamine, 100 U/ml penicillin and 100 μg/mL streptomycin.
3. Phosphate-buffered saline (PBS) buffer (Mg^{2+} and Ca^{2+} free).
4. CsCl-purified DNA plasmids (*see* **Notes 2** and **3**): For our studies, the following plasmids were used: pTKLUC containing the firefly luciferase cDNA cloned downstream of a thymidylate kinase (tk) promoter, p[TRE]$_3$LUC and p[NF]$_3$LUC containing the firefly luciferase cDNA cloned downstream of a thymidylate kinase (tk) promoter and carrying multiple copies of either the AP-1 or NFκB enhancer sequences, respectively, and pSV-β-gal containing the β-gal gene cloned downstream of the SV40 early promoter and enhancer (commercially available from Promega, Madison, WI).
5. Lipofectamine reagent (Gibco-BRL, Grand Island, NY) *(9)*.
6. OptiMEM 1 (serum free medium; Gibco-BRL).

2.2. Analysis of Transfected DNA

2.2.1. Preparation of Cellular Extract

1. Rubber policeman (plunger of a 3-mL sterile syringe).
2. 5X reporter lysis buffer (Promega): Add 4 vol of distilled water to 1 vol of reporter lysis 5X buffer to make a 1X stock (*see* **Note 4**). Prepare fresh as required.
3. Rocking/shaking platform.

2.2.2. Luciferase Assays

1. Luminometer (*see* **Note 5**).
2. Luminometer microtiter plates or borosilicate glass luminometer tubes.
3. Luciferase reaction buffer: 20 mM tricine, 1.07 mM $(MgCO_3)_4Mg(OH)_2$•$5H_2O$, 2.67 mM $MgSO_4$, 0.1 mM EDTA, 33.3 mM DTT, 530 μm ATP containing 270 μM coenzyme A and 470 μM luciferin as substrate (Promega, Madison, WI).

2.2.3. β-Galactosidase Assays

2.2.3.1. ONPG ASSAY

1. β-galactosidase reaction buffer: 100 mM sodium phosphate, pH 7.3, 1 mM $MgCl_2$, 50 mM β-mercaptoethanol, 0.67 mg/mL of *o*-nitrophenol-β-D-galacto-side (ONPG). Store ONPG at –20°C. Make solution fresh as required.
2. Plate reader.
3. Microtiter plates.

2.2.3.2. CHEMILUMINESCENT ASSAY

1. Galacto-light™ or Galacto-light plus™ kit (Tropix Inc., Bedford, MA) (*see* **Note 6**).
2. Galacton™ or Galacton-Plus™ chemiluminescent substrate (Tropix Inc.) (*see* **Note 6**).
3. Light emission accelerator (*see* **Note 6**).
4. Luminometer microtiter plates or borosilicate glass luminometer tubes.

3. Methods

3.1. Cell Culture and Transfection

1. 24 h prior to transfection, plate SMC at a density of 2.5×10^5 cells per 3.5-cm dish in a six-well plate to achieve approx 70% confluency (*see* **Note 7**).
2. Dilute 10 μg of DNA (5 μg each of test plasmid and control plasmid pSV βgal) in to 100 μL of optiMEM 1.
3. Dilute 40 μg of lipofectamine reagent into 100 μL of optiMEM 1.
4. Combine the two solutions together and incubate at room temperature for 45 min (*see* **Note 8**).
5. Dilute the mixture containing the DNA-lipid complexes drop-wise in to 1 mL optiMEM 1. For triplicate wells, scale up the amounts of liposome and DNA appropriately (*see* **Note 9**).
6. Wash the cells to be transfected twice with 2 mL of optiMEM 1, then overlay the mixture containing the DNA-lipid complexes in a total volume of 1 mL onto the cells.

7. Incubate cells at 37°C for 5 h.
8. Wash cells twice in optiMEM 1 to rinse away the DNA-lipid complexes.
9. Add 2 mL of complete medium per well and allow to recover overnight.
10. Replenish cells with fresh complete medium and incubate at 37°C in the absence or presence of the appropriate concentration of the stimulus under investigation until analysis (*see* **Note 10**).

3.2. Analysis of Transfected DNA

3.2.1. Preparation of Cellular Extract

1. Wash cells twice with 2 mL of PBS buffer. Carefully aspirate off the last traces of PBS, then add 200 µL of reporter lysis buffer/well.
2. Incubate at room temperature for 15 min on a rocking platform.
3. Scrape the cells from each well using a rubber policeman and transfer the lysate to a 1.5-mL Eppendorf tube.
4. Pellet cellular debris in a microfuge at 13,000*g* for 30 s at room temperature.
5. Transfer supernatant to fresh tube. Assay immediately or store at –70°C prior to further analysis (*see* **Note 11**).

3.2.2. Luciferase Assays

1. Place 20 µL of extract into microtiter well or luminometer tube (*see* **Note 5**).
2. Initiate the luciferase reaction by injecting 100 µL of luciferase reaction buffer.
3. Measure light output for 30 s in luminometer. If the measured relative light units is outside the linear range, dilute the extract in distilled water and re-assay.

3.2.3. β-Galactosidase Assays

3.2.3.1. ONPG ASSAY

1. Incubate 10–20 µL of cell extract in wells of a microtiter plate with β-galactosidase reaction buffer until a yellow reaction product develops (*see* **Note 12**).
2. Measure absorbance at 405 nm using a plate reader. Measure units of enzyme activity using the formula $U = (380 \times A_{420})$ divided by time (in minutes), where 380 is a constant such that 1 U is equivalent to conversion of 1 nmol of ONPG/minute at 37°C.
3. To normalize for transfection efficiency, divide the luciferase activity in each sample by the amount of β-galactosidase activity such that the value of each sample is expressed as the total number of light counts per unit of β-galactosidase activity. If limited sensitivity is experienced using this method for the detection of β-galactosidase, an alternative method is the chemiluminescent reporter assay (*see* **Subheading 3.2.3.2.**).

3.2.3.2. CHEMILUMINESCENT ASSAY

1. Place 2–20 µL of extract into microtiter well or luminometer tube (*see* **Note 12**).
2. Add 200 µL of reaction buffer to the microtiter well or luminometer tube.
3. Incubate at room temperature for 15–60 min.

4. Place plate or tube in luminometer and inject 300 mL of light emission accelerator. If manual injection is used, the accelerator should be added in the same consistent time frame as the reaction buffer is added (*see* **Note 6**).
5. Measure light output.

4. Notes

1. Primary rabbit aortic SMC used in our studies were prepared from explant cultures of thoracic aorta according to the method of McMurray and coworkers and later modified by Southgate and coworkers *(10,11)*.
2. It is very important that high quality purified form I (covalently closed circular supercoiled) DNA is used. All transfection DNA should be purified through cesium chloride gradients to remove contaminating RNA and nicked or open circular DNA. Dissolve the DNA in sterile TE or water. If inconsistent transfection data is a problem, purify the DNA further using Phenol/chloroform extraction and ethanol precipitation. Alternatively, commercially available DNA purification kits (Qiagen, Chatsworth, CA) can be used to generate pure DNA.
3. The activities of many different types of promoter-luciferase fusion constructs can be assayed following transfection into SMC. In the experiments described here (**Table 1**), the activator binding site, AP-1 and the NFκB enhancer sequences were each placed in a vector proximal to the basal tk promoter fused to the luciferase gene. Measurement of the reporter product provides an estimate of the induction in gene expression directed by the inserted regulatory sequences. Alternatively, to test the functionality of the promoters of heterologous genes, constructs containing luciferase fused downstream of different lengths of promoter fragments can be used. The measurement of luciferase activity will determine the ability of those stretch of sequences to direct transcription. The functionality of *cis*-regulatory elements in the promoter sequences can be determined using deletion mutants or site-directed mutagenesis of the regulatory elements *(1)*.
4. The 1X reporter lysis buffer is useful for the extraction of cells expressing both luciferase and β-gal and does not interfere with the assays of either of these reporters.
5. Different models of luminometers are available. A microplate luminometer with dispenser/injections is highly recommended as it is less time consuming and yields more reproducible results than single-well luminometers.
6. The choice of kit depends upon the type of specialized equipment available for the assay. In the galacto-light chemiluminescent assay, the Galacton chemiluminescent substrate has a half life of approx 4.5 min after the addition of light emission accelerator and is suited for use with luminometers with automatic injectors. Alternatively, the Galacton-Plus chemiluminescent substrate exhibits a half life of approx 180 min and is better suited for use with luminometers without injectors or with scintillation counters.
7. Cells should be healthy and not too sparse prior to start of transfection. Smaller or larger dishes can be used. Adjust for amount of DNA and cells as appropriate.

**Table 1
Activities of the TRE and NFκB Sites in SMC in Response to Growth
Factors and Cytokines[a]**

Construct	Luciferase activity/µU β-gal			
	Control	PDGF	1L-1	PDGF + IL-1
pTKLUC	4.10 ± 1.5	5.30 ± 1.90	4.31 ± 1.50	4.90 ± 1.0
p[TRE]3LUC	18.5 ± 5.1	48.7 ± 14.3	40.0 ± 12.8	81.0 ± 32.2
p[NF]3LUC	157.0 ± 30	211.4 ± 30	221.0 ± 11.4	318.2 ± 41.8

[a]SMC were transfected with plasmids containing the firefly luciferase cDNA cloned downstream of a thymidylate kinase (tk) promoter carrying multiple copies of either the TRE (p[TRE]$_3$LUC) or NFkB (p[NF]$_3$LUC) sequences. An identical plasmid carrying only the tk promoter linked to the luciferase gene was used as a control (pTKLUC). pSV-β-gal was used as an internal control to correct for differences in transfection efficiencies. Following overnight recovery of the cells in complete DMEM, cells were switched to serum-free medium for 10 h, then stimulated with 20 ng/mL of PDGF or 10 ng/mL of IL-1 or 20 ng/mL of PDGF + 10 ng/mL of IL-1. Following 20 h, cells were harvested for luciferase activity. Values are means ± S.E.M of the experiments performed in triplicate and expressed as light counts per microunit of β-gal activity.

8. The amounts of lipofectamine and DNA recommended in this protocol results in up to 30% of positively transfected cells. It is critical to optimize the amounts of DNA and lipid used for each cell type and species used in order to achieve the best transfection efficiency. For example we find that the optimal amount of lipid/DNA activity is different in rabbit SMC vs human SMC. For rabbit SMC, the transfection conditions that resulted in the highest efficiency and lowest toxicity was 40 µg of lipofectamine and 10 µg of DNA vs 10 µg of lipofectamine and 1 µg of DNA for human saphenous vein SMC. Another liposome formulation, called the LipofectAmine Plus Reagent, recently developed by Gibco-BRL has been shown to have advantages over Lipofectamine in cultured cell lines. We have not tested this reagent and do not know whether it leads to improved transfection efficiencies when compared to lipofectamine in SMC.
9. When performing stimulation experiments, it is recommended that transfections should be performed in triplicate. Triple the amount of DNA and lipofectamine and dilute in to water instead of optiMEM. Combine the solutions together and allow the formation of the DNA/lipid complex. After 45 min, dilute the mixture into 3 mL of optiMEM and add 1 mL per well.
10. Assessment of promoter activity may be carried out 24–72 h post-transfection for transient transfection. This time may vary according to the desired treatment of the cells. If the absence of serum is required for stimulation experiments, the cells may be switched to serum-free DMEM following the overnight recovery period.
11. Avoid multiple freeze-thaw cycles of cellular lysates.
12. Purified β-gal should be added to mock-transfected cell lysates and used as a positive control. Mock-transfected cell extracts should be used as a negative control for endogenous enzyme background.

References

1. Ausubel, F., Brent, R., Kingston, R., Moore, D., Seidman, J., Smith, J., and Struhl, K., ed. (1994), *Current Protocols in Molecular Biology.* Wiley, USA.
2. Gould, S. and Subramani, S. (1988) Firefly luciferase as a tool in molecular and cell biology. *Anal. Biochem.* **175,** 5–13.
3. De Wet, J. R., Wood, K. V., DeLuca, M., Helinski, D. R., and Subramani, S. (1987) Firefly luciferase gene: Structure and expression in mammalian cells. *Mol. Cell .Biol.* **7,** 725–737.
4. Alam, J. and Cook, J. (1990) Reporter genes: application to the study of mammalian gene transcription. *Anal. Biochem.* **188,** 245–254.
5. MacGregor, G., GP, N., Fiering, S., Roederer, M., and Herzenberg, L. (1991) Use of E. coli *lacZ* (β-galactosidase) as a reporter gene, in *Gene Transfer and Expression Protocols* (Murray, E., ed.), Humana Press, Totowa, NJ, pp. 217–235.
6. Jain, V. and Magrath, I. (1991) A chemiluminescent assay for quantitation of beta-galactosidase in the femtogram range: application to quantitation of beta-galactosidase in lacZ-transfected cells. *Anal. Biochem.* **199,** 119–124.
7. Young, D., Kingsley, S., Ryan, K., and Dutko, F. (1993) Selective inactivation of eukaryotic beta-galactosidase in assays for inhibitors of HIV-1 TAT using bacterial beta-galactosidase as a reporter enzyme. *Anal. Biochem.* **215,** 24–30.
8. Felgner, P. L. and Ringold, G. M. (1989) Cationic liposome-mediated transfection. *Nature* **337,** 387–388.
9. Hawley-Nelson, P., Ciccarone, V., Gebeyehu, G., and Jessee, J. (1993) Lipofectamine reagent: A new, higher efficiency polycationic liposome transfection reagent. *Focus* **15,** 73–79.
10. McMurray, H., Parrott, D. P., and Bowyer, D. E. (1991) A standardised method of culturing aortic explants, suitable for the study of factors affecting the phenotypic modulation, migration and proliferation of aortic smooth muscle cells. *Atherosclerosis* **86,** 227–237.
11. Southgate, K. and Newby, A. C. (1990) Serum-induced proliferation of rabbit aortic smooth muscle cells from the contractile state is inhibited by 8-Br-cAMP but not 8-Br-cGMP. *Atherosclerosis* **82,** 113–123.

13

Nuclear Run-On Assay to Study Gene Transcription in Vascular Cells

Ulrich Laufs and James K. Liao

1. Introduction

An accurate assessment of gene transcription is important for understanding the mechanism of gene expression. The nuclear run-on assay measures the relative *in situ* transcription rate of specific genes in intact nuclei *(1,2)*. It provides information on the synthesis of a specific gene that occurs as a function of cell state, as opposed to a change in mRNA degradation or transport from the nucleus to the cytoplasm. Within a given experimental condition, the nuclear run-on assay can be used to determine the level of transcription for several different genes. The isolated nuclei contain the full transcription machinery for synthesis of mRNA. Therefore, it is regarded as the gold-standard measurement of overall transcriptional activity of a specific promoter. Other methods of measuring gene transcription, e.g., based on RT-PCR or pulse-labeling of nuclear RNA *(3,4)*, are difficult to perform and are seldom used.

The first step of the nuclear run-on assay is the isolation of intact nuclei of treated cells, because newly synthesized mRNA can be labeled with high specific activity in isolated nuclei compared to intact cells. The nuclei are incubated in the presence of radiolabeled UTP allowing the in vitro transcription of a labeled total mRNA over a defined time. After the transcription reaction, the genomic DNA and cell proteins are digested. The radiolabeled RNA is then isolated and hybridized with denatured DNA, which has been immobilized on a filter membrane. This allows the detection of specific mRNA transcripts. The DNAs usually include cDNA sequences of the gene(s) of interest and of a housekeeping gene that is stably expressed (e.g., GAPDH or β-tubulin) as a standard. Plasmid vector DNA can be used as a control for unspecific binding.

From: *Methods in Molecular Medicine, Vascular Disease: Molecular Biology and Gene Therapy Protocols*
Edited by: A. H. Baker © Humana Press Inc., Totowa, NJ

contr.   IL-1

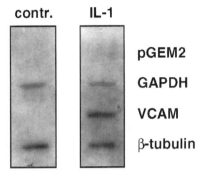

pGEM2

GAPDH

VCAM

β-tubulin

Fig. 1. Example of a nuclear run-on assay. Treatment of human saphenous vein endothelial cells with interleukin-1 (IL-1, 10 ng/mL) for 4 h resulted in a strong gene expression of vascular cell adhesion molecule-1 (VCAM). There was no VCAM gene transcription in untreated control cells (Contr.). The β-tubulin and GAPDH transcription and lack of a pGEM2 band served as internal controls for standardization and nonspecific binding.

After hybridization the membranes are washed and exposed to X-ray film *(5,6)* (**Fig. 1**).

2. Materials

Use DEPC-treated, deionized, distilled water ("RNA water") in all recipes and protocol steps.

2.1. Preparation of DNA Blot

1. DNA inserts of interest.
2. Whatman 3MM filter paper.
3. 0.45-μm nitrocellulose membrane.
4. Slot-blot apparatus (e.g., slot blot system Acrylic: cat. no. 77480, Schleicher and Schuell, Keane, NH) and a vacuum pump.
5. 80°C oven.
6. Sterile 6X SSC.
7. 0.2 N NaOH.

2.2. Preparation of Nuclei from Adherent Cells

1. 15-mL Dounce homogenizer (cat. no. 357544, Wheaton, Millville, NJ).
2. Microscope.
3. Rubber policeman.
4. 15 mL and 50 mL polypropylene centrifuge tubes.
5. Sterile PBS.
6. Lysis buffer: 10 mM Tris-HCl, pH 7.4, 10 mM NaCl, 3 mM MgCl$_2$, autoclave and store at RT. Before use add 0.5% NP-40.

7. Storage buffer: 20 mM Tris-HCl, pH 8.1, 75 mM NaCl, 0.5 mM EDTA, autoclave and store at RT. Immediately before use add 1 mM DTT and 50 % sterile glycerol. For each aliquot of nuclei to be frozen: 49 μL Tris/NaCl/EDTA + 1 μL 0.1 M DTT + 50 μL glycerol.
8. Transcription buffer: 10 mM Tris-HCl, pH 8.0, 5 mM MgCl$_2$, 300 mM KCl, 50 μM EDTA, autoclave and store at RT. Immediately before use place aliquots on ice and add 1 mM DTT, 250 U/mL of RNAse inhibitor (RNasin: *see* **Note 1**), 0.5 mM each recombinant triphosphates (rCTP, rATP, rGTP; *see* **Note 2**), and 200 μCi α-^{32}P UTP per condition (10 mCi/mL stock).

2.3. In vitro Transcription

1. Protective equipment, laboratory facilities, and license to handle ^{32}P-UTP.
2. Shaking water bath.
3. Microfuge, ideally with aerosol-tight safety capsules.
4. Aerosol-tight Eppendorf tubes.
5. Proteinase K buffer: 0.4% SDS, 40 mM Tris-HCl (pH 7.4), 10 mM EDTA, autoclave and store at RT. Before use add 0.4 mg/mL proteinase K.
6. DNase I.
7. Buffered 25:24:1,v,v,v; phenol/chloroform/isoamyl alcohol.
8. Chloroform.
9. 7.5 M ammonium acetate.
10. 100% ethanol (EtOH).

2.4. Hybridization

1. Scintillation counter.
2. Geiger counter.
3. Plastic wrap.
4. X-ray films and cassettes.
5. Plastic bags or 5-mL plastic scintillation vials and roller-bottles.
6. 50X Denhardt's solution: 5 g Ficoll (type 400), 5 g polyvinylpyrrolidine, 5 g bovine serum albumin (fraction V) to a volume of 500 mL of distilled water. Filter sterilize and store in aliquots at –20°C.
7. Prehybridization solution: 50% formamide, 5X SSC, 2.5X Denhardt's solution, 25 mM sodium phosfate buffer, pH 6.5, 0.1% SDS, and 250 ng/mL salmon sperm DNA. Store at 4°C.
8. 10X SSC stock.
9. 10% SDS stock.
10. RNase A.

3. Methods
3.1. Preparation of DNA Blot

1. Soak slot-blotting apparatus in 0.2 N NaOH at room temperature (RT) for 1 h to eliminate RNases, rinse three times with distilled water.

2. Prepare the DNA. It is better to isolate the DNA inserts from plasmid vectors than to just linearize a plasmid vector containing the cDNA of interest. Always include a "housekeeping gene" as positive control and for standardization, e.g., GAPDH or β-tubulin. Use 1 μg of insert DNA per slot. Use 5 μg of linearized plasmid DNA as negative control. Prepare one series of DNAs per treatment condition.
3. Denature each DNA in 50 μL of 0.2 NaOH in an autoclaved Eppendorf tube at RT for 30 min.
4. Add 500 μL of sterile 6X SSC into each DNA solution.
5. During denaturing of DNA (**step 3**) set up the slot-blot apparatus. Use one layer of Whatman 3MM filter paper presoaked in 6X SSC. Presoak 0.45-μm nitrocellulose membrane in 6X SSC and mark its orientation, e.g., cut left upper corner, and lay it onto the wet Whatman filter carefully avoiding air bubbles between the membrane and the filter paper. Assemble top of slot-blot apparatus and lock it tightly with equal pressure on all sides.
6. Apply DNA-SSC solution into slots. Turn on vacuum until all samples are absorbed.
7. Add 1 mL of sterile 6xSSC to each slot and vacuum until all slots are dry.
8. Remove top of slot-blot apparatus and carefully mark the lanes of the DNA slots with a pencil. Air-dry membrane at RT. UV stratalink membrane (optional) and bake it at 80°C for 2 h. Then cut membrane into stripes (*see* **Note 3**).
9. The baked membranes can be stored dry for several weeks.

3.2. Preparation of Nuclei from Adherent Cells

Use sterile solutions and plastics. Keep solutions, cells, and nuclei on ice at all times.

1. Remove medium and place cells on ice. Rinse twice with PBS. Scrape cells with a rubber policeman in PBS. (*see* **Note 4**). Collect cells of each treatment condition in a 50-mL polypropylene centrifuge tube and spin cells down at 162*g* for 5 min at 4°C.
2. Remove supernatant completely. Pellet looks yellowish.
3. Add 12 mL of lysis buffer, lightly resuspend pellet and transfer to autoclaved 15-mL Dounce homogenizer. Keep on ice.
4. Break up cell membrane by stroking up and down for 30–70 cycles. Stroke steadily but do not use force on the handle. Avoid bubbles and foam. Examine 10 μL of nuclei under the microscope every 10 strokes until 70–80 % of nuclei are naked (*see* **Note 5** and **Fig. 2**).
5. Transfer nuclei to 15-mL polypropylene centrifuge tubes and spin nuclei down at 365*g* for 5 min at 4°C. Pellet should be approx one-third of its starting volume (*see* **step 2** above) and appear white.
6. Discard supernatant, wash nuclei by resuspending the pellet in 5 mL lysis buffer and centrifuge at 365*g* for 5 min at 4°C.
7. Repeat **step 6** above.
8. Carefully discard all supernatant and resuspend nuclei in 100 μL of fresh storage buffer and (a) continue with in vitro transcription right away (go to **Subheading 3.3., step 2**) or (b) for storage, snap-freeze in ethanol on dry ice, and store at −70°C or in liquid nitrogen (*see* **Note 4**).

3.3. In Vitro Transcription

1. Thaw nuclei in storage buffer on ice.
2. Add 100 µL ice-cold transcription buffer containing 200 µCi α-^{32}P UTP to each sample (*see* **Note 6**).
3. Incubate at 30°C for 30 min in a shaking water bath (*see* **Note 7**).
4. Add 30 U of RNase free DNase I to each reaction and incubate for 20 min at 30°C in a shaking water bath.
5. Add 200 µL of proteinase K buffer to each reaction and incubate for 30 min at 42°C in a shaking water bath.
6. Phenol/Chloroform extraction (*see* **Note 7**): add 400 µL buffered 25:24:1 phenol/chloroform/isoamyl alcohol to each sample, mix well, microfuge for 5 min, at or below RT. Carefully transfer the aqueous supernatant to a new eppendorf tube. Add 400 µL chloroform, mix well, microfuge for 5 min, and again carefully transfer supernatant to a new Eppendorf tube.
7. Precipitate RNA by adding 200 µL of 7.5 *M* ammonium acetate and 1 mL of 100 % EtOH, mix. Incubate for at least 30 min on dry ice.
8. Microfuge RNA for 30 min at 4°C. Remove supernatant and air-dry pellet. Continue with **Subheading 3.4., step 2**.

3.4. Hybridization

1. Prehybridize each DNA-membrane-strip in 1–5 mL prehybridization solution containing 50% formamide in a plastic bag (if a shaking water bath is used) or coiled into a 5-mL plastic scintillation vial (put vial inside a roller-bottle if hybridization oven is used) at 42 °C for 1–3 h.
2. Completely dissolve the pelleted, radiolabeled RNA (*see* **Subheading 3.3., step 8**) in 1 mL prehybridization solution. Count an aliquot (10 µL) in a scintillation counter. Add an approximately equal amount of radioactivity to each prehydridized blot (e.g., 1×10^7 cpm/mL) (*see* **Note 8**).
3. Hybridize at 42°C for 48 h (*see* **Note 9**).
4. Wash the hybridized membrane strips: 20 min in 2X SSC, 0.1% SDS at 42°C; 20 minutes in 0.2X SSC, 0.1% SDS at 65°C. Check radioactivity using a Geiger counter and adjust the washing conditions accordingly.
5. Place moist membranes in plastic wrap and expose to X-ray film for 12–48 h. The exposure time will vary depending on the experiment.
6. If the background-to-signal ratio is too high or unspecific binding occurs, unravel the strips and incubate in 2X SSC with 10 mg/mL RNase A at 37°C without shaking, and repeat **step 4** above.

4. Notes

1. Recombinant ribonuclease inhibitors work well (usually cheaper).
2. Avoid multiple freeze-thaw cycles or exposure to frequent temperature changes of 5'-triphosphates (rATP, rCTP, and rGTP). These fluctuations can greatly alter stability.

What nuclei should look like:

not sufficient   **sufficient**

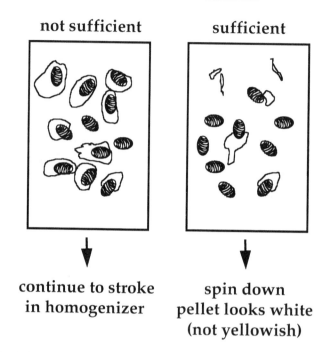

**continue to stroke   spin down
in homogenizer   pellet looks white
(not yellowish)**

Fig. 2. Isolation of nuclei for run-on assay by detergent lysis and Dounce homogenization. Examine 10 μL of nuclei under high-power microscope every 10–20 strokes until 70–80% of nuclei are naked. After centrifugation the pelleted nuclei appear white.

3. It is difficult to detect the location of slots once the nitrocellulose has dried. When cutting the stripes, trim the membrane close to the edge of DNA slots to minimize the volume of the hybridization solution.
4. In our hands, three confluent T-150 flasks of human saphenous vein endothelial or smooth muscle cells are necessary per assay for each treatment condition. Larger amounts of cells can be harvested at the same time and stored in aliquots (storage buffer). Nuclei are stable for up to one year at –70°C or in liquid nitrogen.
5. The most critical step in the nuclear run-on assay is the isolation of nuclei. Nuclei have to be free of membranes and cytoplasmic debris to allow sufficient incorporation of ^{32}P-labeled UTP into nascent transcripts. The suggested protocol combines detergent lysis with Dounce homogenization and has to be adjusted for each cell type. Frequent microscopic control is recommended (**Fig. 2**). Examine 10 μL of nuclei under high-power microscope every 10–20 strokes until 70–80 % of nuclei are naked, 20% nuclei that are half protruding from cell membranes are tolerable. In our hands human saphenous vein endothelial cells, passage 3, require

40–60 strokes of Dounce homogenization, whereas for human saphenous vein smooth muscle cells (passage 3) 30–50 strokes are sufficient.

6. Increasing the amount of ^{32}P-UTP above 200 µCi or prolonging the time of transcription beyond 30 min does not appear to improve the results.

7. Dealing with these high amounts of radioactivity makes the run-on assay cumbersome to perform. Cave: 1 mCi ^{32}P can radiate through thin walls. The most unpleasant step is the isolation of the radioactive total RNA after the in vitro transcription. Although the CsCl-guanidine method gives very good results *(7)*, the risk of contaminating an ultracentrifuge is very high due to the lack of aerosol-tight tubes for most rotors. Also, in many labs ultracentrifuges are localized in rooms that are not licensed and equipped for the use of high amounts of ^{32}P. Therefore, we suggest the chloroform/phenol extraction and ethanol precipitation that works well in our hands *(5,6)*. It is advisable to purchase aerosol-tight eppendorf tubes. For some microfuges aerosol-tight aluminum containers are available (e.g., Eppendorf) that we find very helpful and allow an absolutely contamination-free run-on assay.

8. This is based on the assumption that the overall level of RNA synthesis is not changing as a function of cell state. Under a new set of conditions this has to be confirmed by taking special care to use the same number of nuclei for each cell state analyzed and comparing the transcription rate of the "housekeeping" genes (e.g., GAPDH, β-tubulin).

9. In our experience it is important to hybridize for at least 48 h.

References

1. Marzluff, W. F. (1978) Transcription of RNA in isolated nuclei. *Meth. Cell Biol.* **19,** 317–331.

2. Greenberg, M. E. and Bender, T. P. (1997) Identification of newly transcribed RNA, in *Current Protocols in Molecular Biology*, Wiley, NY, pp. 4.10.1–4.10.11.

3. Elferink, C. J. and Reiners, J. J. (1996) Quantitative RT-PCR on CYP1A1 heterogeneous nuclear RNA: a surrogate for the in vitro transcription run-on assay. *Biotechniques* **20(3),** 470–477.

4. Howard, L. A. and Ortlepp, S. A. (1989) A simplification of the nuclear run-off transcription assay. *BioFeedback* **7,** 156,157.

5. Liao, J. K., Shin, W. S., Lee, W. Y., and Clark, S. L. (1995) Oxidized low-density lipoprotein decreases the expression of endothelial nitric oxide synthase. *J. Biol. Chem.* **270,** 319–324.

6. Laufs, U., La Fata, V., and Liao, J. K. (1997) Inhibition of 3-hydroxy-3-methylglutaryl (HMG) CoA reductase blocks hypoxia-mediated downregulation of endothelial nitric oxide synthase. *J. Biol. Chem.* **272(50),** 31,730–31,735.

7. Chomczynski, P. and Sacchi, N. (1987) Single-step method of RNA isolation by acid guanidinium thiocyanate-phenol-chloroform extraction. *Anal. Biochem.* **162,** 156–159.

14

Electromobility Shift Analysis (EMSA) Applied to the Study of NF-kappa B Binding Interactions in Vascular Smooth Muscle Cells

Todd Bourcier

1. Introduction

The nuclear factor-kappa B (NFκB) family of transcription factors has emerged as a signaling pathway that figures prominently in a cell's initial response to a plethora of inflammatory stimuli. Modified lipids, oxidative stress, bacterial endotoxins, growth factors and cytokines, such as platelet-derived growth factor (PDGF) and interleukin-1 (IL-1), are among the stimuli that free NFκB dimers from their cytosolic inhibitor proteins leading to nuclear translocation of NFκB and transactivation of target genes *(1–3)*. The smooth muscle cells (SMC) of the vasculature express components of this pathway and are activated by these stimuli, promoting dysregulation of gene expression by cells within the atherosclerotic vessel. Indeed, NFκB proteins have been localized within the nuclei of vascular SMC at sites of human atherosclerotic lesions, suggesting a role for NFκB in activation of this cell type in vivo *(4–6)*. NFκB participates in dysregulated gene expression not only by SMC but also by endothelial cells and macrophages, prominent cell types within atherosclerotic lesions, thus much attention has focused on the workings of this signaling pathway within vascular cells and its role in atherogenesis.

The electromobility shift assay (EMSA), also called the gel shift assay, finds utility in identifying specific DNA-binding proteins, such as NFκB and other transcription factors, that exist in the cells' nucleus constitutively or inducibly following a given stimulus. It is quite simple in concept: proteins that bind double-stranded DNA of a specified sequence are identified by mixing nuclear proteins with radiolabeled DNA oligomer; DNA bound to protein is then separated from free, unbound DNA via electrophoresis through a polyacrylamide

From: *Methods in Molecular Medicine, Vascular Disease: Molecular Biology and Gene Therapy Protocols*
Edited by: A. H. Baker © Humana Press Inc., Totowa, NJ

gel under nondenaturing conditions. Unlabeled DNA of identical or mutated sequence is used to compete with the radiolabeled DNA for binding to protein, thus assessing the relative affinity and specificity of binding interactions. A particularly useful aspect of EMSA is the ability to utilize specific antibodies in the binding reaction to identify the proteins that comprise DNA-binding complexes. For example, one could distinguish DNA-binding complexes that contain NFκB dimers p65/p50 (a transactivation-competent dimer) from complexes that contain p50/p50 (a transactivation-silent dimer). This protocol details the steps for performing EMSA on nuclear extracts from human vascular SMC

1. to identify constitutive or inducible NFκB-DNA binding complexes,
2. to assess the relative specificity of the binding interactions, and
3. to identify the NFκB subunits that comprise the DNA-binding complexes by "supershift" analysis.

2. Materials

2.1. Nuclear/Cytosolic Isolation

1. Ice-cold PBS, pH 7.4.
2. Cell scrapers.
3. 2.0-mL microfuge tubes.
4. Low-Salt buffer: 10 mM Hepes, pH 7.9, 1.5 mM MgCl$_2$, 10 mM KCl, 0.5% Nonidet-40, 1 mM DTT, and 0.5 mM PMSF (add last two ingredients fresh). Store at 4°C, stable for several months.
5. High-salt buffer: 20 mM Hepes, pH 7.9, 1.5 mM MgCl$_2$, 420 mM NaCl, 0.2 mM EDTA, 1 mM DTT, and 0.5 mM PMSF (add last two ingredients fresh). Store at 4°C, stable for several months.
6. Glycerol buffer: 20 mM Hepes, pH 7.9, 100 mM KCl, 0.2 mM EDTA, 20% glycerol. Store at 4°C, stable for several months.

2.2. Oligonucleotide Labeling and Purification

1. Double-stranded oligonucleotide containing one or more NFκB-binding elements (e.g., 22 bp NFkB consensus oligonucleotide from Santa Cruz Biotechnology.) (*see* **Note 1**).
2. [γ^{32}P] ATP, 3000 Ci/mmol.
3. 5X kinase buffer: 0.5 mM Tris-HCl, pH 7.50, 50 mM MgCl$_2$, 50 mM DTT (added fresh). Store at –20°C.
4. T4 polynucleotide kinase, store at –20°C.
5. Sephadex G-25 columns (e.g., NAP-5 Columns available from Pharmacia).
6. TE Buffer: 10 mM Tris-HCl, pH 7.4, 1 mM EDTA.

2.3. DNA/Protein Binding Reaction

1. Nuclear extract (*see* **Subheading 3.1.**).
2. ^{32}P-labeled oligonucleotide probe (*see* **Subheading 3.2.**).

3. 10X EMSA buffer: 100 mM Tris-HCl, pH 7.5, 500 mM NaCl, 10 mM EDTA, 50% glycerol (store at –20°C).
4. Poly-deoxyinosine-deoxy-cytidylic acid [poly(dI:dC)] (Boehringer Mannheim): prepare as a 1 mg/mL stock in double distilled water and store at –20°C
5. Bovine serum albumin, Fraction V.
6. Wild-type ,unlabeled oligonucleotide probe.
7. Mutant, unlabeled oligonucleotide probe.
8. Specific antibodies, if supershift analysis is desired.

2.4. Separation of Bound from Free Oligonucleotide Probe

1. 10X TBE buffer: 890 mM Tris, 890 mM boric acid, 20 mM EDTA, pH 8.3. (store at room temperature).
2. 5% polyacrylamide gel, made with 0.5X TBE buffer; 18 cm × 0.75 mm gel works very well for separating free from bound probe.

2.5. Drying of Gel and Autoradiography

1. Three pieces of Whatmann filter paper, cut 3–5 cm larger than the gel.
2. Saran Wrap.
3. Gel dryer.
4. Exposure cassette and autoradiography film.

3. Methods

Human vascular SMC, derived from either saphenous vein or aorta, are grown to confluency in 75 cm^2 Petri dishes. One confluent dish (approx 2×10^5 cells) is used for each experimental group. To validate this technique, I recommend first setting up only two groups: unstimulated cells, and IL-1β-treated cells (10 ng/mL, 2 h incubation).

3.1. Isolation of Nuclear and Cytosolic Fractions

This procedure is modified from that described by Dignam et al. *(7)*. Unless otherwise indicated, all manipulations for this step are performed at 4°C.

1. Following incubations, place culture dishes on ice for 10 min.
2. Wash dishes once with ice-cold PBS.
3. Add 1.0 mL PBS/dish and use a cell scraper to collect the cells.
4. Transfer cells to a prechilled 2.0-mL microfuge tube.
5. Spin tubes for 5 min at 1000g to pellet the cells.
6. Resuspend cell pellet in 80 µL (or 1 original cell volume) of low salt buffer (triturate pellet with pipette, not vortexer).
7. Incubate on ice for 10 min.
8. Spin tubes for 5 min at 13,000g.
9. Remove supernatant and save as the CYTOSOLIC EXTRACT (*see* **Note 2**).
10. Wash nuclear pellet once with 80 µL of low salt buffer.

11. Resuspend nuclear pellet in 40 µL (or 1/2 original cell volume) of high salt buffer (*see* **Note 3**).
12. Incubate on ice for 30 min with gentle agitation.
13. Spin tubes for 5 min at 13,000*g*.
14. Remove supernatant and save as the NUCLEAR EXTRACT.
15. Add 40 µL (or an equal volume) of glycerol buffer to the nuclear extract and mix.
16. Remove an aliquot for protein determination (*see* **Note 4**).
17. Extracts are stored at –80°C and are stable for at least 6 mo (my longest time of storage) for EMSA.

3.2. Labeling and Purification of Oligonucleotide Probe (see Notes 5 and 6)

1. Add the following reactants to a clean 0.5-mL microfuge tube: 3 µL oligonucleotide probe (~40 ng DNA). 2 µL 5X Kinase buffer. 4 µL [γ-^{32}P] ATP (40 µCi). 1 µL T4 polynucleotide kinase.
2. Mix contents well and incubate at 37°C for 30 min.
3. During this time, equilibrate a sephadex G-25 column with 1 vol of TE buffer.
4. Add 90 µL TE buffer to reaction, and load the entire reaction to the equilibrated column.
5. Add 300 µL of TE buffer to column, collect effluent and discard.
6. Add 350 µL TE buffer to column, collect effluent and save as the PURIFIED LABELED PROBE.
7. Count a 2-µL aliquot of probe in 4 mL of scintillation fluid and record the cpm/µL for the reaction (expect 50–80,000 cpm/µL).
8. Store labeled probe at –20°C.

3.3. DNA/Protein Binding Reaction

Described below are three types of EMSA reactions: **Subheading 3.3.1.** tests for DNA-binding proteins in experimental samples; **Subheading 3.3.2.** assesses the relative specificity of the formed complexes; **Subheading 3.3.3.** allows for identification of one or more proteins that comprise a given protein/ DNA binding complex. It is very advisable to run the specificity reaction along with the experimental samples every time EMSA is performed.

3.3.1. Preparing Experimental Sample Reactions

1. To each 0.5-mL microfuge tube, add: 5 µg nuclear extract, 2 µL 10X EMSA buffer (1X final concentration), 2 µg poly (dI:dC) (0.1 µg/µL final concentration), 10 µg bovine serum albumin (0.5 µg/µL final concentration), dH$_2$O to 20 µL final volume, 20,000 cpm labeled probe.

3.3.2. Preparation of Wildtype/Mutant Competitor Reactions

1. Prepare two reactions as described in **Subheading 3.3.1.** using the nuclear extract from a positive control group, omitting addition of labeled probe.

2. Add 20 ng cold wild type probe to one tube, and 20 ng cold mutant probe to the other tube. Mix well and incubate at room temperature for 5 min.
3. Add 20,000 cpm labeled probe to both tubes and mix.

3.3.3. Preparing Antibody "Supershift" Reactions

1. Prepare reaction as described in **Subheading 3.3.1.**, omitting addition of the labeled probe.
2. Add 2 µg of specific antisera to reaction (e.g., anti-human p65, or antihuman p50).
3. Incubate at room temperature for 15 min.
4. Add 20,000 cpm of labeled probe and mix.
5. Incubate all samples at room temperature for 30 min, then place on ice.

3.4. Separating Protein-Bound from Free Oligonucleotide Probe

1. Load samples onto a 5% polyacrylamide gel made with 0.5X TBE buffer (0.5X TBE buffer used as running buffer). Load the first lane with a bromophenol blue marker (dissolved in 5% glycerol/TE buffer) to monitor progress of the gel front. It is not necessary to add loading buffer to the samples due to the presence of glycerol in the reaction buffer.
2. Run the gel at 250 V (with cooling if available), until the bromophenol blue band is ~5 cm from the bottom of the gel. The unbound probe runs just below this band (*see* **Note 7**).

3.5. Gel Drying and Autoradiography

1. Remove gel from apparatus and remove only the top glass plate, leaving the gel resting on the second plate.
2. Transfer the gel to a piece of Whatmann filter paper by placing the filter on top of the exposed gel, and gently peeling it off the glass plate.
3. Place the gel on two additional pieces of filter paper, cover with Saran wrap, and dry the gel for 1 hour at 80°C (*see* **Note 8**).
4. Place the dried gel in an exposure cassette and overlay a sheet of autoradiography film.
5. Expose the film at room temperature and develop the first film after ~16 h (overnight). Expose additional films based on intensity of the first film, but maintain exposure times within films' linear range. Store cassette at –80°C if prolonged exposures are required.

3.6. Interpretation of Results

Figures 1A and **B** depict increased NFkB activity, assessed by EMSA, in human vascular SMC stimulated with IL-1b for 2 h. The DNA binding complexes are retarded in the gel while the free probe migrates with the gels' front. Specificity of binding determined by competition with increasing amounts of wild type or mutant oligonucleotide is shown in **Fig. 1A**. That the wild type oligonucleotide "competed out" the labeled probe at much lower amounts than

A

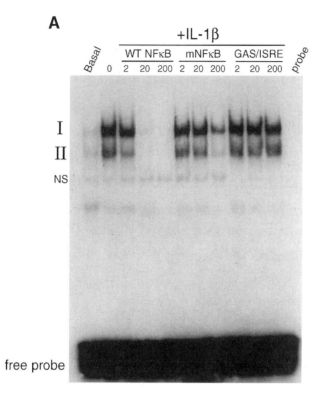

Fig. 1. EMSA detection of NFκB in human VSMC. (**A**) IL-1β-induced NFκB binding complexes from human saphenous vein smooth muscle cells, and competition with
a two-, 20-, or 200-fold excess of unlabeled wild-type (WT) or mutant (m) NFkB
oligonucleotide, or with the consensus GAS/ISRE oligonucleotide, demonstrating
specificity of the induced DNA binding complexes (indicated by I and II). NS represents non specific.

the mutant oligonucleotide identifies the two upper bands as high-affinity binding complexes, and the third lower band as a relatively low affinity binding
complex (*see* **Note 9**). Identifying proteins that comprise the DNA binding
complexes by use of specific antibodies, commonly called "supershifting,' is
depicted in Figure 1B. Simply, if the DNA binding complex is shifted further
upwards (supershifted) when in the presence of antibody, that particular antigen is likely a component of the binding complex (*see* **Note 10**). In the figure,
the upper complex was supershifted by two distinct antisera to p65 and by
antisera to p50, whereas the lower complex was supershifted only by antisera
to p50. Antisera to p49, cRel, RelB, or nonimmune IgG did not supershift any
complex. Thus, p65 and p50 are components of the upper complex and p50,
either in homodimer form or dimerized with unidentified proteins, comprises

B

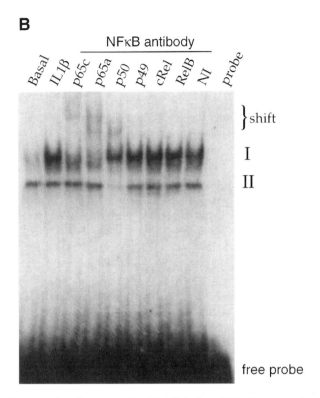

Fig. 1. (B) Rel proteins that comprise IL-1β-induced binding complexes were identified by inclusion of the indicated antibody (2 µg) in the EMSA reaction. Complexes
I, II, and supershifted complexes are indicated on the right. *Probe* indicates EMSA
reaction without nuclear extract.

the lower complex. Taken together, the EMSA method allows detection of
basal and induced DNA binding activities, such as the NFkB family of transcription factors shown herein, the relative specificity of the DNA-protein
interactions, and allows for identification of proteins that comprise the DNA
binding complexes.

4. Notes

1. Diversity in the NFkB binding element located within various enhancers/pro-
   moters (consensus 5'-GGGPuNNPyPyCC-3'), as well as various flanking
   sequences, can influence selectivity in binding various Rel dimers *(8,9)*. Therefore, one should design a double-stranded oligonucleotide that contains the κB
   element identical in sequence to that found in the endogenous enhancer/promoter
   of interest. This issue is less important if your interest is simply to document
   whether a given agonist activates NFkB, for example.

2. Cytosolic extracts are not commonly used to detect activated Rel dimers due to their inability to bind DNA when complexed with IκB proteins. These extracts are useful, however, for immunoblot analyses of NFκB or IκB proteins.

3. Nuclear pellets are somewhat difficult to resuspend; a simple technique is to widen the bore of the pipet by cutting off the tip, thus allowing gentle trituration of the nuclei.

4. Protein concentration of the nuclear extract is performed at this step. The bicinchoninic acid method (BCA method) is not compatible with reducing agents, such as DTT, that are present in the extraction buffers. If you use the BCA method, omit the DTT from the extraction buffers and add it to the samples *after* an aliquot is taken for protein assay. Bio-Rad offers a protein kit that is insensitive to the presence of reducing agents. Using BCA's microplate method, I typically assay 2.5- and 5-μL aliquots of nuclear fractions in a total volume of 100 μl; expect approx 30–50 μg per 2×10^5 smooth muscle cells.

5. The labeling step uses ^{32}P isotope of high specific activity; use appropriate procedures for use, storage, and discarding of radioactive materials.

6. This method of probe purification has yielded quite acceptable results for several DNA probes used in our laboratory. However, if one obtains poor results relative to binding specificity, manifest by multiple 'non-specific' bands, try alternative methods for probe purification such as mini-spin columns. In one rather extreme case, gel purification of a kB-containing probe from the VCAM-1 promoter was required to reduce non-specific interactions in the EMSA.

7. If the bromophenol band runs to the end or off of the gel, then the running buffer will contain the free probe and be radioactive. If better resolution of Rel complexes is desired, one can either run the samples on a longer gel or use a higher percentage polyacrylamide gel.

8. After one hour of drying, gently lift off the plastic cover and expose a corner of the drying gel. If the gel is sticky to the touch, continue drying for another 10 min and recheck the gel. These gels tend to quickly crack as well as avidly stick to film if they are not completely dried.

9. Be aware that all binding complexes can be "competed out" if one adds excessive amounts of cold wild-type oligonucleotide; this is avoided by first titrating the amount of wild type and mutant oligonucleotide, as shown in **Fig. 1A**.

10. It is critical that the antibody be of high quality and recognize only the antigen of interest, and that appropriate species and isotype-matched nonimmune antisera be used to control for binding specificity.

References

1. Siebenlist, U., Franzoso, G., and Brown, K. (1994) Structure, Regulation and Function of NF-kB. Annu. *Rev. Cell Biol.,* **10,** 405–455.

2. Baeuerle, P. A. and Baltimore, D. (1996) NF-kB: Ten years after. *Cell,* **87,** 13–20.

3. May, M. J. and Ghosh, S. (1998) Signal transduction through NF-kB. *Immunology Today,* **19(2),** 80–88.

4. Bourcier, T., Sukhova, G., and Libby, P. (1997) The nuclear factor-kB signaling pathway participates in dysregulation of vascular smooth muscle cells in vitro and in human atherosclerosis. *J. Biol. Chem.*, **272(25),** 15,817–15,824.

5. Brand, K., Page, S., Rogler, G., Bartsch, A., Brandl, R., Knuechel, R., Page, M., Kaltschmidt, C., Baeuerle, P. A., and Neumeier, D. (1996) Activated transcription factor nuclear factor-kappa B is present in the atherosclerotic lesion. *J. Clin. Invest.,* **97,** 1715–1722.

6. Bellas, R. E., Lee, J. S., and Sonenshein, G. E. (1995) Expression of a constitutive NF-kappa B-like activity is essential for proliferation of cultured bovine vascular smooth muscle cells. *J. Clin. Invest.,* **96,** 2521–2527.

7. Dignam, J. D., Lebovitz, R. M., and Roeder, R. G. (1983) Accurate transcription initiation by RNA polymerase II in a soluble extract from isolated mammalian nuclei. *Nucleic Acids Res.*, **11,** 1475–1489.

8. Lin, R., Gewert, D., and Hiscott, J. (1995) Differential transcriptional activation in vitro by NF-kappa B/Rel proteins. *J. Biol. Chem.*, **270,** 3123–3131.

9. Lehming, N., Thanos, D., Brickman, J., Ma, J., Maniatis, T., and Ptashne, M. (1994) An HMG-like protein that can switch a transcriptional activator to a repressor. *Nature,* **371,** 175–179.

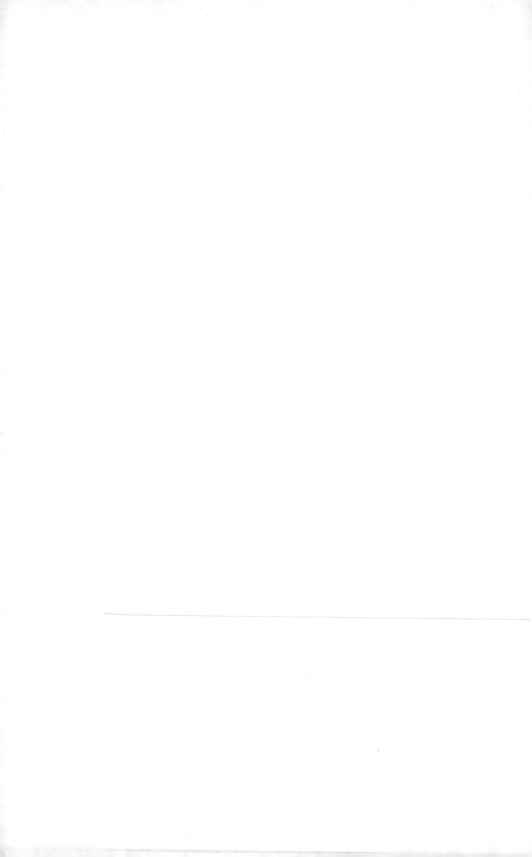

IV

MOLECULAR ANALYSIS OF MRNA EXPRESSION IN VASCULAR CELLS

15

Measurement of Gene Expression in the Vascular Wall by Reverse Transcription-Polymerase Chain Reaction (RT-PCR) Analysis

Joachim Fruebis

1. Introduction

The developments of the polymerase chain reaction (PCR) analysis *(1–3)* and quantitative PCR by Gilliland *(4)* has provided researchers with a unique tool to analyze the expression of various genes in very small amounts of tissue samples. The sensitivity of PCR allows measurement of the expression level of any known gene in a biological sample, in this case, arterial wall tissue. This is achieved by determining the amount of mRNA coding for the target gene product present in the sample. Because PCR requires very little mRNA, a pool of mRNA can be studied for the expression of several genes and can also be used in more specialized PCR-based methods discussed in other chapters (*see* Chapters 7–l0). This represents a major advantage over other methods, such as *in situ* hybridization, RNAase protection, and Northern blot analysis. Although *in situ* hybridization provides information about the localization of gene expression, it cannot give quantitative results, and the large amounts of mRNA required for Northern blot analysis prevents the analysis of small tissue samples. Thus, the main advantages of PCR are its sensitivity, the possibility of obtaining quantitative results, and the ability to analyze a number of genes using the same RNA sample. However, PCR analysis does not offer localization of gene expression, and although quantitative results are obtained, additional studies, in particular the analysis of protein expression, should be performed. This is necessary because gene expression does not necessarily equate to the amount of gene product formed. For example, it can be affected by RNA stability or by the processing of the *de novo* formed protein. For example, interleukin-1 (IL-1) is stored intracellularly and can be released

From: *Methods in Molecular Medicine, Vascular Disease: Molecular Biology and Gene Therapy Protocols*
Edited by: A. H. Baker © Humana Press Inc., Totowa, NJ

without mRNA production. However, the subsequent replenishment of these storage depots requires mRNA synthesis. Thus, mRNA-based PCR data alone might not represent the complete picture. The main difficulties inherent to the technique are

1. the susceptibility of mRNA to degradation (in large part due to RNAases),
2. the fact that PCR analysis is prone to errors resulting from inconsistent yields of the RNA isolation, the RT reaction, or the PCR amplification itself,
3. because of sample contamination leading to erroneous results.

However, by taking appropriate precautions, these difficulties can be controlled. Degradation of mRNA can be prevented by RNAase inhibitors, by keeping samples frozen whenever possible and avoiding unnecessary freeze/thaw cycles (*see* **Subheading 3.1.**) and by adequate experimental techniques to avoid contamination with RNAases. An elegant way to circumvent potential errors of PCR is the use of a semiquantitative determination method. The cDNA coding tor the gene of interest is amplified together with an internal standard gene. Since the internal standard and the target gene are processed in parallel at all times throughout the procedure, errors resulting from pipeting or from inconsistent yields of the RNA isolation will affect both genes to the same degree and the ratio that is used to express the level of target gene expression remains unchanged. Although quantitative results are obtained by this method, which allow for the comparison of expression levels, the data are standardized to a constant but unknown expression level of the internal standard. Thus, it falls short of providing the absolute number of mRNA molecules present in the original sample. RT-PCR can therefore be used to

1. determine gene expression in vessel wall tissue *(5)*,
2. identify genes that show altered levels of expression in atherosclerotic lesions *(6,7)*,
3. isolate new targets for pharmacological or gene-based intervention,
4. follow the appearance of cells such as monocytes and lymphocytes in the artery wall by measuring expression of cell type specific marker molecules, and
5. analyze the effects of atheroprotective drugs and thereby help elucidate mechanisms of action.

2. Materials

2.1. Isolation and Handling of Tissue Samples

1. Diethlypyrocarbonate (DEPC)-treated water: Add 1 mL DEPC (Sigma, St. Louis, MO) to 1 L of distilled water, let sit overnight, and autoclave for 20 min.
2. Phosphate-buffered saline (PBS), 2 mM EDTA: 0.154 M NaCl, 18 mM Na$_2$HPO$_4$, 2.9 mM NaHPO$_4$, and 2 mM EDTA. Use DEPC-treated water to prepare.
3. Preparation trays. Aluminum dissecting pans with dissecting wax (Fisher Scientific, Hampton, NH).
4. Vanna microscissors (Fine Science Tools, Foster City, CA).

2.2. Isolation of Total RNA

1. RNAzol B (Tel-Test Inc., Friendswood, TX).
2. Polytron PT1200 (Fisher Scientific).
3. Chloroform.
4. 75% Ethanol.
5. Isopropanol.
6. 1 mM EDTA, pH 7.0.

2.3. Reverse Transcription (RT) Reaction

1. Superscript II (M-MLV Reverse Transcriptase, Gibco-BRL, Gaithersburg, MD).
2. RT-buffer, included with Superscript enzyme.
3. Dithiothreitol (DTT), 100 mM, included with Superscript enzyme.
4. Oligo dT$_{15}$ primer (Boehringer Mannheim, Indianapolis, IN).
5. Deoxynucleotide triphosphates (dNTPs, 2.5 mM) (Boehringer Mannheim).
6. RNAse inhibitor, 40 u/µL.
7. Bovine serum albumin (BSA), 10 mg/mL.
8. Master mixes should be prepared to ensure identical conditions.

RT master mix (final concentrations in brackets): 3 µL dNTP (0.15 mmol/L), 0.75 µL RNAse inhibitor (30 U/reaction), 0.45 µL BSA (90 µg/mL), 10 µL RT-buffer (1x), 5 µL DTT (10 mM), 1 µL Superscript II RT, (200 U), DEPC water to bring to 22 µL. Multiply the individual volumes by the number of samples plus 1.

2.4. Quantitative PCR using GAPDH as Internal Standard (see *Note 1*)

1. Ampliwax PCR Gem 50 (Perkin-Elmer, Norwalk, CT).
2. *Taq* Polymerase (5 u/µL) (Promega, Madison, WI).
3. MgCl$_2$, 25 mmol/L.
4. 10X PCR buffer without Mg^{2+} (included with *Taq* Polymerase).
5. 10X sample buffer: 50% glycerol, 1 mM EDTA, 0.125% xylene cyanol FF (XC FF). Prepare a 0.25% XC FF solution in 2 mM EDTA, pH 8.0 and combine this solution with an equal volume of glycerol.
6. Master mixes should be prepared to ensure identical conditions. PCR master mix (final concentrations in brackets): 2.0 µL target specific primer (0.24 µmol/L), 1 µL each dNTP (100 µmol/L), 2.0 µL MgCl$_2$ (2 mmol/L), 0.25 µL BSA (100 µg/mL), 2.5 µL 10X PCR buffer w/o Mg^{2+} (1x), 3.75 µL DEPC water to bring total volume to 11.5 µL. Multiply the individual volumes by the number of samples plus 1.
7. *Taq* mix: 0.15 µL *Taq*-Polymerase and 7.35 µL DEPC water.
8. Gene Runner, Primer selection software (Hastings Software, Inc., Hastings, NY).

2.5. Data Analysis

1. Agarose, Nusieve 3:1 (FMC Bioproducts Corp., Rockland, ME).
2. Ethidium bromide.

3. Video camera, solid-state black and white (Cohu, San Diego, CA).
4. Optimas 4.0 imaging software (Bothwell, WA).

3. Methods
3.1. Isolation and Handling of Tissue Samples

The main concern when isolating tissues for RT-PCR analysis should be to avoid sample contamination and RNA degradation (*see* **Note 2**).

1. Following *in situ* perfusion, transfer the tissue to an RNAase-free preparation tray, pinned out, and keep submerged in a bath of ice-cold PBS. Clean and dissect tissue into segments of interest.
2. Immediately transfer to sterile polypropylene tubes.
3. Snap freeze in liquid nitrogen and keep at –70°C until required.

3.2. Isolation of Total RNA

We have tested a number of protocols to isolate RNA and selected RNAzol for its convenience, reliability, and good yield of intact RNA. Total RNA is isolated and discriminated for mRNA using oligo dT primers during the RT reaction. The RNA isolation procedure is performed according to the manufacturer's protocol in a room different from the one used for the animal work. RNAzol contains both denaturing guanidiniumthiocyanate and reducing β-mercaptoethanol and therefore prevents RNA loss due to RNAase release.

1. Add 1 mL of RNAzol™ per 50 mg of tissue and homogenize three times for 20 s on setting 4. Transfer solution to a 1.5-mL Eppendorf tube.
2. Add 0.1 mL chloroform per 1 mL of RNAzoL™ and shake for 15 s, do not vortex.
3. Incubate sample for 10 min on ice.
4. Centrifuge 15 min at 12,000g at 4°C.
5. Transfer the RNA containing aqueous upper phase to a fresh tube and add an equal volume of isopropanol. Incubate on ice for 15 min.
6. Centrifuge for 15 min at 12,000g at 4°C. RNA forms a white-yellow precipitate.
7. Discard supernatant and wash RNA once with 75% ethanol by vortexing. Use at least 0.8 mL of ethanol per 50–100 μg RNA.
8. Centrifuge for 8 min at 7500g at 4°C.
9. Dry pellet briefly under vacuum for 10–15 min, do not dry completely.
10. Dissolve RNA in 50 μL of 1 mM EDTA, pH 7.0.
11. Determine the concentration of the total RNA by measuring the absorption at 260 nm. An OD of 1 corresponds to 40 μg/mL RNA. The quality of the RNA is examined by measuring the ratio of 260/280 nm and also visually after separation by denaturing agarose gel. Pure RNA preparations have ratios of 2.0. Contaminations with protein or organic solvents will lower this ratio and will also lead to inaccurate determinations.

3.3. RT Reaction

Samples of 2 µg total RNA are reverse transcribed into cDNA in 50 µL reaction mixtures using 200 U of recombinant M-MLV reverse transcriptase (Superscript Il:, Gibco BRL) and oligo dT_{15} as primer. The reaction is carried out in the RT-buffer supplied with the enzyme in 0.5-mL PCR tubes.

1. Aliquot 2 µg of RNA into a 0.5-mL PCR tube.
2. Add 6 µL of oligo dT_{15} containing 150 pmol and adjust the total volume to 28 µL using DEPC water.
3. Heat at 72°C for 5 min to denature the RNA. Cool down to 37°C and add 22 µL of RT master mix pre-warmed up to 37°C. (Because concentrations vary from product to product, the final concentrations are shown and volumes should be adjusted accordingly to give a final volume of 22 µL.)
4. Incubate samples for 60 min at 42°C (use the PCR cycler or a thermo block).
5. Inactivate the enzyme by heating the samples to 94°C for 10 min. Snap freeze the RT-products (RTP) on ice and store at –70°C.

3.4. Quantitative PCR using GAPDH as Internal Standard

PCR is performed on an Ericomp Twinblock Easycycler and is carried out in a total volume of 25 µL. To obtain maximum fidelity, hot start conditions are applied, using ampliwax beads (Perkin-Elmer). A control reaction without addition of cDNA is included in each PCR-run to test for possible contamination (*see* **Note 3**). The PCR profile starts with a 5-min denaturing phase at 88°C, followed by a 5-min annealing phase at 63°C. The subsequent cycles consist of a 1-min elongation phase at 72°C, a 45-s denaturing phase at 94°C, and a 1-min annealing phase. The PCR reaction is concluded by a 10-min elongation phase, again at 72°C. The annealing temperature is chosen according to the composition of the primer (*see* **Note 4**). To obtain quantitative data on the expression level of the tested gene, a second primer specific for the chosen internal standard is added. GAPDH was selected as internal standard because it is ubiquitous and has a constant level of expression compared to the expression level of the target gene. Thus, in each PCR-reaction a 465 bp PCR product of GAPDH is coamplified and used as an internal standard. If GAPDH is found to be expressed at higher levels than the target genes, GAPDH primers are added delayed. This measure ensures that GAPDH amplification does not reach the plateau phase earlier than the target gene. The fully quantitative analysis of GAPDH expression requires the cloning of a competitor cDNA. This can be achieved following general cloning procedures and using commercially available cloning kits.

1. Aliquot 4.0 µL cDNA RT product into each PCR tube already containing one wax bead.

2. Add 11.5 μL PCR master mix. Since concentrations vary from product to product, the final concentrations are shown and the volumes should be adjusted accordingly to give a final volume of 11.5 μL.
3. Heat to 65°C to melt the wax, centrifuge for 30 s to form a solid wax layer covering the reaction mix and cool on ice.
4. Add 7.5 μL of *Taq* mix.
5. Start the PCR program, put the machine into hold mode as soon as the annealing temperature (88°C) is reached, and insert the tubes. Resume the cycler.
6. After completion of eight cycles the machine enters into an extended annealing phase (10 min). After completion, put the machine on hold, remove the tubes, spin for 30 s, and cool on ice.
7. Add 2.0 μL of the GAPDH primers to a final concentration of 0.24 μmol/L.
8. Put the reaction tubes back into the machine and resume the PCR program; the machine enters into a second denaturing phase at 88°C, followed by an additional 27 cycles, and a final elongation step (10 min at 72°C).
9. Immediately after completion of the reaction, remove samples from the cycler, spin for 30 s, and put on ice. Flip over the wax lid with the pipet tip and remove 22.5 μL. Transfer the PCR product into a new tube, which already contains 2.5 μL 10X sample buffer. Vortex and store at 4°C until analyzed by gel electrophoresis.

3.5. Quantitative PCR to Determine the Expression of the Internal Standard GAPDH

A precondition for the use of GAPDH or any other gene (e.g., β-actin, transferritin) as internal reference is to show that its expression in the relevant sample is indeed constant and not, for example, affected by the experimental conditions tested. To confirnn this precondition, fully quantitative determination of GAPDH expression using competitive PCR is performed. PCR is done following a similar protocol as described in **Subheading 3.4.**, however, in addition to now 2.5 μL of RTP, an equal volume containing a competitor cDNA is added and, because only one primer is included in the reaction, the volume of DEPC water is increased by 1 μL. The competitor cDNA (also called mimic) is identical to the GAPDH PCR product, except for a 102 bp deletion. Five increasing concentrations of competitor (between 5 and 40 pg/μL) are chosen after an initial wide-range analysis (*see* **Note 1**). The target primer in this experiment is GAPDH specific.

3.6. Data Analysis

1. Run 10 μL of the PCR product on a 3% agarose gel. Ethidium bromide is added to the nonpolymerized gel after heating, adding 2.5 μL to a 40 mL gel (*see* **Note 5**).
2. Run for 100 min at 70 V.
3. Analyze gel on a transillumintor at 302 nm.
4. Capture electronic images using a solid-state black and white video camera (**Fig. 1**).

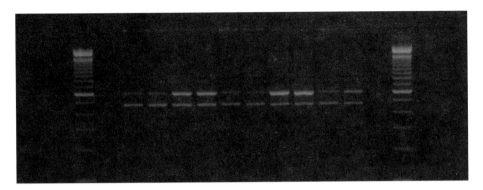

Fig. 1. VCAM-1 gene expression in the vascular wall of NZW rabbits. The expression of VCAM-1 was determined in aortic wall tissue isolated from control, cholesterol-fed and cholesterol-fed, probucol-treated NZW rabbits using quantitative RT-PCR as described. The expression of GAPDH served as internal standard. RT-PCR was performed on combined medial and intimal tissue and also on intimal tissue only. A strong upregulation of VCAM-1 can be seen after cholesterol feeding and is even greater in intimal tissue only. Probucol treatment leads to a strong inhibition of VCAM-1. Each lane shows gene expression in aortic tissue isolated from one rabbit. The upper band represents the PCR product of VCAM-1 (567 bp), the lower band the PCR product of GAPDH (465 bp). The DNA ladder used as standard shows bands in 100 bp intervals, the prominent band corresponds to 600 bp. The fluorescence intensity of the bands was determined using Optimas 4.0 imaging software.

Lane	Treatment	Tissue	VCAM-1	GAPDH	Ratio	VCAM-1 (%)
1	Control chow	Intima + media	5.42	16.00	0.34	96
2	Control chow	Intima + media	6.97	19.01	0.37	104
3	Cholesterol-fed	Intima + media	30.74	17.27	1.78	505
4	Cholesterol-fed	Intima + media	32.16	19.21	1.67	475
5	Cholesterol-fed + probucol treated	Intima + media	4.48	13.66	0.33	93
6	Cholesterol-fed + probucol treated	Intima + media	4.17	11.38	0.37	104
7	Cholesterol-fed	Intima	38.82	13.51	2.87	815
8	Cholesterol-fed	Intima	40.24	12.36	3.26	924
9	Cholesterol-fed + probucol treated	Intima	6.12	12.60	0.49	138
10	Cholesterol-fed + probucol treated	Intima	11.99	10.63	1.13	320

5. Assess the intensity of each band using Optimas 4.0 imaging software (or equivalent software). Each image analysis is performed twice by the same observer.
6. Gene expression is determined in triplicate. Expression is calculated as the ratio of target gene divided by the expression of GAPDH (*see* **Fig. 1**).

4. Notes

1. Competitive PCR requires the use of a competitor cDNA at a concentration range starting just below and ending just above the expression level of the target gene. Since this is unknown, initially a wide range analysis needs to be done to estimate the expression level. We use an initial range of competitor cDNA stretching over a 1000,000-fold concentration difference. The result of this experiment allows to set a much more narrow range of competitor, close to the actual concentration required to achieve a 50% competition.
2. To minimize RNAase activity liberated during cell lysis and from severed tissue and to prevent contamination, a number of measures are taken. Gloves are worn throughout the procedure and changed frequently, water to prepare buffers is treated with DEPC before use. Glassware and plastic ware are treated following the standard procedures to remove contaminations and to make them RNAase free. All procedures are performed on ice.
3. A further control that needs to be performed is to verify that the number of amplification cycles used for a typical sample/primer combination does not exceed the exponential phase of the reaction. This can be tested by repeatedly interrupting the PCR reaction ancl removing a small aliquot. The amount of PCR product formed after increasing cycle numbers is determined by gel electrophoresis and UV densitometry. Within the limits of the exponential phase of the reaction, both the reference and the target gene amplification should proceed in parallel without displaying a decrease in yield.
4. Selection of the annealing temperature (AT) is done using the described computer program (Gene Runner), the method is based on the AT/GC method. As a first measure to eliminate unspecific PCR products that might appear, the AT should be raised.
5. Ethidium bromide is added to the nonpolymerized gel after heating, adding 2.5 μL to a 40 mL gel. Precautions should be taken when handling ethidium bromide.

References

1. Mullis, K. B. and Faloona, F. A. (1987) Specific synthesis of DNA in vitro via a polymerase-catalyzed chain reaction. *Meth. Enzymol.* **155,** 335–350.
2. Mullis, K., Faloona, F., Scharf, S., Saiki, R., Horn, G., and Erlich, H. (1986) Specific enzymatic amplification of DNA in vitro: the polymerase chain reaction. *Cold Spring Harbor Symposia on Quantitative Biology,* Cold Spring Harbor, NY, **51 Pt 1,** 263–273.
3. Saiki, R. K., Scharf, S., Faloona, F., Mullis, K. B., Horn, G. T., Erlich, H. A., and Arnheim, N. (1985) Enzymatic amplification of beta-globin genomic sequences

and restriction site analysis for diagnosis of sickle cell anemia. *Science* **230(4732),** 1350–1354.

4. Gilliland, G., Perrin, S., Blanchard, K., and Bunn, H. F. (1990) AnalysNis of cytokine mRNA and DNA: detection and quantitation by competitive polymerase chain reaction. *Proc Natl Acad Sci USA* **87(7),** 2725–2729.

5. Fruebis, J., Gonzalez, V., Silvestre, M., and Palinski, W. (1997) Effect of probucol treatment on gene expression of VCAM-l, MCP-l and M-CSF in the aortic wall of LDL receptor-deficient rabbits during early atherogenesis. *Arteriosclerosis, Thrombosis, and Vascular Biology* **17,** 1289–1302.

6. Witztum, J. L. and Steinberg, D. (1991) Role of oxidized low density lipoprotein in atherogenesis. *J. Clin. Invest.* **88,** 1785–1792.

7. Berliner, J. A., Navab, M., Fogelman, A. M., Frank, J. S., Demer, L. L., Edwards, P. A., Watson, A. D., and Lusis, A. J. (1995) Atherosclerosis: Basic mechanisms. Oxidation, inflammation, and genetics. *Circulation* **91,** 2488–2496.

16

Northern Blot Analysis to Quantify Gene Expression in Vascular Diseases

Mingyi Chen and Tatsuya Sawamura

1. Introduction

To understand the molecular mechanisms of vascular diseases, studies are designed to process gene function from the discovery of relevant genes to examination of their expression and association with disease. Once a gene has been cloned, Northern blot analysis can directly monitor the gene expression at the mRNA level. Therefore, it is the most expedient strategy for investigating the potential relationship between specific gene expression and disease.

In Northern blot analysis, total or poly(A)$^+$ mRNA is run on a denaturing agarose gel and detected by hybridization to a radiolabled probe following transferral to a nitrocellulose or nylon membrane. A positive signal with poly(A)$^+$ mRNA demonstrates that the gene of interest is expressed under the conditions tested. Northern blot analysis can also quantify specific messages compared to an internal standard gene such as β-actin, GAPDH, or ubiquitin of which the expression levels do not change under different conditions. Most of the highly expressed genes can be observed in total RNA, while some of the rare messages must be detected using poly(A)$^+$ mRNA. In general, the experimental procedures are performed in three steps.

1. Acid guanidium isothiocyanate-phenol-chloroform method for total RNA preparation from vascular tissue or cultured cells.
2. Isolation of mRNA by oligo(dT)-cellulose chromatography.
3. Blotting, northern hybridization with probes and signal analysis.

From: *Methods in Molecular Medicine, vol. 30: Vascular Disease: Molecular Biology and Gene Therapy Protocols*
Edited by: A. H. Baker © Humana Press Inc., Totowa, NJ

2. Materials

1. DEPC treated water: Add diethyl pyrocarbonate (DEPC) to deionized water to a final concentration of 0.1%. Incubate overnight at room temperature, then autoclave for 20 min before use.
2. Guanindine isothiocyanate (GI) extraction buffer (contained in RNA isolation kits, e.g., TRIZOL Reagent from Gibco-BRL, Grand Island, NY, ISOGEN from Wako, Osaka, Japan, RNA isolation kit from Stratagene La Jolla, CA or equivalent).
3. 20X MOPS buffer: Add 83.72 g of MOPS (free acid) and 8.23 g of sodium acetate to 400 mL of DEPC-treated water and stir until completely dissolved. Add 20 mL of DEPC treated 0.5 M EDTA and adjust the pH to 7.0 with 10 N NaOH. Bring the final volume to 500 mL with DEPC-treated water and autoclave for 20 min.
4. 20X SSC buffer: Add 87.7g of NaCl, 44.1 g of sodium citrate to 400 mL of DEPC treated water. Adjust the pH to 7.2 with 10 N NaOH. Bring the final volume to 500 mL with DEPC-treated water and autoclave for 20 min.
5. mRNA binding buffer: 0.01 M Tris-HCl, pH 7.5, 0.5 M LiCl, 0.1% SDS, 1 mM EDTA in DEPC treated water.
6. mRNA wash buffer: 0.01 M Tris-HCl, pH 7.5, 0.15 M LiCl, 0.1% SDS, 1 mM EDTA in DEPC treated water.
7. mRNA elution buffer: 0.01 M Tris-HCl, pH 7.5, 0.05% SDS, 1 mM EDTA in DEPC treated water.
8. Agarose/formaldehyde RNA electrophoresis gel: Prepare a 1.1% gel by combining 1.5 mL of 20X MOPS, 27 mL of DEPC-treated water and 0.33 g of agarose, mix well and boil to dissolve the agarose, and cool to 55°C prior to addition of 1.6 mL of 37% of formaldehyde. Mix thoroughly and pour a 0.6-cm-thick electrophoresis gel.
9. RNA loading buffer: Mix 4.32 mL of deionized formamide, 0.48 mL of 20X MOPS, 1.26 mL of 37% formaldehyde, 0.48 mL of glycerol, 0.48 mL of saturated bromophenol blue (BPB), and 1.68 mL of DEPC-treated water for a total volume of 9.0 mL and mix well. Dispense into 1.0 ml aliquots and store at –20°C in Eppendorf tubes for future use. Apply 10 μL for each RNA sample.
10. Prehybridization/hybridization solution: 0.05 M Tris-HCl, pH 7.5, 1% SDS, 1.0 M NaCl, 10% Dextran sulfate, and 250 μg/mL of yeast tRNA.
11. Stringency wash solution I: 2X SSC, 0.1% SDS.
12. Stringency wash solution II: 0.2X SSC, 0.1% SDS.
13. Chloroform.
14. Isopropanol.
15. 75% of ethanol.
16. 0.1 M NaOH.
17. 1 mg/mL ethidium bromide.
18. Filter papers: ADVANTEC TOYO (Tokyo, Japan), and Whatman 3MM (England).
19. UV-crosslinker (Stratalinker, Stratagene).

3. Methods

3.1. Acid Guanidium Isothiocyanate-Phenol-Chloroform Method of Total RNA Extraction Protocol (1,2) (see Note 1 and also Chapter 4)

When the normal or diseased vascular tissues are collected, they should be immediately processed for RNA purification after removal from the body, or quickly frozen in liquid nitrogen and kept in –80°C for future use (*see* **Note 2**).

1. Homogenize the tissue samples in GI extraction buffer in a volume of 1.0 mL/ 100 mg of tissue. If cultured cells are used for the extraction of RNA, directly lyse cells in the culture dish by adding GI extraction buffer to a volume of 1.0 mL/ 10 cm^2 of dish area.
2. Incubate the homogenized samples or cultured cell extract in GI extraction buffer at room temperature for 5 min.
3. Add a 20% volume of chloroform to GI extraction buffer and shake vigorously or vortex for 30 s.
4. Subject the samples to centrifugation at no more than 12,000g for 15 min at 4°C. RNA is exclusively separated in the clear colorless upper aqueous phase while the DNA and proteins are left in the white interphase and lower red phenol-chloroform phase.
5. Collect the aqueous phase and mix with isopropanol at 50% volume of GI extraction buffer and incubate at room temperature for 10 min.
6. Centrifuge at no more than 12,000g at 4°C for 10 min (*see* **Note 3**).
7. Remove the supernatant and wash the RNA pellet once with the same volume of 75% of ethanol as GI extraction buffer used.
8. Briefly dry the RNA pellet and dissolve in DEPC-treated water with or without 0.2% of SDS (*see* **Note 4**).
9. Pipet several times and incubate for 10 min at 55°C to completely dissolve.
10. Quantify the concentration and purity of eluted RNA by spectrophotometry by reading the absorbancies at A_{260} and A_{280} (1 A_{260} unit = 40 µg/mL of RNA). Absolutely pure RNA will exhibit A_{260} / A_{280} ratios of 2.0. However, if the RNA obtained has a ratio in the range 1.7–2.0, it will be suitable for Northern blotting analysis. (*see* **Notes 5** and **6**).

3.2. mRNA Purification by Oligo(dT)-Cellulose Chromatography (3)

The poly(A)$^+$ mRNA can be directly isolated from homogenized tissues or cells lysates, or indirectly from total RNA preparations by the method of oligo(dT)-cellulose chromatography. In this method, homogenized tissues or cells are mixed with the mRNA binding buffer (*see below*). Or, total RNA can also be directly applied to mRNA binding buffer.

1. Prepare the oligo(dT)-cellulose by resuspending 0.5 mL of dry powder in 1.0 mL of 0.1 *M* NaOH and transferring it onto the column.

2. Wash the column with 1.0 mL of DEPC-treated water several times until the pH is neutral, and briefly rinse with 2–3 mL of binding buffer.
3. Load the mixed solutions onto the oligo(dT)-cellulose column and incubate at room temperature for several minutes. This ensures efficient hydrogen-bond formation between poly(A) tail on the mRNA molecules and oligo(dT) attached to cellulose.
4. Centrifuge briefly to collect the oligo(dT)-cellulose:mRNA complexes.
5. Wash the pellet several times with 3 mL of mRNA binding buffer (high salt) and wash buffer (low salt) sequentially.
6. Elute the mRNA in a small volume of elution buffer. The concentration and purity of mRNA in the final elute can also be determined by spectrophotometry as the method described in total RNA purification (*see* **Subheading 3.1., step 8**) (*see* **Notes 5–7**).

3.3. Analysis of RNA by Northern Hybridization (4,5)

3.3.1. Agarose/Formaldehyde Gel Electrophoresis of RNA

1. Pour a 0.6-cm-thick gel (*see* **Subheading 2.**).
2. Prepare the RNA samples by mixing with 10 μL of RNA loading buffer and heat at 65°C for 10 min.
3. Load the RNA samples (*see* **Note 8**).
4. Electrophorese in 1X MOPS buffer until the bromophenol blue has migrated to two-thirds of the gel.
5. The integrity of the samples can be confirmed by staining the RNA with ethidium bromide for the presence of the 28S and 18S RNA bands. Add 20 μL of 1 mg/mL ethidium bromide stocking solution to 100 mL DEPC-treated water and soak the gel for 15 min with gentle shaking.
6. Wash with 10X SSC for 30 min to reduce background.
7. Visualize under UV transillumination and perform photography.

3.3.2. Transfer of RNA to Hybridization Membrane and Fix by UV Exposition (see **Fig. 1**)

1. Rinse the gel in DEPC-treated water three times to remove the formaldehyde.
2. Presoak in 10X SSC for 45 min. Also, prewet the hybridization membrane and filter papers in DEPC-treated water and completely soak in 10X SSC until needed (*see* **Note 9**).
3. Set several pieces of presoaked thick ADVANTEC TOYO filter paper in a clean plastic container half-filled with transferring buffer (10X SSC). Sometimes, completely saturated blotting pads or sponges can be alternatively applied. In addition, apply two pieces of wet Whatman 3MM filter papers on the top of thick ones.
4. Place the gel on the top of the filter papers with the bottom side of the gel up.
5. Using gloved hands, place the nylon membrane on the top of the gel and then cover with another two pieces of Whatman 3MM filter paper prewet with 10X of SSC (*see* **Note 10**).

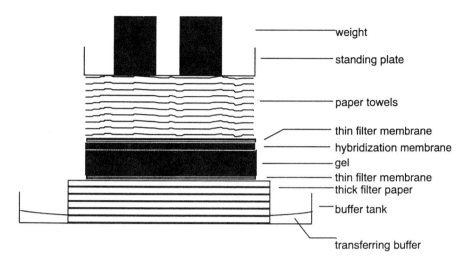

Fig. 1. Transfer RNA to hybridization membrane. RNA in the gel is blotted onto hybridizing membrane when the transfer buffer moves from the bottom tank through the paper towels mediated by capillary action.

6. Place dry blotting paper towels to 5–10 cm thickness on the filter paper and compress with a 250–500 g of weight.
7. Allow the transfer to proceed for 1–16 h at room temperature ensuring most of the RNA is transferred to the hybridization membrane by an action of capillary suction.
8. Remove the membrane and air-dry for 5 min.
9. UV-crosslink the RNA to the membrane with the RNA side up.

3.3.3. Hybridization of Probe

1. Prehybridize the membrane with hybridization buffer at 60°C for 3 h.
2. Hybridize at 65°C overnight following addition of a radiolabled probe (*see* **Note 11**).
3. Wash hybridized membranes twice with stringency wash solution I at 65°C for 30 min each, and with stringency wash solution II at 65°C for 30 min.
4. Autoradiograph at room temperature overnight.
5. Analyzed by densitometry using a suitable computer system (e.g., NIH image, a free software on Macintosh).

In order to confirm the integrity of the RNA samples applied, the membrane can be rehybridized to some standard genes such as actin, GAPDH, or ubiquitin in the same procedures just shown (*see* **Fig. 2**).

3.4. Potential Value of Results

A typical figure applying the strategy of Northern blot analysis to study LOX-1 gene expression on vascular tissues is illustrated (*see* **Fig. 2**). LOX-1, an endothelial-cell-specific oxidized LDL receptor, which is highly expressed

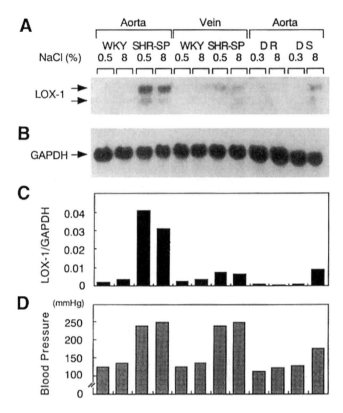

Fig. 2. Northern blot analysis to examine LOX-1 gene expression in the aorta and vein of SHR-SP, WKY, DS (Dahl salt-sensitive), and DR (Dahl salt-resistant) rats. Evidently, LOX-1 gene is markedly enhanced in hypertensive and stoke-prone SHR rats (7).

in vascular tissues, was recently cloned (6). It is characterized as avidly binding , internalizing , and phagocytosing ox-LDL and therefore may play a role in the pathogenesis of atherosclerosis (6). More recently, a study applying Northern blotting was performed to examine LOX-1 gene expression in the aortas and veins of SHR-SP (hypertensive and stoke-prone), WKY (normal), DS (Dahl salt-sensitive), and DR (Dahl salt-resistant) rats (7). RNA was extracted from the aortas and veins of the rats, and poly(A)$^+$ mRNA was purified. After transferring to a nylon membrane, the blot was hybridized to a probe of rat LOX-1. The results demonstrated that LOX-1 gene was markedly upregulated in SHR rats compared to normal WKY rats (7). Therefore, it is tended to suggest that the highly expressed LOX-1 on vascular endothelium of SHR-SP rats may mediate the ox-LDL induced impairments of endothelium-dependent vasodilatation, which at least can partially explain the hypertensive state and tendency of atherosclerosis.

4. Notes

1. In the course of RNA isolation and analysis, a ribonuclease-free environment should be strictly applied. For all of the experimental manipulations, wear disposable gloves to prevent RNase contamination from the hands. Glassware should be baked at 200°C overnight. Sterile disposable plasticware is highly recommended. Nondisposable plasticware should be merged in 0.1 N NaOH/ 1 mM EDTA or 20% H_2O_2 for 2 h, and then thoroughly rinsed with DEPC-treated water before use.

2. RNA can be easily degraded by endogenous RNAses in the vascular tissue, therefore, in order to obtain enough RNA, the samples of vascular tissue should be as fresh as possible. It is highly suggested to homogenize the vascular tissues immediately after removing from the body. However, if the liquid-nitrogen-frozen sample has to be used, it should be homogenized during the frozen state before it is thawed to prevent degradation by RNases.

3. After phase separation, RNA collection should be strictly limited to the clear aqueous phase by a gentle and accurate operation. Sometimes only collect the upper two-thirds of the aqueous phase. Be sure not to disturb the interphase and phenol-chloroform phase. Otherwise, it will decrease the purity of RNA by contaminating with protein or phenol, which can interfere with the following steps of experiment.

4. If the isolated RNA is not to be used for RT-PCR, in vitro transcription or any other conditions in which specific enzymes are applied, 0.2% of SDS is highly recommended for the final dissolving solution, otherwise, it must be omitted to prevent the inactivation of enzymes.

5. During the quantification ofthe RNA or mRNA concentration by spectrophotometry (especially, when the RNA samples are directly measured without dilution and then recovered), the cuvettes should be RNase-free to prevent contamination. Therefore, it is recommended to wash the cuvettes thoroughly with 0.1 N NaOH, 1 mM EDTA followed by a brief rinsing with nuclease-free water.

6. If the ratios of A_{260}/A_{280} are lower than 1.65, it may be due to protein or phenol contamination. An additional phenol:chloroform extraction on the purified RNA should be introduced to obtain a higher A_{260}/A_{280} ratio although it may cause a reduction in the RNA concentration. Also, RNA can be precipitated again by 0.1 vol of 3 M sodium acetate, pH 5.2, and 1.0 vol of isopropanol at –20°C overnight. After centrifugation at >12,000g for 10 min, wash the RNA pellet with 1.0 mL of 75% ethanol, dry at room temperature for several minutes, and then resuspend in DEPC-treated water with or without 0.2% of SDS (*see* **Note 4**).

7. Sometimes, the mRNA may need to be concentrated by precipitation prior to be used for Northern blot analysis. Add 1/10 vol of 3 M sodium acetate, pH 5.2, and 1.0 vol of isopropanol in –20°C overnight. After centrifugation at >12,000g for 10 min, wash the RNA pellet with 1.0 mL of 75% ethanol, dry at room temperature for several minutes, and resuspend again in DEPC treated water with or without 0.2% of SDS (*see* **Note 4**).

8. The amount of RNA applied is determined by transcript abundance. Generally, 0.2–10 µg of total RNA is required for a highly expressed gene while at least 3 µg of poly(A)$^+$ mRNA may be needed for a rare message.

9. Before setting the membrane on the gel, mark the back of the membrane to indicate which is the RNA side. Always put the RNA side up during the course of fixation by UV and during hybridization by probe.

10. In order to transfer RNA evenly and efficiently to the membrane with lower background, remove any bubbles between the membrane and the gel. Whenever the hybridization membrane is set on the gel, it should not be moved again in order to prevent false signals.

11. Radiolabeled probes may be generated by random-prime labeling (e.g., kit 6054 by Takara Biomedicals, Shiga, Japan) to a specific activity of 10^9 cpm/µg DNA using [^{32}P]dCTP (6000 Ci/mmol). After the labeling reaction, the probe is purified by ethanol precipitation. Mix with 1/10 vol of ammonium acetate and 2.2 vol of 100% ethanol, incubate at –20°C for 30 min, and then spin down at >12,000g at 4°C for 10 min. Discard the supernatant and wash the pellet with 0.5 mL of 100% ethanol at once. Then, redissolve the cDNA probe in water again. Alternatively, just pass through a Biospin column (Bio-Rad) to remove unincorporated radioactive [^{32}P]dCTP. The probe can be denatured by boiling or alkalizing with NaOH at final concentration of 0.1 M. Boil the DNA solution for 5 min and immediately chill on ice to denature.

References

1. Chomczynski, P. and Sacchi, N. (1987) Single-step method of RNA isolation by acid guanidinium thiocyanate-phenol-chloroform extraction. *Anal. Biochem.* **162(1)**, 156–159.
2. Chomczynski, P. (1993) A reagent for the single-step simultaneous isolation of RNA, DNA and proteins from cell and tissue samples. *Biotechniques*, **15(3)**, 532–534.
3. Chirgwin, J. M., et al. (1979) Isolation of biologically active ribonucleic acid from sources enriched in ribonuclease. *Biochemisrty,* **18(24)**, 5294–5299.
4. Sambrook, J., Fritsch, E. F., and Maniatis, T. (1989) *Molecular Cloning: A Laboratory Manual,* 2nd ed., Cold Spring Harbor Laboratory Press, Cold Spring Harbor, NY.
5. Ausubel, F. M., Brent, R., Kingston, R. E., Moore, D. D., Seidman, J. G., Smith, J. A., et al., eds. (1993) *Current Protocols in Molecular Biology,* Vol. 2, Greene Publishing Associates, Inc., Wiley, New York, NY.
6. Sawamura, T., Kume, N., Aoyam, T., Moriwaki, H., Hoshikawa, H., Aiba, Y., et al. (1997) An endothelial receptor for oxidised low-density lipoprotein. *Nature (London)* **386,** 73–77.
7. Nagase, M., Hirose S., Sawamura T., Masaki T., and Fujita T. (1997) Enhanced expression of endothelial oxidized low-density lipoprotein receptor (LOX-1) in hypertensive rats. *Biochem. Biophy. Res. Commun.* **237,** 496–498.

17

Localization of Gene Expression in Human Atherosclerotic Lesions by *In Situ* Hybridization

Lee D. K. Buttery and Julia M. Polak

1. Introduction

The technique of *in situ* hybridization was developed in the late 1960s *(1)* and is based on the ability of a single-stranded sequence of nucleotides to hybridize specifically to a complementary sequence to form stable double-stranded duplexes or hybrids. Incorporating a readily detectable label into the nucleotide sequence permits it to be used as a probe to identify specific complementary target sequences within cells or tissues and thereby derive useful information on the site(s) of expression of a particular gene. Although this technique can be adapted to detect any nucleotide sequence, this chapter is concerned with the detection of mRNA. The advantage of *in situ* hybridization for detecting mRNA over other methods such as Northern blotting is that this technique allows morphological identification of a specific mRNA species in a particular cell or a subpopulation of cells within a tissue. This can yield useful information on sites of synthesis, turnover, and, when combined with a method such as immunocytochemistry, storage of the transcribed protein.

Although there are numerous variations on this technique that have been adapted to suit specific applications *(2,3)*, all protocols require attention to three main factors:

1. Sensitivity, which is influenced by accessibility of the target sequence, preservation of tissue morphology and choice of probe.
2. Specificity, which is dependent on the stringency conditions imposed on the technique and the adoption of rigorous controls.
3. Signal resolution, which is determined by the method of probe labeling and detection.

From: *Methods in Molecular Medicine, Vascular Disease: Molecular Biology and Gene Therapy Protocols*
Edited by: A. H. Baker © Humana Press Inc., Totowa, NJ

The method presented in this chapter describes the detection of mRNA in tissue sections using complementary single-stranded RNA probes incorporating either isotopic or nonisotopic labels. Although the protocols can easily be applied to detecting mRNA in most tissues, we have indicated in the **Notes** section various options that have proved especially useful to performing *in situ* hybridization in a friable tissue such as the atherosclerotic lesion (*see* **Fig. 1**).

2. Materials
2.1. Probe Preparation

1. 5X Transcription buffer: 200 mM Tris-HCl, pH 8.0, 30 mM MgCl$_2$, 50 mM dithiothreitol (DTT), 10 mM spermidine, 5 U/μL RNasin, 0.05% (w/v) bovine serum albumin (BSA, RNase free). Store in aliquots at –20°C.
2. Nucleotides for isotopic labeling: 5 mM each of unlabelled nucleotides (ATP, GTP, and UTP) and 25 μCi/mL ^{32}P-CTP (or other isotope). Add fresh (to transcription buffer) from frozen aliquots (stored according to manufacturer's instructions).
3. Nucleotides for or nonisotopic labeling: 5 mM each of unlabeled nucleotides—ATP, GTP, CTP, and digoxigenin-UTP, 2.5 mM. Add fresh (to transcription buffer) from frozen aliquots (stored according to manufacturer's instructions).
4. RNase-free water: deionized water treated for 12 h with 0.1% (v/v) diethylpyrocarbonate (DEPC). Store at room temperature protected from light. Prepare all buffers for probe preparation and hybridization in DEPC-treated water. For all other stages preparation of buffers/reagents with DEPC-treated water is not necessary.
5. Tris-EDTA buffer: 10 mM Tris-HCl, 0.1 mM EDTA, pH 8.0. Store at room temperature.
6. Phenol:chloroform (1:1): saturated with Tris-EDTA buffer. Store at 4°C.
7. Chloroform:isoamyl alcohol (24:1): Store at 4°C.
8. 7 M ammonium acetate. Store at room temperature.
9. Ethanol: graded series prepared with deionized water (99%, 90%, 70%, 50%, v/v). Store at room temperature.
10. Probe hydrolysis buffer: 0.4 M NaHCO$_3$, 0.6 M Na$_2$CO$_3$. Store aliquots at –20°C.
11. Neutralizing buffer: 3 M sodium acetate, pH 6.0, 10% (v/v) glacial acetic acid. Store at room temperature.
12. RNA polymerase: T3, T7, or SP6—50 U/mL.

2.2. Tissue Preparation

1. Phosphate-buffered saline (PBS): 0.1 M phosphate buffer, 0.15 M NaCl, pH 7.4.
2. Fixatives: paraformaldehyde, 1% or 4% solution (w/v) in PBS. Store aliquots at –20°C.
3. PBS:sucrose washing buffer: PBS containing 15% (w/v) sucrose and 0.1% (w/v) sodium azide. Store at room temperature.
4. Mounting medium (Tissue Tek, Miles Inc., Elkhart, IN).

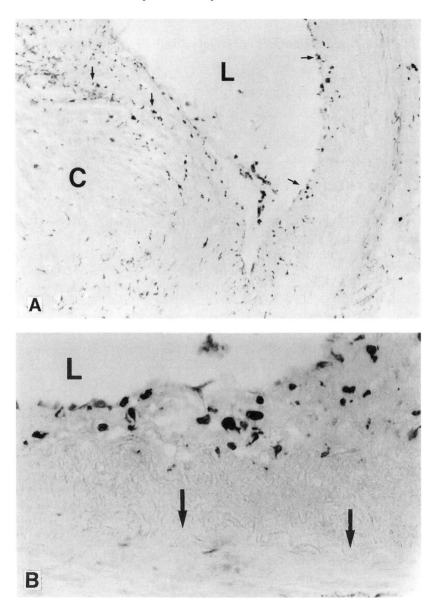

Fig. 1. *In situ* hybridization in human atherosclerotic lesions. Frozen cryostat sections of human atherosclerotic artery were hybridized with a digoxigenin-labeled human inducible nitric oxide synthase (iNOS) mRNA probe. **(A)** Low-power photomicrograph illustrating labeling of numerous mononuclear cells in and around the atherosclerotic lesion (*see arrows*). L = lumen, C = oxidized lipid/ceroid core. **(B)** High-power photomicrograph demonstrating strongly labeled mononuclear cells within the thickened intima (arrows denote the internal elastic lamina). L = lumen.

2.3. Tissue Pretreatment

1. PBS:Triton: 0.2% (v/v) Triton X-100 in PBS. Store at room temperature protected from light.
2. Proteinase K solution (1 µg/mL) in Tris-EDTA: Add proteinase K fresh from –20°C aliquots (10 mg/mL).
3. Glycine (proteinase K inactivation) buffer: 0.1 *M* glycine in PBS. Store at room temperature.
4. Acetylation buffer: 0.25% (v/v) acetic anhydride in 0.1 *M* triethanolamine, pH 8.0. Store aliquots at –20°C.

2.4. Hybridization

1. Deionized formamide: mix 100 mL of formamide with 5 g of mixed bed ion-exchange resin at room temperature for 30 min and filter through Whatman filter paper in deionized water.
2. 20X standard saline citrate (SSC): 3 *M* NaCl, 0.3 *M* sodium citrate, pH 7.0.
3. 100X Denhardt's reagent: dissolve 10 g of Ficoll, 10 g of polyvinylpyrrolidone, 10 g of BSA in 500 mL of DEPC-treated water and store in aliquots at –20°C.
4. Yeast tRNA.
5. Salmon sperm DNA. Store at –20°C in 10-mg/mL aliquots.
6. Hybridization buffer: 50% (v/v) deionized formamide, 4X SSC, 0.125 mg/mL tRNA. Can be prepared fresh or store in aliquots at –20°C. Add denatured salmon sperm DNA (heated to 80°C for 2 min) fresh to the hybridization buffer to a final concentration of 100 µg/mL.
7. Dimethyldichorosilane (Sigma, Poole, UK).

2.5. Posthybridization Washes

1. 2X SSC: Prepare from a 20X SSC stock with deionized water. Store at room temperature.
2. 2X SSC/0.1% SDS: Prepare from a 20X SSC stock and 10% (w/v) SDS stock with deionized water. Store at room temperature.
3. 0.1X SSC/0.1% SDS: Prepare from 20X SSC stock and 10% (w/v) SDS stock with deionized water. Store at room temperature.
4. RNase solution: 10 µg/mL RNase A in 2X SSC. Prepare fresh.
5. Ethanol: graded series (70, 90, and 99%, v/v) prepared with deionized water containing 0.3 *M* ammonium acetate.

2.6. Autoradiography

1. Nuclear track emulsion (Ilford, K5).
2. Kodak D19 developer.
3. Kodak F24 fixer.

2.7. Digoxigenin Detection Buffers

1. Buffer 1: 100 m*M* Tris-HCl, 150 m*M* NaCl, pH 7.5. Prepare fresh.
2. Buffer 2: 100 m*M* Tris-HCl, 100 m*M* NaCl, 50 m*M* $MgCl_2$, pH 9.5. Prepare fresh.

3. Buffer 3: 1 mM levamisole, 0.34 mg/mL nitroblue tetrazolium salt (NBT), 0.17 mg/mL 4-chloro-3-indolylphosphate (BCIP) in buffer 2. Prepare fresh.

3. Methods

3.1. Synthesis of cRNA Probes for In Situ Hybridization

All reactions should be performed in RNase-free Eppendorf plastic tubes (1.5 mL) and aliquots dispensed using RNase-free Gilson polypropylene pipet tips. As has been indicated, all solutions for probe synthesis and hybridization should be RNase-free (made using DEPC-treated water). All glassware should be baked at 250°C for at least 4 h.

1. At room temperature add the following:

5X transcription buffer	2 μL
400 mM DTT	1 μL
1.0 mg/mL linearized vector	1 μL
α^{32}P-CTP (25 mCi/mL)	5 μL
Digoxigenin-UTP (2.5 mM)	2 μL
RNA polymerase (T3, T7, or SP6 – 50 U/mL)	1 μL

   Make up to 10 μL with DEPC-treated water. Incubate for 1–2 h at 37°C (*see* **Note 1**).
2. Terminate the transcription by removing the template. Add 200 μL of DEPC-treated water containing 1 μg/mL RNase-free DNase and incubate for 10 min at 37°C.
3. Purify the probe by adding 200 μL of phenol:chloroform (1:1, v/v) *(4)*. After shaking vigorously, centrifuge at 11,500g for 5 min, and pipet the aqueous supernatant into a fresh tube and add an equal volume of chloroform:isoamyl alcohol (24:1, v/v) .
4. After mixing and centrifugation at 11,500g for 5 min, decant the aqueous layer into a fresh tube, and add 0.5 of a volume of 7 M ammonium acetate and 3 vol of 99% ethanol. Leave the labeled probe to precipitate overnight at –20°C.
5. Centrifuge for 15 min at 11,500g and decant and discard the supernatant.
6. Dry the pellet under vacuum and then resuspended in 50 μL of DEPC-treated water or Tris-EDTA buffer.
7. At this point the probe size and incorporation of label can be checked/determined (*see* **Note 2**).

3.2. Adjusting the Probe Length

Mild alkaline hydrolysis of a cRNA transcript (to ~500 bp) can improve the signal by increasing penetration and access of the probe to the target sequence (*see* **Note 3**).

1. Add one volume of probe hydrolysis buffer to the probe, carefully mix and incubate at 60°C for the amount of time given by the following equation;

$$t = (L_o - L_f)/kL_oL_f$$

where t = time in minutes, L_o = starting length (kb), L_f = desired length (kb), k = rate constant for hydrolysis (0.11 scissions/kb/min).

2. Stop the hydrolysis by adding 10 μL neutralizing buffer.
3. Precipitate and determine the incorporation as in **Subheading 3.1.** and *see* **Note 2**.

3.3. Tissue Preparation and Pretreatment

1. Immerse the dissected tissue of interest in 1–4% solution of paraformaldehyde for 6–8 h at room temperature or overnight at 4°C (*see* **Note 4**).
2. Wash the tissues thoroughly in several changes of PBS:sucrose over 2–3 d.
3. Prepare cryostat blocks by orientating the tissues on cork mats, surrounding it in mounting medium, and rapidly freezing it in melting isopentane suspended over liquid nitrogen (*see* **Note 5**).
4. Section the tissues (5–10 μM) in a cryostat at –25°C and thaw mount onto treated slides and leave to air-dry for 1 h at room temperature (*see* **Note 6**).
5. Rehydrate the sections by immersing in PBS:triton for 15 min and wash in PBS (2 × 5 minutes).
6. Place the slides in a prewarmed (37°C) proteinase K solution for 10–30 min (*see* **Note 7**).
7. Inactivate the proteinase K by immersing the slides in glycine buffer for 5–10 min.
8. Briefly (2–3 min) postfix the slides in 4% paraformaldehyde and then wash in PBS (1 × 5 min).
9. Acetylate sections by immersing in acetic anhydride for 10 minutes at room temperature (*see* **Note 8**).
10. Rinse slides in 2X SSC or DEPC-treated water, dehydrate through graded ethanol concentrations (50, 70, 90, 99% ×2) and leave to air-dry.

3.4. Hybridization

1. Dilute the probe 1:10 in hybridization buffer to give a final probe concentration of 1–10 ng (*see* **Note 9**).
2. Prepare sufficient hybridization buffer to cover the section (10–30 μL), cover the section with a coverslip coated with dimethyldichlorosilane or a piece of parafilm (*see* **Note 10**) and place the slides in a humidified chamber at 42°C overnight (~16–20 h) (*see* **Note 11**).

3.5. Posthybridization Washes

1. Carefully remove the coverslips. (If using parafilm they can be easily lifted off the section, whereas to remove glass coverslips the slide must be immersed in 2X SSC and the coverslips allowed to float off.)
2. Wash the slides in 2X SSC/0.1 SDS at room temperature (4 × 5 min).
3. Wash the slides in 0.1X SSC/0.1% SDS at 42°C (2 × 10 min).
4. Wash the slides briefly in 2X SSC to remove all traces of SDS.
5. Remove nonspecifically bound single-stranded RNA probe by immersing the slides in RNase solution for 10 min at 37°C.
6. Briefly wash in 2X SSC and dehydrate through graded ethanol concentrations (70, 90, and 99% ×2) containing 0.3 *M* ammonium acetate and leave to dry at room temperature.

3.6. Autoradiography

All procedures are performed in a "dark room" illuminated by a safe light fitted with a Kodak Wratten Series II (red) filter and a 25 W bulb.

1. Remove the photographic emulsion (Ilford K5) from its light tight container and dilute with warm (45°C) double-distilled water 1:1 (v/v). Divide the diluted emulsion into aliquots (10 mL each, in nylon scintillation vials). Empty one 10-mL aliquot into a slide-dipping chamber and partially immerse in a 45°C water bath. Place the remaining aliquots in a light-tight box and store at 4°C.
2. After allowing to settle, dip a clean, blank slide into the emulsion to check for bubbles. (When ready, the emulsion should coat the slide evenly with no lumps or bubbles.)
3. Warm the experimental slides to 45°C on a hotplate and then dip briefly in the emulsion and place vertically in a drying rack and leave to dry for approx 1 h in complete darkness (*see* **Note 12**).
4. Place the dry, emulsion-dipped slides in a light-tight slide box together with a small perforated bag of desiccant/silica gel, seal, and store at 4°C until the appropriate exposure time has elapsed. It is advisable to select two or three different times of exposure for each slide.
5. Allow sealed slide boxes to warm for 15 min at room temperature. Under safe-light conditions develop slides by immersion in Kodak D19 developer at 20°C for 3 min, followed by a brief rinse in distilled water and fixing for 5 min in Kodak F24 fixer. After thorough washing in tap water lightly counterstain in Harris's heamatoxylin, dehydrate through graded ethanol concentrations (50, 70, 90, 99% ×2), clear (xylene or similar agent ×2) and mount (Pertex/DPX or similar compound) (*see* **Note 13**).
6. For exposure to film, dry the slides as for emulsion-dipping and place face up in an X-ray film cassette and in complete darkness lay a sheet of Hyperfilm β Max over the slides (emulsion coated side of the film facing the slides) (*see* **Note 14**).
7. Seal the cassette and store at 4°C for the appropriate exposure time.
8. Develop the films in D19 developer at 20°C for 5 min, wash in tap water and fix in Kodak F24 fixer for 5 min. After washing thoroughly leave films to dry in a drying cabinet.

3.7. Immunological Detection of Digoxigenin-Labeled Hybrids

1. After posthybridization washes (**Subheading 3.5., steps 1–6**, but without dehydration) immerse the slides (or spot blots) in digoxigenin buffer 1 for 5 min at room temperature.
2. Incubate the sections in buffer 1 containing 2% normal sheep serum and 0.05% BSA for 30 min at room temperature.
3. After blotting the slides (without washing), incubate the sections in buffer 1 containing 1% normal sheep serum and polyclonal alkaline phosphatase-conjugated sheep antidigoxigenin-Fab fragments diluted 1:500 for 2 h at room temperature.
4. After a brief wash in buffer 1, equilibrate the sections in buffer 2 for approx 20 min.

5. Incubate the sections in buffer 3 in a light-tight box for the appropriate development time (*see* **Note 15**).
6. After color reaction has proceeded to completion, the reaction is stopped by immersion in Tris-EDTA buffer.
7. Mount the slides in 1:1 (v/v) Tris-EDTA:glycerol.

4. Notes

1. After 1 h we generally add a further aliquot (1 µL) of RNA polymerase and incubate for the time remaining (1 h).
2. In order to assess incorporation of the radiolabeled nucleotide and hence transcription efficiency, spot 1 µl of the probe onto 2×1 cm^2 pieces of filter paper marked A and B. Wash filter B in 0.5 M Na$_2$HPO$_4$ (6×5 min), then distilled water (2×1 min) and finally 99% ethanol (2×1 min). After air drying, measure the cpm emitted using a scintillation counter. Incorporation of the radiolabeled nucleotide into the probe is given by the following equation;

$$\% \text{ incorporation} = (\text{cpm filter B/cpm filter A}) \times 100$$

The total yield of probe can then calculated according to the amount of limiting nucleotide in the labeling reaction. For example:

$$^{32}\text{P-CTP limiting nucleotide} = 12.5 \text{ m}M$$

For 100% incorporation = 0.125 nmol of CTP incorporated

Assuming equal incorporation for all four nucleotides = 0.5 nmoles of NTPs incorporated

The average MW of a ribonucleotide is 330 thus,

$$330 \times 0.50 \text{ nmol of NTPs incorporated} = 165 \text{ ng}$$

165 ng of probe = 100% incorporation

From the percentage incorporation of the labeling reaction the amount (ng) of probe is determined. For digoxigenin-labeled probes we generally perform spot blot analysis. Dilute a small aliquot (1 µL) of probe (1:20, 1:50, 1:100, etc.) and spot 2–3 µL on Hybond N (Amersham International, Buckinghamshire, UK) and nucleic acid immobilize using a UV lamp (e.g., Stratalinker). Develop the filter as described in **Subheading 3.7.** From this an "optimum" dilution of probe is selected. To determine probe concentration in nanograms, a digoxigenin-labeled standard (Boehringer Mannheim, Lewes, UK) is included in the spot blot analysis. This labeling method in many instances is much more convenient (and more economical) than isotopic hybridization and also removes the "hazards" of working with radioactivity. It is also advisable to run 1 µL of probe on an agarose gel to check the probe is the correct size.
3. Some workers have reported that probe hydrolysis does not improve significantly hybridization and is therefore an unnecessary step (*5*). Moreover, designing

shorter probes in the first instance can negate the need to adjust probe length. We have included a protocol to reduce probe length and probes are typically reduced to 300–500 bp.

4. Good preparation of tissue is essential for a clear demonstration of mRNA's *in situ*. Where possible, we collect tissue directly at the time of surgery (transporting in sterile PBS on ice). To ensure adequate tissue fixation we generally dissect samples to sizes no greater than 1 cm × 1 cm × 0.5 cm. Larger pieces of tissue can be used but will require longer periods of fixation. Choice of fixative can also be important if the tissue is to be used for additional investigations such as immunocytochemistry or combined *in situ* hybridization—immunocytochemistry *(3)*. For example, we have worked extensively on determining the distribution and localization of NO synthase within the vasculature and have found that tissues fixed in a 1% solution of paraformaldehyde give good results for both *in situ* hybridization and immunocytochemistry *(3,6)*. Conversely, whereas NO synthase mRNA is readily detected in tissues fixed in 4% paraformaldehyde, immunostaining for NO synthase is comparatively poor.

5. We have described a method for preparing cryostat blocks. However, it is also possible to use paraffin-embedded tissues. If using paraffin-embedded section slides these have to be dewaxed in xylene (or similar clearing agent) and rehydrated through graded ethanol concentrations to DEPC-treated water. Good preparation of blocks can alleviate potential problems with sectioning. For large pieces of tissue (1 cm × 1 cm) we often prepare a mould made from autoclave tape (wrapped around the cork tile), and this produces an evenly shaped block and minimizes air bubbles. For orientating blood vessels transversely, a small pin inserted carefully down the lumen holds the tissue in the correct orientation preventing it from moving when the mounting medium is poured over the tissue. Also, when sectioning, gloves should be worn, and the surface onto which slides are placed should be RNase free (lay slides on aluminium foil). Slides should be marked with pencil for identification (do not use pen as the mark will be erased in subsequent ethanol treatments).

6. Prior to treatment of slides to improve section adhesion, load the clean glass slides into metal slide racks wrapped in aluminum foil and bake at 250°C for at least 4 h. After baking and cooling, handle the slides wearing gloves. We usually treat slides with Vectabond™ (Vector Laboratories) which chemically damages the surface of the glass slide and thereby improves section adhesion. Poly-L-lysine coated slides can also be used; however we have found that nonspecific binding is increased especially at the margins of the tissue and in lumen of blood vessels, which is particularly problematic for investigating hybridization of probes to the adventitia and intima. The problem seems to be more prominent in the case of immunological detection of digoxigenin-labeled probes.

7. Precise incubation times for each tissue being investigated should be derived by performing a time course and assessing hybridization signal and tissue integrity. It may also be necessary to titrate proteinase K to determine a suitable concentration. Such procedures are often worthwhile particularly with friable tissues such

as atherosclerotic blood vessels where prolonged digestion can result in the section breaking up or floating away completely.

8. Acetylation is a common step to minimize nonspecific binding of the probe by electrostatic attraction. Numerous comparisons between hybridization seen with or without acetylation suggest that under the conditions used by us there is no significant advantage to acetylation and thus this step can easily be omitted.

9. For qualitative investigation of mRNA *in situ* we generally use probe at two or three different concentrations to determine an "optimum" concentration that gives the clearest hybridization signal. This concentration can then be used for all subsequent investigations. Suitable controls should be included to assess hybridization;

    a. Label the sense probe and apply to sections in the same way as the antisense probe. Any hybridization in these negative control sections can be considered nonspecific.

    b. RNase pretreatment destroys the target mRNA. Prior to proteinase K treatment, incubate sections in RNase (100 µg/mL) in 2X SSC prewarmed at 37°C for 30 min. After washing, incubate the slides in 2X SSC (2 × 3 min) to remove RNase. While treating with RNase care should be taken to avoid contact with the test slides.

    c. Chemography is used to evaluate false labeling caused by chemical reactions between substances in the tissue and the emulsion. Treat unlabelled sections with all solutions used in the hybridization method and hybridization buffer containing no probe and finally dip in emulsion along with sections hybridized with probe.

    d. Inappropriate probe or tissue not expected to be present or contain the mRNA of interest serves as a good indicator of specificity and background.

10. To prevent evaporation of the probe during hybridization the section is covered. Silane-coated coverslips are often used for this; however, dimethyldichlorosilane used in the preparation of the coverslips is very toxic and preparation has to be performed in a fume cupboard. As an alternative we find that a piece of parafilm cut a little larger than the size of the section is equally as good as a silane-coated coverslip. Moreover, a small fold at one corner enables the "coverslip" to be easily lifted off the section and minimizes the damage to the section that can occur when floating off coverslips in buffer. Whichever type of coverslip is used, care should be taken to avoid air bubbles, although any bubbles that do form can usually be removed by pressing gently on the coverslip with a pair of fine forceps.

11. Humidified chambers are easily created using a tupperware box with lid lined with filter paper and containing a horizontal slide support (two 10-mL pipets). The filter paper is soaked with 5X SSC, coverslipped slides placed on the supports, and the box sealed and placed in an incubator. The temperature for hybridization may have to be determined for each probe. For this it is common to perform hybridization reactions from 37–57°C at 5°C intervals. In all applications we find 42°C to be optimum for hybridization.

12. The emulsion can be used more economically if the tissue sections are mounted on the extreme end of the microscope slide. Thus, only a few centimeters depth of emulsion is needed. When dipping, it is important to dip slides to the same depth and at the same speed in an attempt to obtain a layer emulsion of the same thickness on each slide. Keep sets of slides to be developed at different exposure times in separate boxes and clearly label the box with dipping date. With friable tissue, the dipping process can damage the section, resulting in poor-quality preparations. As an alternative to dipping the slide/section into the emulsion, dipped coverslips can be used. In this method the coverslip is dipped and dried in the same way the slide would be. The dipped coverslip is then loosely mounted onto the slide secured by superglue along its top edge and with the bottom edge overhanging the end of the slide by approx 2 mm. After exposure the coverslip is developed by gently lifting the bottom free edge and inserting a small piece of orange stick to secure the coverslip, exposing the emulsion to developer, etc. Throughout the procedure the coverslip remains secured by superglue along its top edge, and, thus, once mounted, should be perfectly apposed with the tissue and in the same position as during the exposure period. Obviously extreme care needs to be taken with this method, because breakage of the coverslip renders the slide useless. Because the bottom edge of the coverslip needs to be raised, the section needs to be mounted higher up the slide. However, the benefits of clearer signal and tissue integrity make it a worthwhile method.

13. When developing slides, care should be taken not to damage the delicate emulsion layer, which, at this stage, is rehydrated and in gel form. Do not shake the slides during development/fixation. Keep all solutions at 18–20°C as sudden changes in temperature can also damage the emulsion layer.

14. Exposing radiolabeled slides to film and subsequent investigation macroscopically is useful for ascertaining the "global" distribution of hybridization signal and identifies specific areas for more detailed microscopic analysis.

15. To check color development, slides can be periodically removed from the light-tight container and viewed microscopically and, if necessary, replaced for further incubation.

References

1. Gall ,J. G. and Pardue, M. L. (1969) Formation and detection of RNA-DNA hybrid molecules in cytological preparations. Proc. Natl. Acad. Sci. USA **63,** 378–383.
2. Wilkinson, D. G. (ed.) (1994) The theory and practice of in situ hybridization, in *In Situ Hybridization: A Practical Approach*, Oxford University Press, pp. 1–13.
3. Gordon, L. and Bishop, A. E. (1996) Modern morphological techniques in molecular cell analysis, in *Clinical Gene Analysis and Manipulation: Tools, Techniques and Troubleshooting*, (Jankowski, J. A. Z. and Polak, J. M., eds.), Cambridge University Press, pp. 113–150.
4. Maniatis, T., Fritsch, E. F., and Sambrook, J. (eds.) (1989) *Molecular Cloning, A Laboratory Manual.* Cold Spring Harbor Press.

5. Martinez-Montero, J. C., Herrington, C. S., Stickland, J., Sawyer, H., Evans, M., Flannery, D. M., and McGee, J. O. (1991) Model system for optimizing mRNA non-isotopic in situ hybridization: riboprobe detection of lysozyme mRNA in archival gut biopsy specimens. *J. Clin. Pathol.* **44,** 835–839.
6. Buttery, L. D. K., Springall, D. R., Chester, A. H., Evans, T. J., Standfield, N., Parums, D. V., et al. (1996) Inducible nitric oxide synthase is present within human atherosclerotic lesions and promotes the formation and activity of peroxynitrite. *Lab. Invest.* **75,** 77–85.

18

RNase Protection Assays for Quantitation of Gene Expression in Vascular Tissue

Nengyu Yang, Shuli Wang, and James E. Faber

1. Introduction

Ribonuclease protection assay (RPA) is a sensitive solution hybridization method for quantitation of specific RNAs *(1–3)*. The method is based on the ability of single-strand specific ribonuclease to degrade single-stranded RNA while leaving intact fragments of labeled antisense RNA probe, which are annealed to homologous sequence in the sample RNA. After ribonuclease digestion, the hybridized portion of the probe ("protected fragment") can be visualized via electrophoresis of the mixture on a denaturing polyacrylamide gel followed by autoradiography.

RPA has many advantages over Northern assays. RPA is 10–100 times more sensitive, owing in part to more complete hybridization in solution than on filters, digestion of unlabeled probe to reduce background, lack of losses during gel blotting, and no effect of partial degradation of the target RNA (providing it does not include the region homologous to the probe). Thus, most low abundance transcripts can be detected without poly(A$^+$) selection. RPA is able to differentiate cross-hybridization with multigene families and comigrating mRNA, and can be used to map intron/exon splices and transcription initiation and termination sites. Disadvantages are that no transcript size information is obtained, sample RNA is digested during assay eliminating the "strip and reprobe" option of Northern, and RPA is less sensitive than quantitative RT-PCR. The probe (radio- or nonisotopically labeled) must be for the antisense sequence, usually completely homologous to the target sequence, and only several hundred bases in length.

RPA provides a wide dynamic range of linear relationship between mRNA amount and band intensity. Since multiple probes can be used simultaneously

From: *Methods in Molecular Medicine, Vascular Disease: Molecular Biology and Gene Therapy Protocols*
Edited by: A. H. Baker © Humana Press Inc., Totowa, NJ

in the same RPA reaction, the probe for the gene of interest can be used together with another probe for internal control, such as cyclophilin, providing convenience and better accuracy. By simultaneously measuring a cellular RNA that one must show does not change with the stimulus or intervention, variation from slight differences in RNA isolation or assay procedures among samples can be normalized. In addition, RPA, unlike Northern blot analysis, can assay as much as 100 µg of RNA per reaction, which allows detection of low-abundant mRNAs.

As an example of use of RPA for analysis of rare transcripts, we present here expression of α-adrenergic receptor (α-AR) mRNA in rat vascular tissue. Vascular smooth muscle cells (SMCs) express up to five of the six α1 and α2-AR genes *(4)*. However, the distribution and abundance among vessel types, tissues, and species is poorly defined. These G protein-coupled receptors mediate sympathetic regulation, including constriction of vessels *(4)*. Previous α-AR mRNA and receptor binding studies using intact arteries such as rat aorta have interpreted results to reflect SMC expression. However, besides the medial layer, which is composed primarily of SMCs, the thin intimal layer is composed of endothelial cells, while the thick adventitia of such large arteries contain predominately (>99%) fibroblasts *(5)*. Because the adventitia comprises approximately one-third of the vessel dry weight, it is possible that adventitial cells could also express α-ARs and complicate conclusions about SMC expression reported in previous studies. We employed RPA to examine the expression of α-AR 1A, 1B, 1D, and 2D mRNAs in both adventitial and medial layers of adult rat thoracic aorta (α_{2B} and α_{2C} are not expressed in this vessel). We find that mRNA for α_{1A} and α_{2D} subtypes are more abundant in adventitia (8 and 12 times higher, respectively) than in media. By contrast, α_{1B} and α_{1D} transcripts are more abundant in media (5 and 11 times higher, respectively) than in adventitia.

1.1. Overview of RNase Protection Assay

An excess (about fivefold) of usually radiolabeled antisense probe is hybridized in solution with cell RNA containing the target RNA (or poly A^+ RNA if necessary). Excess unhybridized single-stranded probe molecules and cell RNA are degraded by a mixture of single-strand specific RNases (e.g., A, T1, ONE) that are selective for different base mismatches. The RNases are then inactivated, usually by proteinase K/SDS, and recovered in a separate tube by phenol-chloroform extraction and ethanol precipitation of the extract. The protected fragments are then resolved by denaturing PAGE.

1.1.1. Isolation of Total RNA

To preserve mRNA levels, tissues should be obtained in a way to prevent nonspecific RNA degradation and exposure to endogenous RNases and to minimize cellular damage and release of endogenous RNases. Preservation is aided by rapid gentle surgical dissection under a pool of 4°C sterile saline, followed by snap-freezing in liquid nitrogen, storage at –80°C, pulverization in liquid nitrogen, and immediate homogenization of frozen powder in an RNase denaturant. Many methods and kits with proprietary extraction solutions are available that vary in the purity and yield of total cellular RNA obtained. We have found satisfactory results using the acid guanidinium thiocyanate-phenol-chloroform method *(6)*.

1.1.2. In Vitro Synthesis of Antisense RNA Probe and Sense-Strand RNA

The most practical way of preparing the antisense riboprobe and sense strand for assay calibration is to subclone the particular coding segment (usually 100–500 bp) of the target gene into a commercial plasmid vector possessing a broad multicloning site flanked by promoter and transcription initiation sites for T7 and SP6 RNA polymerases (e.g., Promega's [Madison, WI] pGEM plasmids). Purified subcloned plasmid is then completely linearized with one of two selected restriction enzymes to yield the desired DNA template for either riboprobe or RNA sense synthesis, blunt ended if necessary, and used in an in vitro transcription reaction employing either T7 or SP6 in the presence of high concentrations of all four unlabeled rNTPs (for which one is present in less abundance when its radiolabeled specie is used to make the riboprobe). The DNA template is degraded with DNase I and the high specific activity continuously labeled riboprobe is then gel purified to eliminate nonfull length transcripts, DNA template and unincorporated nucleotides (sense strand purification is usually not necessary). Sense strand is then carefully quantitated by OD_{260} absorbance. It is also useful to verify by gel electrophoresis that purified probe and sense consist of full-length transcripts (for sense by including tracer nucleotide in the synthesis reaction).

1.1.3. Construction of Standard Curve

The most accurate way to quantitate the RPA requires construction of a standard curve for the targeted gene of interest using known amounts of in vitro-generated (exogenous) sense-strand RNA hybridized with excess of labeled riboprobe. The sense molar concentration range should span, in 100-fold excess, the expected cellular (endogenous) concentration of the target. Importantly, amounts of sense should be mixed with a constant amount of total RNA (the same amount planned for assay of endogenous target mRNA) obtained from "null" cells or tissue lacking expression of the target gene. This allows use of a constant amount of RNase during the digestion step. The common use of yeast tRNA as "carrier" RNA for this purpose may not provide a background for nonhomologous binding of riboprobe that optimally mimics cellular total RNA, which can lead to inaccuracies. However, the availability of a tissue or cell type from which to obtain the appropriate null carrier RNA may be limited and may still not accurately mimic the RNA background of the targeted tissue. Experimental samples are run concurrent, but separate from the standard curve samples, and the intensity of the labeled protected fragment for the experimental sample is compared to the standard curve to estimate the absolute amount of the target mRNA present in the sample of total tissue RNA. The effects of variation among reaction tubes and gel lanes can be minimized by addition of the experimental sample RNA into each standard curve assay tube if the exogenous sense strand has been synthesized about 30 bases shorter (or just sufficient to be detected as separate from endogenous target). This has the additional advantage of eliminating construction of a separate sense curve with carrier RNA, but requires that RNA from the target tissue be not limiting (a problem with vessels from small animals).

1.1.4. Semiquantitative RPA

This can also be used to determine fold-differences among different samples that do not require standard curves (*see* **Subheading 3.8.**). An internal "control" riboprobe, such as cyclophilin, is added to all samples in addition to the target riboprobe. Prior RPAs must be conducted to establish that the cyclophilin concomitant RPA does not influence the intensity of the target band and that the cyclophilin riboprobe is in molar excess. The cyclophilin signal can then be used, provided it does not change with the intervention, to normalize for variation in assay conditions, RNA loading, and film exposure time. If cyclophilin message is affected by the intervention or differs among the tissues being compared, this can also be used productively to analyze specific differences in the target levels. If an internal control is not used, companion aliquots of sample RNA can be run on an ethidium bromide gel for quantitation of 28 and 18S rRNA, scanned, and used to correct for variations in RNA loading among samples *(7)*. The RPA should be tested for specificity using cells or tissues known to be positive and negative for expression of the target gene. In closely related gene sequences, absence of cross-reactivity (yielding an indistinguishably sized protected fragment) should be demonstrated for the given riboprobe *(7)*.

1.1.5. The Assay

RNA from the target tissue and sense RNA are aliquoted, carrier RNA added to bring each tube up to the same amount of total RNA, and a constant amount of riboprobe in slight molar excess is added. Two-to-three concentrations of sense spanning the expected range of the endogenous transcript level should be run to demonstrate that conditions of molar excess of probe were maintained in each assay tube (the intensity of the bands should increase linearly *[7]*). After hybridization, single-stranded RNA is digested with specific RNases, the RNases degraded, and the protected double-stranded hybrids extracted and precipitated. Hybrids are then resolved on a gel and exposed to film for subsequent densitometry. Alternatively, the samples can be TCA precipitated and counted directly, although the latter will not detect other protected fragments that may represent hybridization to nontarget mRNAs, or differentiation of sense protected fragments if done in the same reaction tube. After plotting band optical density against sense concentration to obtain the standard curve, the density of the endogenous RNA band can be directly read from the curve for molar amount of target mRNA present in the original sample total cellular RNA (if the size of sense fragments was made to equal that of the target mRNA protected fragments). This molar amount can then be converted to number of transcripts per cell, when the cell number from which the original sample RNA has been obtained.

2. Materials

2.1. Vascular Tissues Preparation and Total RNA Extraction

All procedures and solutions should be as close to sterile (RNase-free) as possible.

2.1.1. Artery Tissue Preparation

1. PBS: 137 mM NaCl, 2.68 mM KCl, 7.98 mM Na$_2$HPO$_4$, 1.47 mM KH$_2$PO$_4$, pH 7.2. Autoclave and store at 4°C.
2. Modified Hank's balanced salt solution (HBSS): HBSS (BRL) with extra addition of 16 mM NaHCO$_3$ and 1 mM CaCl$_2$. Filter through 0.45-μm sterile filter system and store at –20°C.
3. Collagenase (CLS2, Worthington, Freehold, NJ). Store at –20°C.
4. Trypsin inhibitor (SI, Worthington). Store at –20°C.
5. Elastase (ESL, Worthington). Store at 4°C.
6. Enzyme solution: 1 mg/mL collagenase and trypsin inhibitor, 0.25 mg/mL elastase in modified HBSS. Stable for several days at 4°C if sterile.

2.1.2. RNA Preparation (see **Note 1**)

1. Diethylpyrocarbonate (DEPC)-treated water: Mix 1 L of distilled, deionized water with 1 mL DEPC (Sigma, St. Louis, MO) and stir overnight at room temperature (RT). Autoclave (loosen cap to allow removal of DEPC breakdown products) and store at RT.
2. 10% N-lauroyl sarcosine: Dissolve 10 g of N-lauroyl sarcosine (Sigma) in 100 mL of DEPC-treated water, filter (0.45-μm sterile filter) and store at RT.
3. 0.25 M sodium citrate: Dissolve 7.35 g of citric acid in 80 mL of DEPC-treated water and adjust the pH to 7.0 with 1 N HCl, q.s. to 100 mL. Store at RT.

4. 2 M sodium acetate, pH 4.0: Add 10 mL of DEPC-treated water to 27.2 g sodium acetate, adjust the pH to 4.0 with glacial acetic acid, q.s. to 100 mL. Autoclave and store at RT.

5. Solution D (denaturant): 4 M guanidinium thiocyanate, 25 mM sodium citrate, pH 7.0, 0.5% sarcosine. Store at RT. Add 78 µL of 2-mercaptoethanol (Sigma) to 10 mL of solution D. After adding 2-mercaptoethanol, solution D can be stored for 1 mo at RT.

6. Phenol: phenol (Boehringer Mannheim, Indianapolis, IN) needs to be saturated in DEPC-treated water, pH 6.6. Store at 4°C.

7. Chloroform/isoamyl alcohol: Mix 24:1 and store in a dark bottle.

8. Isopropanol.

9. 75% ethanol: Add 25 mL of DEPC-treated water to 75 mL of 100% ethanol.

10. Glacial acetic acid.

2.2. Riboprobe Synthesis and Purification

2.2.1. Probe Synthesis

1. TE buffer: 10 mM Tris-HCl, pH 8.0, 1 mM EDTA. Autoclave and store at RT.

2. 100% Ethanol.

3. 5X transcription buffer (Promega, Madison, WI): 200 mM Tris-HCl, pH 7.5, 30 mM MgCl$_2$, 10 mM spermidine, and 50 mM NaCl. Store at –20°C.

4. RNasin ribonuclease inhibitor (Promega). Store at –20°C.

5. Dithiothreitol (DTT): Dissolve 46.3 mg of DTT (BRL) in 10 mL of DEPC-treated H$_2$O to make 300 mM stock solution. Store at –20°C in small aliquots.

6. ATP, GTP and UTP mixture (AUG): Prepare by mixing equal volumes each from 10 mM ATP, GTP, and UTP stocks (Promega). Store at –20°C in small aliquots.

7. 100 µM CTP. Made from 10 mM CTP stock (Promega) by 100X dilution with DEPC-treated H$_2$O. Store at –20°C in small aliquots.

8. ^{32}P-CTP (Amersham, Piscataway, NJ). 800 Ci/mmol. Store at –20°C.

9. T3 or T7 RNA polymerase (Promega). Store at –20°C.

10. RQ1 RNase-free DNase (Promega). Store at –20°C.

11. Proteinase K (BRL): 20 mg/mL in DEPC-treated H$_2$O and store at –20°C in small aliquots.

12. 10% SDS: Dissolve 10 g of SDS in 100 mL DEPC-treated H$_2$O. Store at RT.

13. 500 mM EDTA: Dissolve 18.6 g of EDTA in DEPC-treated H$_2$O and adjust the pH to 8.0 with 10 N NaOH, q.s. to 100 mL. Autoclave and store at RT.

14. Century marker templates (Ambion, Austin, TX). Store at –20°C.

2.2.2. Riboprobe Purification

1. 10X Tris borate electrophoresis buffer (TBE): 108 g Tris base, 55 g boric acid, and 40 mL of 0.5 M EDTA. q.s. to 1 L. Autoclave and store at RT.

2. Urea. Store at RT.

3. 40% acrylamide:bisacrylamide solution, 19:1 (National Diagnostics, Atlanta, GA). Store at 4°C.

4. 6% polyacrylamide gel/8M urea: Dissolve 48 g of urea in 15 mL of 40% poly-acrylamide gel and 10 mL of 10X TBE, q.s. to 100 mL with DEPC-treated H_2O. Store at 4°C.

5. 10% Ammonium persulfate: Dissolve 100 mg of ammonium persulfate (Sigma) in 1 mL of DEPC-treated H_2O. Make fresh.

6. N,N,N',N' Tetramethylethylenediamine (TEMED) (Sigma). Store at 4°C.

7. Formamide (Boehringer Mannheim). Store at 4°C.

8. Bromophenol blue (Sigma): Stock is 100 mg/mL. Dissolve 100 mg of bromophenol blue in 1 mL of DEPC-treated H_2O. Store at 4°C.

9. Xylene cyanol FF (Sigma). Stock is 100 mg/mL. Dissolve 100 mg of xylene cyanol FF in 1 mL of DEPC-treated H_2O. Store at 4°C.

10. 1 M Ammonium acetate: Dissolve 7.7 g of ammonium acetate in 100 mL DEPC-treated H_2O. Autoclave and store at RT.

11. Elution buffer: 0.5 M ammonium acetate, 1 mM EDTA, 0.1% SDS. Store at RT.

12. Loading buffer: 80% formamide, 10 mM EDTA, pH 8.0, 1 mg/mL bromophenol blue, and 1 mg/mL xylene cyanol FF. Stored at –20°C in small aliquots.

2.3. Hybridization, RNase Digestion, and Detection of Protected Fragments

1. 1 M PIPES (Sigma), pH 6.4: Add 80 mL of DEPC-treated H_2O to 30.2 g of PIPES and adjust the pH to 6.4 with 1 N HCl, q.s. to 100 mL. Autoclave and store at RT.

2. 4 M NaCl: Dissolve 23.3 g of NaCl in DEPC-treated H_2O, q.s. to 100 mL. Autoclave and store at RT.

3. Hybridization buffer: 80% formamide, 40 mM PIPES, pH 6.4, 400 mM NaCl, and 1 mM EDTA. Store at –20°C in small aliquots.

4. 3 M sodium acetate, pH 5.2: Add 60 mL of DEPC-treated water to 40.8 g of sodium acetate, adjust the pH to 5.2 with glacial acetic acid, q.s. to 100 mL. Autoclave and store at RT.

5. 1 M Tris-HCl, pH 7.4: Dissolve 12.1 g of Tris base in DEPC-treated H_2O and adjust the pH to 7.4 with HCl, q.s. to 100 mL. Autoclave and store at RT.

6. RNase digestion buffer: 300 mM NaCl, 10 mM Tris-HCl, pH 7.4, 5 mM EDTA. Store at RT.

7. RNase A (Boehringer Mannheim): 20 µg/mL. Store at –20°C.

8. RNase T1 (Boehringer Mannheim): 250 U/mL. Store at –20°C.

9. TE-saturated phenol/chloroform/isoamyl alcohol: Mix equal volumes of TE buffer and phenol. After separation of TE buffer and phenol, remove the upper aqueous. Then mix one part of lower phenol phase with 1 part of 24:1 chloroform:isoamyl alcohol.

10. Yeast tRNA (BRL): 10 mg/mL in DEPC-treated water. Store at –20°C in small aliquots.

2.4. Specialized Materials and Equipment

1. Glassware. Wash well, and bake at 180°C for 8 h (or autoclave and dry).

2. Spectrophotometer.

3. Cassette with double intensifying screens.
4. Geiger counter.
5. Film developer.
6. Liquid scintillation counter.
7. Densitometry scanner.
8. Radiation protection shield.
9. Small tissue homogenizer (e.g., Omni International small tissue homogenizer, Atlanta, GA).
10. Compression mortar (e.g., Fisher Bessman pulverizer).

3. Methods

3.1. Thoracic Aorta Tissue Preparation (As An Example)

1. Perfuse rat with 4°C PBS after CO_2 asphyxiation and decapitation.
2. Dissect the rat thoracic aorta in pool of 4°C PBS.
3. Gently remove the fat and loosely adherent connective tissue.
4. Place the aorta in 4°C PBS after several rinses to remove blood.
5. Transfer the aorta into enzyme solution and incubate at 37°C for approx 23 min.
6. Separate the media and adventitia with fine forceps under a dissection microscope. Remove endothelial cells by gently rubbing with a cotton-tipped applicator after opening the lumen with microscissors (examine several vessels with silver nitrate stain to verify removal). Do step 6 in 4°C PBS in presence of RNase inhibitor (vanadyl ribonucleoside complexes, GIBCO-BRL, 10 mM).
7. Rinse in cold PBS, immediately freeze in liquid nitrogen, then store at –70°C.

3.2. RNA Extraction

Although the RPA can tolerate partially degraded RNA, extreme care should be taken when handling samples to avoid RNA degradation. Gloves should be worn at all times. Glassware should be washed well and baked at 180°C for at least 8 h. Sterile disposable plasticware should be used whenever possible. All solutions except Tris-buffer should be treated with 0.1% DEPC overnight, following by autoclaving as described in **Subheading 2.1.2., step 1**. Tris solutions should be made with DEPC-treated and autoclaved water.

1. Place frozen thoracic aorta media or adventitia in a compression mortar precooled with liquid nitrogen, then hammer several times to create fine tissue powder.
2. Transfer the powder to a dry-ice chilled 15-mL polypropylene tube containing solution D (1 mL/30–50 mg tissue). Place tube in wet ice and homogenize for 8–10 s at high speed.
3. Add one-tenth volume of 2 M sodium acetate, pH 4.0, mix well.
4. Add an equal volume of DEPC-water saturated phenol. Close lid and briefly vortex.
5. Add one-fifth volume of chloroform:isoamyl alcohol (24:1).
6. Vortex for 30 s, place tube in ice for 15 min.
7. Centrifuge the samples at 8000g for 20 min at 4°C.

8. Transfer the top aqueous phase to a new polypropylene tube. Be careful not to remove any of the organic phase or white interface.
9. Repeat **steps 4–8**.
10. Add an equal volume of isopropanol to the aqueous phase of each sample. Vortex to completely mix.
11. Place the samples at –20°C for at least for 1 h.
12. Centrifuge at 8000g for 20 min at 4°C.
13. Remove as much of the supernatant as possible from each sample. Be careful not to disturb the small white RNA pellet on the bottom and side wall of the tube.
14. Air-dry the pellet.
15. Resuspend pellet in 500 µL of solution D, making sure the pellet is completely dissolved.
16. Transfer the RNA solution to an eppendorf tube and add 500 µL of isopropanol. Vortex for a few seconds.
17. Place the sample at –20°C for at least 1 h.
18. Spin at 16,000g for 20 min at 4°C.
19. Remove the supernatant. Be careful not to remove the RNA pellet.
20. Add 500 µL of 4°C 75% ethanol.
21. Vortex until the RNA pellet is dislodged from the bottom of the tube.
22. Spin at 16,000g for 10 min at 4°C.
23. Remove as much of the supernatant as possible. Do not disturb RNA pellet.
24. Air-dry the pellet (do not let RNA pellet overdry).
25. Resuspend the pellet in 100 µL of DEPC-water (volume not critical).
26. Vortex sample several times to dissolve RNA completely, then brief spin.
27. Determine the concentration of RNA at OD_{260}. Make sure the ratio of OD_{260}/OD_{280} is > 1.7.
28. Store the sample at –70°C.

3.3. Linearization of Plasmid cDNA Template for Antisense Riboprobe Synthesis (see Notes 2–4)

RPA requires use of an antisense RNA probe. cDNA clone inserts, genomic DNA fragments, and oligonucleotides cannot be used as probes. To make antisense RNA probes, specific cDNA fragments derived from restriction enzyme digestion or PCR or RT-PCR products need to be cloned into a plasmid vector with bacteriophage promoter. This allows synthesis of RNA transcripts using T3, T7, or SP6 RNA polymerase. We inserted restriction enzyme-fragments (α_{1B} and α_{1D}) and PCR fragments (α_{1A} and α_{2D}) into pGEM-3Z, pGEM-4Z (Promega) or pBluescript SK$^+$ (Stratagene, La Jolla, CA) vectors (*8,9*). The antisense RNA probes used in this study were synthesized using linearized plasmid as template.

1. Digest DNA plasmid with restriction enzymes: α_{1A} plasmid with *Xba*I; α_{1B} plasmid with *Hin*dIII; α_{1D} plasmid with *Nco*I and α_{2D} plasmid with *Xho*I.
2. Extract with phenol/chloroform, precipitate with 100% ethanol, wash DNA pellet with 75% ethanol, then dry DNA per standard protocol.

3. Resuspend DNA in DEPC-treated water and determine the concentration. Adjust concentration to 250 ng/μL. Store at –20°C.

3.4. Antisense Riboprobes and Sense Synthesis and Purification

3.4.1. Riboprobe and Sense Synthesis

1. Add the following in order given. Final reaction volume is 20 μL.

DEPC-treated H_2O	Balance
5X transcription buffer	4 μL
300 mM DTT	0.75 μL
40 U/mL RNasin	0.5 μL
DNA template	1 μL (0.25 μg)
10 mM each of AUG NTPs	4 μL
100 mM CTP	1 μL*
^{32}P-CTP	2.5 μL
RNA polymerase (T3 or T7)	1 μL (10–20 U)[‡]

2. Vortex for 2 s, then brief spin. Make sure no bubbles form.
3. Incubate at 37°C for 45 min.
4. Add 2 μL of RQ1 RNase-free DNase. Vortex for 2 s and spin briefly. Be careful not to leave bubbles in reaction cocktail.
5. Incubate at 37°C for 20 min.
6. For α-AR or cyclophilin probe synthesis, 20 μL of loading buffer is added to the reaction tube, then purified (*see* **Subheading 3.4.2.**). For synthesis of RNA marker (or cold sense), continue the following steps (for sense, omit ^{32}P-CTP from above and add 10 mM CTP).
7. Add 180 μL of DEPC-treated H_2O.
8. Add 20 μL of 2 M sodium acetate, pH 4.0. Close lid and vortex for 5 s.
9. Add 200 μL of DEPC-treated H_2O saturated phenol. Close lid and vortex for 5 s.
10. Add 40 μL of chloroform:isoamyl alcohol (24:1). Close lid and vortex for 20 s.
11. Centrifuge at 16,000g for 5 min at 4°C.
12. Transfer the aqueous phase to new tube. Be careful not to take any of the organic phase.
13. Add 1 μL (10 μg) of yeast tRNA and 500 μL of 100% ethanol. Vortex for 5 s.
14. Place tube at –20°C for 1 h or on dry ice for 30 minutes.
15. Centrifuge at 16,000g for 20 min at 4°C.
16. Remove as much of supernatant as possible. Do not disturb the pellet.
17. Add 500 μL of 75% ethanol. Vortex for 10 s.
18. Centrifuge at 16,000g for 5 min at 4°C.
19. Remove as much of supernatant as possible. Do not remove white pellet.
20. Air-dry pellet. Do not overdry.
21. Add 100 μL of DEPC-treated H_2O. Vortex several times to dissolve pellet.

---

*For synthesis of cyclophilin riboprobe, 10 mM CTP is used.

[‡]T7 RNA polymerase for α_{1A}, α_{1B}, α_{1D}, cyclophilin antisense probes and RNA marker synthesis; T3 RNA polymerase for α_{2D} probe synthesis.

22. Count 1 μL in a counting vial or eppendorf tube (dependent on the scintillation counter).
23. Store RNA marker at –70°C. Can be used for at least 2 wk.

3.4.2. Probe Purification (see **Note 5**)

1. Wash gel electrophoresis apparatus (e.g., Model v16–4 [BRL]). Glass plates, side spacer (0.75-mm thick) and comb (0.75-mm thick and 8-mm wide) should be washed with detergent and hot water, rinsed several times with tap water, distilled and deionized water, and finally with 100% ethanol.
2. Set glass plates on a rack, such as pipet tip box. Make sure the plates are level.
3. Make 50 mL of 6% polyacrylamide gel/8 M urea (enough for size 16 × 20 cm, 0.75-mm thick gel) in a clean beaker. Add 250 μL of 10% ammonium persulfate and 25 μL of TEMED. Swirl gently to mix well.
4. Fill the gel solution space between the two glass plates with a disposable pipet. Insert the comb. Clamp both spacer sides with large clamps.
5. After complete polymerization (about 45 min), remove clamp and set in the electrophoresis apparatus.
6. Add 1X TBE into both top and bottom tanks. Make sure there are no leaks.
7. Mark the wells with a marker pen before removing comb.
8. Flush wells with 1X TBE using a needle and syringe before loading gel.
9. Heat the probe (from **Subheading 3.4.1., step 6**) at 85°C for 3 min, then load into two wells. (If more than one probe is to be purified, it is best to skip two well spaces to avoid crosscontamination).
10. Run for 1–2 h at 200 V. (Running time is dependent on the size of probe, e.g., α_{1A}, α_{1D}, and cyclophilin run for 1 h; α_{1B} and α_{2D} run for 2 h).
11. Remove gel from electrophoresis apparatus. Disassemble the plates. Make sure the gel is only attached to one plate. Wrap the gel with plastic wrap. The TBE buffer in the bottom tank should be collected into a radioactive waste jar.
12. Place the gel (gel face up) in a plastic box with a right angle and low sides (box aids alignment of gel and film). Put gel into one corner of the box.
13. Overlay the film onto the gel in the dark room. Film edge should be against the same box corner as the gel. A designated corner of the film can be bent for orientation. Expose film for 1 min (time may be varied).
14. Develop film.
15. Remove the plastic wrap. Put the developed film underneath the gel to use as a guide. The position of gel and film should be the same as in **step 13**.
16. Excise the full-length RNA band denoted by the film with a clean scalpel. In general, the strongest top band is the full-length probe. After the band is cut out, the gel can be reexposed to make sure the probe is excised correctly. Dispose the gel in radioactive waste.
17. Transfer excised gel to a microfuge tube, add 300 μL of elution buffer. Make sure the gel is completely submerged in elution buffer.
18. Incubate the tube with shaking at room temperature overnight.
19. Transfer the probe to a new tube, and take 1 μL for scintillation counting.
20. Store the purified probe at –70°C. Probe can be used for 1 wk.

3.5. Size of Antisense Probe

Each synthesized antisense probe consists of two fragments, one from the specific insert and the other from vector sequence. After hybridization with sample RNA and digestion with RNase A and T1, the size of the protection band is the same as that of the specific insert: α_{1A}: 252 bp (179 bp + 73 bp, specific + vector sequence); α_{1B}: 340 bp (306 bp + 34 bp); α_{1D}: 159 bp (117 bp + 42 bp); α_{2D}: 432 bp (340 bp + 92 bp); cyclophilin: 179 bp (103 bp + 76 bp).

3.6. Hybridization

1. Aliquot required amount of total tissue RNA to new microfuge tubes (for aorta media and adventitia: 50 µg for α_{1A} and α_{1B}, 30 µg for α_{1D}, and 80 µg for α_{2D}). If tubes are to be compared, add tRNA to all tubes to equalize total RNA per tube. Adjust to 200 µL with DEPC-H_2O, then add one tenth volume 3 M sodium acetate, pH 5.2 and two volumes of 100% ethanol. Vortex for 5 s.
2. Incubate at –20°C for 1 h or dry ice for 30 min.
3. Centrifuge at 16,000g for 10 min at 4°C.
4. Discard the supernatant. Do not disturb the RNA pellet.
5. Add 300 µL of 75% ethanol. Vortex for 5 s.
6. Centrifuge at 16,000g for 5 min at 4°C.
7. Remove as much supernatant as possible. Do not remove pellet.
8. Air-dry the RNA pellet. Do not overdry.
9. Resuspend in 30 µL of hybridization buffer containing 2×10^5 cpm of probe (one of the α-AR probes) and 1×10^4 cpm of cyclophilin probe to serve as internal control. RNA should be dissolved completely (facilitated by vortexing and/or pipet trituration).
10. Briefly spin the samples. Incubate for 5 min at 85°C to denature the RNA.
11. Transfer tubes immediately to a 55°C incubator or water bath (incubator avoids condensation in hybridization tube). Incubate overnight.

3.7. RNase Digestion and Protected Fragment Detection

1. Remove the tubes from incubator and cool to room temperature.
2. Prepare RNase working solution. Dilute RNase A and RNase T1 in RNase digestion buffer to 20 µg/mL and 250 U/mL, respectively (*see* **Note 6**).
3. Add 300 µL of RNase working solution to each hybridization tube. Vortex and spin briefly.
4. Incubate for 30 min in 37°C water bath.
5. Add 20 µL of 10% SDS and 4 µL of proteinase K. Vortex and spin briefly.
6. Incubate for 20 min in 37°C water bath.
7. Add 300 µL of TE-saturated phenol/chloroform/isoamyl alcohol. Vortex for 30 s.
8. Centrifuge at 16,000g for 5 min at 4°C.
9. Remove the supernatant to a new microfuge tube. Be careful not to take any of the interface or organic phase.
10. Add 1 µL of 10 mg/mL yeast tRNA and 600 µL of 100% ethanol.

11. Transfer tubes to –20°C freezer for 30 min or dry ice for 15 min.
12. Centrifuge at 16,000g for 10 min at 4°C.
13. Remove supernatant. Do not disturb pellet. Geiger counter can be used to monitor.
14. Air-dry the pellet. Do not overdry.
15. Resuspend the pellet in 10 µL of loading buffer. Vortex several times to completely dissolve.
16. Prepare a 6% polyacrylamide /8 *M* urea gel solution as in **Subheading 3.4.2., steps 1–8**. Use 0.75-mm thick comb with 4 mm wide wells.
17. Heat the samples at 85°C for 5 min. Briefly spin and transfer tubes to ice.
18. Load the samples onto the gel. For RNA marker and the undigested probe, 10^3 cpm is loaded onto the gel.
19. Run the gel at 200 constant volts until the xylene cyanol FF dye is near the bottom 2 cm.
20. Disassemble the gel. Make sure the gel remains on one glass plate. Overlay 0.3-mm Whatman filter paper (the paper is slightly larger than the gel) and peel the filter slowly. Make sure the gel is attached to the filter.
21. Cover the gel with plastic wrap (do not wrap). Place the gel in a gel dryer. Dry for 45 min at 85–90°C.
22. Place the dried gel in the cassette (gel face up) and fix with Scotch Tape.
23. Put X-ray film on the gel in the dark room and close cassette.
24. Place cassette in –70°C freezer. Expose film overnight.
25. Develop film. Depending on the strength of the signal for protected band, reexpose the film for more or less time.
26. Scan the protected bands. Be sure to use same scan size for every sample, including background scanning.

3.8. Results

Figure 1 shows representative RPAs for α_{1A} and α_{2D} adrenergic receptor (AR) mRNA in adult rat thoracic aorta media and adventitia, and intact thoracic vena cava. Semiquantitative analysis was used to compare relative levels of expression (*see* **Fig. 2**). This was accomplished (using NIH Image1 software) by subtracting the densitometric value for lane background from the α-AR protected fragment and normalizing this value with the cyclophilin protected fragment (use top band of cyclophilin [CP] doublet) from 12-h exposure to avoid overexposure of CP evident in **Fig. 1** (*see* **Notes 7–11**). The remainder was multiplied by a "CTP factor" (different for each probe). This accounts for differences among probes in specific activity (number of cytosine bases in each protected fragment), where the α_{1D} CTP factor was set to 1.0; this product was divided by the CP-specific densitometric value from a 12-h exposure (α-AR signals were for 50-h exposures); the quotient is then expressed as a percentage of CP mRNA level. Both adult rat aorta media, composed of smooth muscles cells, and adventitia (composed of fibroblasts) *(5)* express all four transcripts but with strikingly different relative abundances. α_{1D} and α_{1B} are

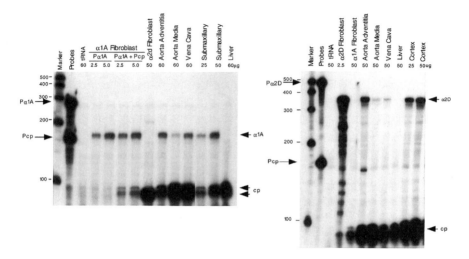

Fig. 1. RNase protection assay (RPA; 50 h exposure) for freshly isolated vascular tissue (rat thoracic aorta and vena cava), showing protected fragments (right-hand arrows) for α_{1A} (left) and α_{2D}-adrenergic receptor (AR), together with cyclophilin (cp). Assayed amounts of total tissue RNA given in micrograms. Positive and negative controls are rat1 and 3T3 fibroblasts stably expressing α_{1A}- and α_{2D}-ARs, respectively, and several non-vascular tissues (submaxillary gland, liver, cerebral cortex). As shown, inclusion of cp probe has no effect on α_{1A}-AR mRNA detection (verified for all other RPAs). Cp densitometry determined for 12-h exposures (to avoid overexposure) and used as internal control. Note in contrast to medial smooth muscle cells (SMCs), adventitia (fibroblasts) expresses relatively abundant α_{1A} and α_{2D}; vena cava, where adventitial cells and SMCs cannot be separated, expresses both. Left and right lanes: 1: molecular weight marker, 2: probes only, 3: yeast tRNA; left lanes 4–7: α_{1A}-AR probe alone or with cp probe together.

dominant in media, whereas α_{1A} and α_{2D} are dominant in adventitia; α_{2B} and α_{2C} were not detected. We have confirmed these findings with quantitative RT-PCR *(10)*.

These data represent the first comparison of α-AR expression across the vascular wall, and demonstrate the necessity of separating media and adventitia in radioligand binding, mRNA, or immunoblot analysis of α-ARs in vascular tissues. It is known that the α_{1D}-AR mediates adult aorta constriction *(11)*. However, the role of these other α-ARs is unknown. Even more suprising than the unexpected expression of multiple $\alpha1$-AR subtypes by medial SMCs was the multiple expression by adventitia. This presumably reflects adventitial fibroblasts, since we detected no mRNA or immunohistochemical protein for α-smooth muscle actin, nor desmin or SM1 myosin heavy chain in Westerns of adventitia *(12)*. To our knowledge, only neonatal cardiac fibroblasts has been

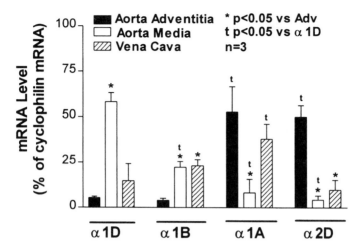

Fig. 2. Freshly isolated aorta adventitial and medial layers express four α-AR mRNAs, but with different abundances. Quantitation by transmission scanning densitometry, with normalization to cp and correction for differences in background, exposures time, mg RNA assayed and specific activity among probes (*see* **Subheading 3.8.**). Relative levels for thoracic vena cava were 16 ± 9, 23 ± 3, 38 ± 8, and 10 ± 5 for the four α-AR mRNAs, respectively. Values are mean ± SEM for $n = 3$ independent RPAs for each mean from three different RNA extractions each obtained from 5–10 pooled rat thoracic aorta medial and adventitial and vena cava segments (from 230 g rats). Statistics by ANOVA and Bonferroni *t*-correction.

examined for α1-AR subtype expression, and no expression was detected *(13)*. It is possible that the adventitial fibroblast expresses α-ARs because of its differentiation from a mesenchymal precursor cell similar to or common with the SMC precursor cell. However, whether these adventitial α-ARs mediate sympathetic influences over adventitial function, for example matrix expression or wall remodeling, is unknown.

4. Notes

1. The quality, purity, and integrity of total RNA directly affects the RPA results. When handling samples, extreme care should be taken to prevent RNA degradation. The purity of RNA (ratio of OD_{260}/OD_{280}) should be greater than 1.7. If the ratio is less than 1.7, repeat the phenol/chloroform extraction and ethanol precipitation. In general, phenol/chloroform extraction of tissue RNA preparation must be done at least twice.
2. It is very important to confirm the orientation of the riboprobe plasmid construct by restriction enzyme digestion or sequencing. The riboprobe to be transcribed by bacteriophage RNA polymerase must be complementary to the target RNA. Only the antisense probe will produce protected bands.

3. The plasmid DNA template should be completely linearized with a restriction enzyme and purified by phenol/chloroform extraction and ethanol precipitation. The selection of enzyme for cleavage depends on the construct orientation and desired size of the probe (100–600 bp; around 300 bp works best). This restriction site is always downstream of the bacteriophage promoter that is used for probe synthesis. The site can be within, at the end, or beyond the end of the inserted cDNA of the target gene. It is best to choose an enzyme that will yield a probe about 30 bases longer than the protected duplexed fragment, to allow differentiation of probe from protected band. If the template is cleaved with an enzyme that leaves 3' overhangs, the 3' overhangs must be blunt-ended with Klenow DNA polymerase. This will prevent spurious initiation of phage RNA polymerase binding and transcription, which would yield labeled sense RNA and cause high background.

4. The selection of RNA polymerase type for antisense probe synthesis also depends on construct orientation. For example, the α_{1A} cDNA fragment was ligated into the *Bam*HI/*Eco*RI site of pBluescript SK$^+$ vector in the forward orientation. The T7 promoter then drives α_{1A} antisense probe synthesis using T7 RNA polymerase. The α_{2D} cDNA fragment was ligated into the *Sac*I/*Sac*II site of SK$^+$ in the reverse orientation. T3 RNA polymerase is then used for antisense probe synthesis.

5. It is necessary to purify the full-length probe away from incomplete RNA transcripts and DNA template by polyacrylamide gel electrophoresis to reduce background. The purified probe should be stored at –70°C and used within 7 d (within 3 d for best results). Background will increase with longer storage.

6. The concentrations of RNase A and RNase T1 often need to be optimized. The concentrations in this protocol are sufficient for most targets. Insufficient digestion will produce high background; and over-digestion will give weak protected bands. Elimination of nonspecific probe hybridization with yeast tRNA is a good indication that ribonuclease concentration/time are sufficient. Also, the presence of a very weak band for the probe alone in tRNA and other lanes (higher band than the protected fragment) can provide a useful check that RNase digestion is not excessive. A mixture of RNase A and T1 exhibits a wide concentration range over which single-stranded RNA and mismatched hybrids are effectively degraded. However, A-U rich regions often separate ("breath") between strands during RNase digestion, yielding less full-length protected fragments. Duplex separation can be lessened by reducing temperature or increasing buffer salt concentration, although the latter will decrease RNase activities. Use of increased concentration of RNase T1 (or no RNase A), because it cleaves only at G residues, may be helpful. Often, other RNases (e.g., RNase ONE, T2) can be used to detect single-base mismatches or may be advantageous in certain circumstances.

7. We use the cyclophilin gene as an internal control because cyclophilin mRNA is in two- to 10-fold higher abundance in SMCs (but still relative "low") than α-AR mRNAs. The gene is highly conserved. A high concentration of cold CTP is used for cyclophilin probe synthesis to produce a lower specific activity probe. The

principle underlying the RPA requires that probe be in molar excess of the target RNA in the RNA sample. Thus, to avoid cyclophilin protected band from becoming overexposed on an overnight film exposure, we use a low specific activity probe rather than over-diluting the probe. Probe excess can be confirmed by including several dilutions of sense or tested RNA and noting that protected band intensity increases linearly (the sense dilution range should bracket your target band in intensity).

8. For quantification of the same target mRNA in different tissues, it is best to use the same amount of RNA for each tissue and run on the same gel. After scanning and normalization with cyclophilin, the relative abundance can be calculated (*see* **Subheading 3.8.**).

9. For quantification of different target mRNAs, the amount of RNA used, probe size and specific activity, and film exposure time need to be optimized. The relative amounts of target mRNAs can be calculated with the formula [(target – background) × CTP factor/CP] × 100 (after first normalization of the target band densitometry value with the cyclophilin value minus its background), where target is the densitometry value for the specific protected band; background is the densitometry value taken from the lane using the same scanning size rectangle; CTP factor is the number of cytosines in each probe (setting the probe factor for the most abundant target to 1.0; in our studies, α_{1D}-AR probe CTP factor is set at 1.0 and the α_{1A}, α_{1B}, and α_{2D} probes are set at 0.84, 0.77 and 0.89); CP is the densitometry value of cyclophilin probe minus background which was loaded with the same amount of cpm in every experiment. Densitometry values for CP protected fragment and CP probe bands are taken from 12-h film exposures (overexposure causes film saturation and invalidates densitometry values). For accuracy, all experiments need to be done at least three times with independent assays against RNA samples from different animal groups or cell lines.

10. Internal "assay" control. Inconsistency in the "loading" of RNA among samples in the same run, or between different runs (experiments) introduces experimental errors from unequal efficiency of isolation of RNA from tissue samples, and from errors in OD_{260} quantitation and pipeting of RNA. As well, all of the remaining RPA steps can vary among samples and runs to some degree. These effects can be controlled for by simultaneously measuring the level of expression of a "control" gene in addition to the target gene, and using this value to normalize the experimental value. An ideal control gene is one which is not changed by the experimental variable. Thus at the outset several possible control genes should be tested in each experimental situation. Constitutively expressed "housekeeping" genes (i.e., essential cell proteins) such as β-actin, GAPDH, rRNAs, and cyclophilin have most often been used, although their constancy must still be demonstrated.

11. Internal control for "nonspecific" change. A second often equally important purpose of an internal control is to distinguish whether a change in target gene expression reflects an unique event or instead simply occurs because of a nonspecific change in overall mRNA or certain mRNA species. For example, trophic

stimuli can cause an increase in cell size or cell number (note in RPA that normalization of loaded RNA to a constant cell number or tissue mass may be more appropriate in certain situations *[7]*). Thus, many mRNA signals may be increased. The control gene for nonspecific changes should be expressed at levels (abundant, moderate, rare) similar to that of the target gene. Also, since rRNAs are transcribed by a distinct polymerase, they would not represent a good "nonspecific" control. Cyclophilin is a ubiquitous cytoplasmic protein involved in protein folding that is in low abundance in rat vascular tissue and in many tissues (although this varies). As such, cyclophilin is more appropriate to use as an internal control when studying expression of rare mRNA species, both as an "assay" and "nonspecific" control since it has been found to be unaffected by many experimental stimuli *(14)*. As a final note, evidence has accumulated that other commonly used control genes are often modulated by many treatments. However, many papers are still published that do not demonstrate statistical constancy for the internal control used. This becomes even more important when the changes in target mRNA are only severalfold or less.

References

1. Melton, D. A., Krieg, P. A., Rebagliati, M. R., Maniatis, T., Zinn, K., and Green, M. R. (1984) Efficient in vitro synthesis of biologically active RNA and RNA hybridization probes from plasmids containing a bacteriophage SP6 promoter. *Nucleic Acids Res.* **12,** 7035–7056.
2. Sambrook, J., Fritsch, E. F.m and Maniatis T. (1989) *Molecular Cloning: A Laboratory Manual*, 2nd ed. Cold Spring Harbor Laboratory, Cold Spring Harbor, NY.
3. Gilman, M. (1989) In: *Current Protocols in Molecular Biology*, (Ausubel, F., et al., eds.), Vol. 2, Wiley, New York, NY, pp. 4.7.1–4.7.8.
4. Leech, C. J. and Faber, J. E. (1996) Different α-adrenoceptor subtypes mediate constriction of arterioles and venules. *Am. J. Physiol.* **270** (*Heart Circ. Physiol.* **39**), H710–H722.
5. Rhodin, J. A. G. (1980) Architecture of the vessel wall. In: *Handbook of Physiology. The Cardiovascular System. Vascular Smooth Muscle.* American Physiological Society, Bethesda, MD, pp. 1–32.
6. Chomczynski, P. and Sacchi, N. (1987) Single-step method of RNA isolation by acid guanidinium thiocyanate-phenol-chloroform extraction. *Ann. Biochem. Exp. Med.* **162,** 156–159.
7. Chen, L., Xin, X., Eckhart, A. D., Yang, N., and Faber, J. E. (1995) Regulation of vascular smooth muscle growth by α_1-adrenoceptor subtypes in vitro and in situ. *J. Biol. Chem.* **270,** 30,980–30,985.
8. Xin, X., Yang, N., Eckhart, A. D., and Faber, J. E. (1997) α_{1D}-Adrenergic receptors and mitogen-activated protein kinase mediate increased protein synthesis by arterial smooth muscle. *Mol. Pharmacol.* **51,** 764–775.
9. Yang, N., Xin, X., Eckhart, A. D., and Faber, J. E. (1997) CRE-like response element regulates expression of rat α_{2D}-adrenergic receptor gene in vascular smooth muscle. *Am. J. Physiol.* **273** (*Heart Circ. Physiol.* **42**), H85–H95.

10. Faber, J. E., Yang, N., and Erami, C. (1999) Angioplasty injury reduces α-adrenergic receptor (AR) expression in neointima, media and adventitia. *FASEB J.* **13,** 416.12 (abstract).
11. Piascik, M. T., Guarino, R. D., Smith, M. S., Soltis E. E., Saussy, D. L. Jr, and Perez, D. M. (1995) The specific contribution of the novel alpha-1D adrenoceptor to the contraction of vascular smooth muscle. *J. Pharm. Exper. Thera.* **275,** 1583–1589.
12. Yang, N., Erami, C., and Faber, J. E. (1999) Adventitial fibroblasts (AFBs) express functional α1-adrenergic receptors (ARs), and modulate to myofibroblasts (myoFBs) in primary culture and after angioplasty in vivo. *FASEB J.* **13,** 426.13 (abstract).
13. Stewart, A. F., Rokosh, D. G., Bailey, B. A., Karns, L. R., Chang, K. C., Long, C. S., et al. (1994) Cloning of the rat alpha 1C-adrenergic receptor from cardiac myocytes. alpha 1C, alpha 1B, and alpha 1D mRNAs are present in cardiac myocytes but not in cardiac fibroblasts. *Circ. Res.* **75(4),** 796–802.
14. Clements, M. L., Banes, A. J., and Faber, J. E. (1997) Effects of mechanical loading on vascular α_{1D}- and α_{1D}-adrenergic receptor expression. *Hypertension* **29,** 1156–1164.

V

MOLECULAR METHODS TO STUDY APOPTOSIS AND PHENOTYPIC CHANGES IN VASCULAR CELLS AND TISSUE

19

Detection of Apoptosis in Atherosclerosis and Restenosis by Terminal dUTP Nick-End Labeling (TUNEL)

Mark Kockx, Johannes Muhring, and Michiel Knaapen

1. Introduction

Kerr and Wyllie *(1)* have introduced the term apoptosis to separate this special form of cell death from necrosis. When a cell receives a signal to die an apoptotic death, it goes through a series of morphological changes that can be easily observed with the light microscope. Starting from shrinkage of the cell membrane, to condensation of nuclear chromatin, cellular fragmentation, and finally the engulfment of the apoptotic bodies by neighboring cells. Although the term apoptosis was introduced only 30 years ago, typically apoptotic morphology has been described by embryologists in the beginning of this century. Embryologists recognized the need for some mechanism to counterbalance cellular proliferation during the development of organs and limbs. Apoptosis, however, is not limited to cell death during embryonic development. In recent years, apoptosis has been implicated in cell deaths caused by ionized radiation, steroid treatment, chemotherapy, ischemia–reperfusion, and in atherogenesis.

The initial description of apoptosis was based on morphological features. Several useful biochemical and immunohistochemical detection methods were subsequently introduced. Andrew Wyllie in 1980 described fragmentation of nuclear DNA into multiples of 180 bp as the result of endonuclease activation *(2)*. When fragmented DNAs were electrophoresed in an agarose gel, they separated into a characteristic DNA ladder pattern *(2–4)*. Gavrieli et al. described another widely used method in which DNA breaks in apoptotic nuclei were marked by dUTP-biotin transferred to the free 3'-end of the cleaved DNA *(5)*. Because terminal deoxynucleotidyl transferase was used to transfer dUTP-biotin

From: *Methods in Molecular Medicine, Vascular Disease: Molecular Biology and Gene Therapy Protocols*
Edited by: A. H. Baker © Humana Press Inc., Totowa, NJ

by nick end labeling, a more convenient acronym, TUNEL, was used to describe this procedure.

Recently, the detection of DNA fragmentation by the use of the TUNEL technique or *in situ* nick translation has become a standard technique for the detection of apoptosis in tissue sections (*see* **Note 1**). This technique is particulary interesting in those diseases that are characterized by low values of cell replication and cell death (e.g., the formation of atherosclerotic plaques and cell loss during ischemic and nonischemic cardiomyopathy), which are characterized by the slow progressive nature of the lesions. In the present chapter we discuss the TUNEL technique when used for the study of cardiovasular tissues.

2. Materials

2.1. Tissue Handling

1. Immediately fix tissues in 10% formaldehyde solution (*see* **Note 2**).
2. Embedded in paraffin.
3. 3-Aminopropyltriethoxysilane (APES, Sigma, St. Louis, MO).
4. Cut 5-μm sections and mounted on APES coated glass slides and dry at 37°C.

2.2. Solutions

1. 3% H_2O_2 (v/v).
2. 3% citric acid.
3. Proteinase K stock solution (1 mg/mL): dissolve 10 mg of proteinase K in 10 mL of 0.05 M Tris-HCl, pH 7.6 and divide in to aliquots. Store at –20 °C.
4. Proteinase K working solution: dilute 20 μL of the above stock solution in 1 mL of 0.05 M Tris-HCl, pH 7.6 just before use.
5. Tris-cacodylate buffer: 1 M sodium cacodylate, 125 mM Tris-HCl, 1.25 mg/mL bovine serum albumin, pH 6.6.
6. Terminal deoxynucleotidyl transferase (Tdt) solution: 750 μL of distilled water (dH_2O), 1 μL of 10 mM dATP, 200 μL of Tris-cacodylate buffer, 50 μL of 25 mM CoCl$_2$, 2.5 μL of 1 mM FITC-dUTP and 2 μL (= 50 U) of Tdt enzyme stock (Boehringer Mannheim, Germany).
7. Blocking reagent (Amersham Pharmacia Biotech, Buckinghamshire, UK): 5 mg/mL in phosphate-buffered saline, pH 7.6.
8. Sheep antiFITC-peroxidase conjugate (Boehringer Mannheim): 1/300 dilution in blocking reagents.
9. Amino-ethyl carbazol (AEC) solution: dissolve 400 mg of AEC in 100 mL of *N,N*-dimethyl formamide. For a working solution, dissolve 2.5 mL of the stock in 25 mL of 0.1 M sodium acetate, pH 5.6, and add 50 μL of 30 % H_2O_2. Filter before use.
10. Haematoxylin.
11. Glycerine jelly.

3. Methods

3.1. Detection Methods

1. Deparaffinise sections three times for 3 min each in toluene.
2. Immerse in ethanol three times for 3 min each and finally place in dH_2O.
3. Treat with 3% H_2O_2 for 15 min.
4. Wash three times in dH_2O.
5. Treat with 3% citric acid for 1 h (*see* **Note 3**).
6. Wash three times in dH_2O.
7. Treat with proteinase K working solution for 30 s to 10 min (*see* **Note 4**).
8. Wash at least four times in dH_2O for 5 min each.
9. Incubate in Tdt solution 1 h at 37°C (*see* **Note 5**).
10. Wash at least four times in dH_2O for 5 min each.
11. Incubate with blocking reagent for 1 h.
12. Incubate in sheep anti FITC-peroxidase conjugate for 1 h.
13. Wash twice in phosphate-buffered saline, pH 7.6, for 5 min each.
14. Treat sections with AEC solution for 10 min (*see* **Note 6**).
15. Wash twice in dH_2O.
16. Counterstain in haematoxylin.
17. Wash in tap water and mount in glycerine jelly.

3.2. Final Comments

All these findings are of considerable interest in the interpretation of TUNEL data obtained for atherosclerotic plaques and other pathological processes (*6–13*). The reported values of TUNEL-labeled cells in atherosclerotic plaques range from 30–60%, which would indicate that these plaques are in an imminent state of collapse. However, if the TUNEL technique is combined with morphological criteria, low values were obtained for human and experimental atherosclerotic plaques (*11–13*). The values that we obtained for atherosclerotic plaques if we combine TUNEL with morphological criteria were approx 2% (*11*). The same is true for the values that were found for apoptotic cell death in ischemic and nonischemic cardiomyopathy. Initially values of 20–30% were found counting the TUNEL labeled nuclei (*14*). However, if the TUNEL labeling was combined with morphological criteria, the values drop to 0.1% (*15*). Schwartz and Bennett remarked that the main message of the TUNEL technique, applied on atherosclerotic plaques, is not the rate of apoptosis but the fact that apoptosis is occurring (*16*). This would be true if the TUNEL technique only detects apoptosis or apoptotic nuclear remnants but not if the TUNEL technique also detects nuclei showing RNA synthesis and splicing, which could lead to very different conclusions in the study of cardiovascular diseases as remarked by Newby and George (*17*). Therefore, the TUNEL technique should always be combined with additional techniques, such as markers of transcription and morphological criteria.

4. Notes

1. Classically it was stated that DNA breakdown is a late event in necrosis and that oligonucleosomal DNA cleavage is a hallmark of apoptosis. In cell cultures it was demonstrated that the TUNEL but not the ISEL technique can differentiate between apoptotic and necrotic cell death *(18)*. However, other authors state that these techniques cannot differentiate between apoptotic and necrotic cell death *(19)*. Recent studies have indeed demonstrated that oligonucleosomal DNA fragmentation also occurs during necrosis as an early event but appears to be triggered by proteolytic mechanisms different from those described in apoptosis *(20)*. However, this result indicates that techniques based on detection of oligonucleosomal-sized DNA fragments may not reliably differentiate between apoptosis and necrosis.

2. It has been demonstrated that fixation and especially the prefixation time (fixation delay) can influence the percentages of TUNEL-labeled nuclei in tissue sections *(21,22)*. In tissues that were left for 15 min and then fixed, there was a dramatic increase in the number of labeled cells *(22)*. This problem is especially relevant for human cardiovascular tissues obtained during autopsy or cardiovasular surgery. In general, the variable fixation delay could result in major differences in the TUNEL labeling. It was demonstrated that nonapoptotic nuclei that show signs of active RNA synthesis are more sensitive to this aspecific labeling *(23)*. This could explain why some authors found high TUNEL labeling in atherosclerotic plaques, while the underlying media showed only few labeled nuclei. Fixation delay could induce proteolytic cleavage of nuclear proteins as well as cellular DNA. To our understanding the result of fixation delay is an increase in fragmented DNA strands that could be labeled by the TUNEL technique (*see* **Fig. 1**). For some reason nuclei that show more RNA synthesis are more sensitive for DNA fragmentation by fixation delay.

3. Besides RNA synthesis other phenomena can interfere with the TUNEL technique. Previously we have reported that the TUNEL technique can also label nonnuclear structures in atherosclerotic plaques by aspecific binding of the nucleotides to small calcium containing vesicles in the plaques *(24)*. This technical problem can be avoided by pretreating the tissue sections by calcium-chelating agents (e.g., citric acid 3% for 1 h).

4. In most protocols of the TUNEL technique the tissue sections are pretreated with proteinase K to make the DNA more accessible. However, we have found that this step is the reason for most aspecific labeling and can be omitted without a loss of sensitivity. It must be remarked that the TUNEL technique is not specific for the execution phase of apoptosis, the technique is only selective (rather than specific) for apoptotic nuclei because these contain a far greater degree of DNA fragmentation than nonapoptotic nuclei. However, if proteinase K is used, nonapoptotic nuclei can easily become labeled *(25)*. Nevertheless, not all nuclei show the same sensitivity for this aspecific labeling. As already explained in **Note 2** most of the aspecifically labeled nuclei show signs of RNA synthesis. We think that this is a consequence of the important conformational changes that

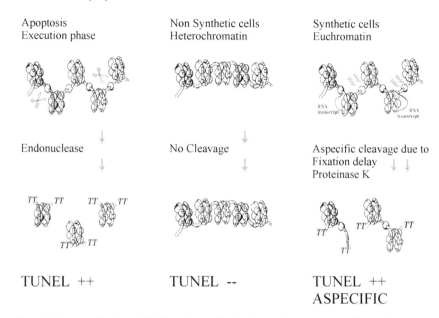

Apoptosis
Execution phase

Non Synthetic cells
Heterochromatin

Synthetic cells
Euchromatin

Endonuclease

No Cleavage

Aspecific cleavage due to
Fixation delay
Proteinase K

TUNEL ++

TUNEL --

TUNEL ++
ASPECIFIC

Fig. 1. Tunel technique/pitfalls. In the final phase of apoptotic cell death (execution phase) the nuclear DNA is cleaved in oligonucleosomal-sized DNA fragments containing hydroxylated 3' ends. The TUNEL uses Tdt, which adds labeled nucleotides to the free 3' ends. This results in a tail (of labeled nucleotides/TT), which can be visualized. In nonapoptotic nuclei the number of five 3'OH ends is below the detection limit. However, breaks in the DNA can be artificially induced by delay in fixation or proteinase K pretreatment. This happens far more frequent in highly synthetic cells.

occur in DNA structure during transcription *(26)*. In the past, several groups have even employed a modification of the nick translation method for DNA labeling to allow the *in situ* detection of sites of active gene transcription *(27,28)*. These methods rely on the use of DNAse to partially digest DNA to produce single-strand breaks, which are subsequently filled with a DNA polymerase, thereby incorporating a radiolabeled or nonisotopic nucleotide. By the judicious use of DNAse it is possible to label only actively transcribing genes, since inactive chromatin is relatively protected from digestion by its tight struture and the presence of associated proteins. It is therefore possible that the proteinase K pretreatment itself induces single-strand breaks in the DNA by digesting the associated proteins (*see* **Fig. 1**).

5. The enzymatic reaction which is used to add nucleotides to the free 3'OH ends can be performed by Tdt or the Klenow fragment of DNA polymerase I. The method using Tdt was originally described as the TUNEL technique by Gavrieli et al. *(5)*, whereas the other method using DNA polymerase I was described by Iseki *(29)* and its application in detecting apoptosis by Fehsel *(30)* and Wijsman et al. *(31)* as *in situ* end-labeling (ISEL or ISNT). In our experience both methods

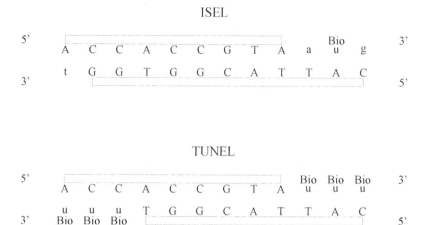

Fig. 2. The TUNEL technique versus ISEL. The way of incorporating the labeled nucleotides is different in the two techniques. In the ISEL technique the nucleotides are incorporated at the 3' OH end of sticky DNA ends in a template dependent way. The TUNEL technique labels all types of DNA fragments in a template independent way. a = dATP, g = dGTP, uBio = dUTP-biotin.

are highly sensitive and rather specific in detecting apoptosis. The method of nucleotide incorporation is however different in both methods (*see* **Fig. 2**). In the ISEL technique nucleotides are incorporated at the 3'OH end of sticky DNA ends in a template-dependent way. This technique cannot label the blunt ends of DNA. The TUNEL technique labels all types of DNA fragments in a template-independent way. In our experiments the TUNEL technique gives a stronger signal of the apoptotic nuclei. An explanation could be that in the TUNEL technique all the incorporated nucleotides are conjugated and will be detected by the antibody raised against the conjugate.

6. The TUNEL stained sections can be subsequently stained by the desired immunohistochemical labeling. Therefore, it is necessary to use the water insoluble diamino carbazol (DAB) instead of the water soluble amino-ethyl carbazol (AEC) in the last step of the TUNEL technique. The water insoluble poly-DAB complexes remain present on the apoptotic nuclei during a subsequent immunohistochemical stain. It is even possible to use a microwave pretreatment of the TUNEL stained paraffin sections. However it is not always possible to charactarize the cell type of the apoptotic cells since most apoptotic cells loose their differentiation markers during the process of apoptosis.

References

1. Kerr, J. F. R., Wyllie, A. H., and Currie, A. R. (1972) Apoptosis: a basic biological phenomenon with wide ranging implications in tissue kinetics. *Brit. J. Cancer* **26,** 239–257.

2. Wyllie, A. H. (1980) Glucocorticoid-induced thymocyte apoptosis is associated with endogenous endonuclease activation. *Nature* **284,** 555,556.

3. Arends, M. J., Morris R. G., and Wyllie, A. H. (1990) Apoptosis: the role of the endonuclease. *Am. J. Pathol.* **136,** 593–608.

4. Wyllie A. H., Morris, R.G., Smith, A., and Dunlop D. (1984) Chromatin cleavage in apoptosis : association with condensed chromatin morphology and dependence on macromolecular synthesis. *J. Pathol.* **142,** 67–77.

5. Gavrieli, Y., Sherman, Y., and Ben-Sasson, S. A. (1992) Identification of programmed cell death in situ via specific labeling of nuclear DNA fragmentation. *J. Cell. Biol.* **119,** 493–501.

6. Isner, J. M., Kearney, M., Bortman, S., and Passeri, J. (1995) Apoptosis in human atherosclerosis and restenosis. *Circulation* **91,** 2703–2711.

7. Geng, Y. J. and Libby, P. (1995) Evidence for Apoptosis in Advanced Human Atheroma. *Am. J. Path.* **147,** 251–266.

8. Han, D. K. M., Haudenschild, C. C., Hong, M. K. Tinkle, B. T., Leon, M. B., and Liau, G. (1995) Evidence for apoptosis in human atherogenesis and in a rat vascular injury model. *Am. J. Pathol.* **147,** 267–277.

9. Björkerud, S. and Björkerud, B. (1996) Apoptosis is abundant in human atherosclerotic lesions, especially in inflammatory cells (macrophages and T cells), and may contribute to the accumulation of gruel and plaque instability. *Am. J. Pathol.* **149,** 367–380.

10. Mallat, Z., Ohan, J., Lesèche, G., Tedgui, A. (1997) Colocalization of CPP-32 with apoptotic cells in human atherosclerotic plaques. *Circulation* **96,** 424–428.

11. Kockx, M. M., De Meyer, G. R. Y., Muhring, J., Bult, H., Bultinck, J., and Herman, A. (1996) Distribution of cell replication and apoptosis in atherosclerotic plaques of cholesterol-fed rabbits. *Atherosclerosis* **120,** 115–124.

12. Kockx, M. M., De Meyer, G. R. Y., Muhring, J., Jacob, W., Bult, H., and Herman, A. G. (1998) Apoptosis and related proteins in different stages of human atherosclerotic plaques. *Circulation* **97,** 2307–2315.

13. Hegyi, L., Skepper, J. N., Cary, N. R., and Mitchinson, M. J. (1996) Foam cell apoptosis and the development of the lipid core of human atherosclerosis. *J. Pathol.* **180,** 423–42.

14. Narula, J., Haider, N., Virmani, R. et al. (1996) Apoptosis in myocytes in end-stage heart failure. *N. Engl. J. Med.* **335,** 1182–1189.

15. Olivetti, G., Abbi, R., Federico Quaini, F., et al. (1997) Apoptosis in the failing human heart. *N. Engl. J. Med.* **336,** 1131–1141.

16. Schwartz, S. M. and Bennett, M. R. (1995) Death by any other name. *Am. J. Pathol.* **147,** 229–234.

17. Newby, A. C. and George, S. J. (1998) Proliferation, migration, matrix turnover and death of smooth muscle cells in native coronary and vein graft atherosclerosis. *Curr. Opin. Cardiol.* **11,** 574–582.

18. Gold, R., Schmid, M., Girgerich, G., Breitschopf, H., Hartung, H.P., Toyka, K.V., and Lassmann H. (1994) Differentiation between cellular apoptosis and necrosis by the combined use of in situ labeling and nick translation techniques. *Lab. Invest.* **71,** 219–225.

19. Mundle, S. and Raza, A. (1995) The two in situ techniques do not differentiate between apoptosis and necrosis but rather reveal distinct patterns of DNA fragmentation in apoptosis. *Lab. Invest.* **72,** 611,612.

20. Dong, Z., Saikumar, P., Weinberg, J. M., and Venkatachalam, M. A. (1997) Internucleosomal DNA cleavage triggered by plasma membrane damage during necrotic cell death: involvement of serine but not cysteine proteases. *Am. J. Pathol.* **151,** 1205–1213.

21. Tateyama, H., Toyohiro, T., Hattori, H. , Murase, T., Li, W. X., and Eimoto, T. (1998) Effects of prefixation and fixation times on apoptosis detection by in situ End-labeling of fragmented DNA. *Arch. Pathol. Lab. Med.* **122,** 252–255.

22. Hall, P. A., Coates, P. J., Ansari, B., and Haywood D. (1994) Regulation of cell number in the mammalian gastro-intestinal tract : the importance of apoptosis. *J. Cell. Science* **107,** 3569–3577.

23. Kockx, M. M., Muhring, J., Knaapen, M. W. M., and De Meyer, G. R. Y. (1998) RNA synthesis and splicing interferes with DNA in situ end labeling techniques used to detect apoptosis. *Am. J. Pathol.* **152,** 885–888.

24. Kockx, M. M., Muhring, J. , Bortier, H., De Meyer, G. R. Y., and Jacob, W. (1996) Biotin or Digoxigenin conjugated nucleotides bind to matrix vesicles in atherosclerotic plaques. *Am. J. Pathol.* **148,** 1771–1777.

25. Hegji, L., Hardwick, S. J., and Mitchinson, M. J. (1997) Letter to the editor. *Am. J. Pathol.* **105,** 371–373.

26. Roychoudhury, R., Jay, E., and Wu, R. (1976) Terminal labeling and addition of homopolymer tracts to duplex DNA fragments by terminal deoxynucleotidyl transferase. *Nucleic Acid Res.* **3,** 101–116.

27. Murer-Orlando, M. L. and Peterson, A. C. (1985) In situ nick translation of human and mouse chromosomes detected with biotinglated nucleotide. *Exp. Cell Res.* **157,** 322–334.

28. Adolph, S. and Hamaster, H. (1985) In situ nick translation of metaphase chromosomes with biotin-labelled d-UTP. *Hum. Genet.* **69,** 117–121.

29. Iseki, S. (1986) DNA strandbreaks in rat tissues as detected by in situ nick translation. *Exp. Cell Res.* **167,** 311–326.

30. Fehsel, K., Kolb Bachofen, V., and Kolb H. (1991) Analysis of TNF alpha-induced DNA strand breaks at the single cell level. *Am. J. Pathol.* **139,** 251–254.

31. Wijsman, J. H., Jonker, R. R., Keijzer, R., van de Velde, C. J., Cornelisse, C. J., and van Dierendonck J. H. (1993) A news method to detect apoptosis in paraffin sections: in situ end-labeling of fragmented DNA. *J. Histochem. Cytochem.* **41,** 7–12.

20

In Vitro Detection of Apoptosis in Isolated Vascular Cells

Shiu-Wan Chan and Martin R. Bennett

1. Introduction

Apoptosis is a programmed cell death process in which surplus or damaged cells are eliminated through a highly regulated procedure. The first description of apoptosis relied upon morphological differences among apoptotic, necrotic, and healthy cells (*1*). Indeed, there are usually a number of features of apoptotic cells, whatever their lineage, that allows rapid identification. Morphologically, the cells are seen to undergo shrinkage followed by membrane blebbing, chromatin condensation, and nuclear fragmentation. Eventually, the cells cleave off into apoptotic bodies to be phagocytosed by bystander neighboring cells or professional phagocytic cells such as macrophages.

Apoptosis is characterized by the inhibition or cleavage of a range of intracellular proteins. For example, the putative inactivation of an aminophospholipid translocase results in cell membrane composition changes as the cells translocate the membrane phospholipid phosphatidyl serine (PS) from the cytoplasmic face to the membrane surface (*2,3*). The breakdown of the cytoskeleton proteins fodrin and actins (*2,4,5*) may result in cell shrinkage and membrane blebbing. These changes occurring at the membrane surface may account for the alteration in cell permeability seen in apoptotic cells, including an increased permeability to certain dyes such as trypan blue and propidium iodide (PI). However, in contrast to necrosis, membrane function is retained until relatively late in apoptosis. The cell membrane changes *per se* do not distinguish apoptotic from necrotic cells, but do allow the identification of dead cells. As a late event in apoptosis, nuclear DNA is degraded into oligonucleosomal-sized fragments by a caspase-activated deoxyribonuclease (*6,7*). These changes are brought about by the activation of one or a number of cysteine

From: *Methods in Molecular Medicine, Vascular Disease: Molecular Biology and Gene Therapy Protocols*
Edited by: A. H. Baker © Humana Press Inc., Totowa, NJ

protease(s) (caspases), which are responsible for the PS externalization *(8)*, DNA fragmentation *(6,7,9)*, and cleavage of specific death substrates, e.g., poly(ADP-ribose) polymerase (PARP) *(10)*, U1-70 kD small nuclear ribonucleoprotein *(11,12)*, DNA-dependent protein kinase *(13)*, fodrin *(14)*, actins *(4, 5)*, and nuclear lamins *(15)*, eventually leading to apoptosis of the cells. The morphological changes, DNA degradation, cell membrane changes, caspase, and death substrate cleavage are all defined processes in apoptosis and can all serve as useful markers in the detection of apoptosis.

A number of methods are available to detect apoptosis and to dissect the mechanisms of apoptosis. Morphologically, apoptosis can be detected by phase contrast or electron microscopy. Other markers such as DNA degradation, cell membrane changes and cleavage of apoptosis-associated substrates can be detected by agarose gel electrophoresis/TdT-mediated dUTP nick end labeling (TUNEL), Annexin V binding/trypan blue exclusion, and Western blot. On the other hand, cell free apoptosis assays, in which a cytosolic extract is added directly to induce apoptosis in isolated nuclei, offer useful tools to dissect the role of individual factors in apoptosis *(16)*.

2. Materials

2.1. Morphology

2.1.1. Phase Contrast Morphology

1. 100% methanol fixative.
2. Acid dye mix: 0.1% (w/v) eosin, 0.1% (w/v) formaldehyde, 0.4% (w/v), sodium phosphate (dibasic), 0.5% w/v potassium phosphate (monobasic).
3. Basic dye mix: 0.4% methylene blue, 0.4% azure A, 0.4% (w/v) sodium phosphate (dibasic), 0.5% (w/v) potassium phosphate (monobasic).

2.1.2. Propidium Iodide and Hoechst 332589 (HO258) or 33342 (HO342) Staining

1. 4% (w/v) paraformaldehyde fixative.
2. PBS, pH 7.2.
3. 10 µg/mL PI: Prepare from a stock solution of 10 mg/mL in PBS.
4. HO258 or HO342: Dissolve 0.1 mg of HO258 or HO342 in 1 mL of distilled water.

2.1.3. Electron Microscopy

1. 0.1 M sodium cacodylate buffer, pH 7.4.
2. Glutaraldehyde/paraformaldehyde fixative: 2% (v/v) glutaraldehyde, 2% (v/v) paraformaldehyde, 0.02% $CaCl_2$ in 0.M sodium cacodylate buffer.
3. 2% (v/v) glutaraldehyde: Dilute in 0.1 M sodium cacodylate buffer.
4. 1% (w/v) osmium tetroxide in 0.1 M sodium cacodylate buffer.
5. 0.1 M maleate buffer, pH 5.2.

6. 2% (w/v) uranyl acetate: Make in 0.1 M maleate buffer, pH 5.2 (*see* **Note 1**).
7. 0.1 M maleate buffer, pH 6.0.
8. Ethanol.
9. Propylene oxide.
10. Epon resin.
11. Reynold's lead citrate stain.

2.2. DNA Degradation

2.2.1. Agarose Gel Electrophoresis

1. DNA lysis buffer: 150 mM NaCl, 25 mM EDTA, 0.125% SDS.
2. TE: 10 mM Tris-HCl, 1 mM EDTA, pH 8.0.
3. 6X DNA sample loading buffer: 0.25% bromophenol blue, 30% glycerol, 10 mM EDTA, pH 8.0.
4. 50X TAE: 242 g Tris base, 57.1 mL of glacial acetic acid, 100 mL of 0.5 M EDTA, pH 8.0, make up to 1 L with dH$_2$O.
5. 1.5% agarose: 1.5 g agarose in 100 mL of 1X TAE buffer.
6. 3 M sodium acetate, pH 5.2.
7. Ethidium bromide, 0.5 μg/mL.
8. Proteinase K (Boehringer Mannheim, Indianapolis, IN), 50 mg/mL in water.
9. RNase A, DNase-free (Boehringer Mannheim), 500 μg/mL.
10. Phenol/chloroform (1:1).
11. Chloroform.

2.2.2. Incorporation of Labeled Nucleotides (TUNEL)

A number of TUNEL assays are available commercially as kits. These include the *In Situ* Cell Death Detection Kit used here (Boehringer Mannheim), ApopTag Plus (Oncor), and the Apoptosis Detection System (Promega, Madison, WI).

1. 4% paraformaldehyde in phosphate-buffered saline (PBS), pH 7.4.
2. 0.3% H$_2$O$_2$ in methanol.
3. 0.1% Triton X-100 in 0.1% sodium citrate.
4. Solution 1 (terminal deoxynucleotidyl transferase from calf thymus, 10X) from the kit.
5. Solution 2 (nucleotide mixture in reaction buffer, 1X) from the kit.
6. Converter-POD (horseradish peroxidase conjugated antifluorescein antibody Fab fragment) from the kit.
7. DAB (3,3'-diaminobenzidine) (Sigma [St. Louis, MO] Fast DAB Tablet Set).
8. Harris haematoxylin solution modified (Sigma).
9. Destain: 0.25% HCl, 50% MeOH.
10. Mounting medium: 10% glycerol in PBS.
11. 10 mg/mL PI in PBS.
12. Fluorescent Mounting Medium (Dako).

13. DNase I, 1 mg/mL to 1 µg/mL.
14. Eight-well chamber slides (Nunc Lab-Tek II, Naperville, IL).

2.3. Flow Cytometry

1. Trypsin-EDTA (Sigma).
2. Soybean trypsin inhibitor (Sigma): 1 mg/mL in complete medium.
3. Fetal calf serum (FCS): 2% in PBS.
4. Ethanol: 70% ice-cold.

2.4. Cell Membrane Changes

2.4.1. PS/Annexin V Binding

1. 10X binding buffer: HEPES buffered saline solution supplemented with 25 mM CaCl$_2$.
2. Annexin V-FITC antibody, 10 µg/mL (e.g., R&D systems).
3. PI, 50 µg/mL.

2.4.2. Trypan Blue Exclusion

1. EBSS (Earle's balanced salt solution).
2. 0.4% (w/v) trypan blue solution (Sigma).

2.5. Cleavage of Apoptosis-Associated Substrates

1. 2X protein sample buffer : 0.125 M Tris-HCl, pH 6.8, 4% SDS, 10% β-mercapto-ethanol, 20% glycerol, 0.004% bromophenol blue.
2. Transfer buffer: 2.93 g glycine, 5.81 g Tris-HCl, 0.375 g SDS, 150 ml methanol, make up to 1 L with dH$_2$O, pH 9.2.
3. 10X TBS: 100 mM Tris-HCl, 9% NaCl, pH 7.4.
4. Blocking buffer: 5% Marvel (nonfat dried milk) in 1X TBS.
5. Incubation buffer: 5% Marvel and 0.1% Tween-20 in 1X TBS.
6. Wash buffer: 0.1% Tween 20 in 1X Tris-buffered saline (TBS).
7. Bradford Reagent (Bio-Rad, Hercules, CA).
8. 8% SDS-PAGE gel (Bio-Rad Mini-Protean II Electrophoresis Cell).
9. ECL kit (Amersham, Buckinghamshire, UK).
10. Mouse monoclonal antiPARP antibody, clone C-2-10 (BIOMOL).
11. Peroxidase conjugated antimouse antibody.
12. Immobilon-P membrane (Millipore).
13. BioRad Trans-Blot SD Semidry Transfer Cell.

2.6. Cell Free Apoptosis Assay

1. Buffer A: 150 mM NaCl, 1 mM KH$_2$PO$_4$, 1 mM EGTA, 1 mM Na$_3$VO$_4$, 5 mM MgCl$_2$, 10% glycerol, pH 7.2.
2. Cell lysis buffer: 0.3% Triton X-100 in buffer A.
3. Bio-Rad DC protein assay.
4. Hoechst (Sigma): 10 µM in formalin.
5. Peptide inhibitors: e.g., Ac-YVAD-CHO, Ac-DEVD-CHO or zVAD-fmk (Bachem).

3. Methods

3.1. Morphology

3.1.1. Phase Contrast Morphology

Light microscopy definitively identifies the exact mode of cell death in cultured cells. Apoptosis is characterized under the light microscope by chromatin condensation, nuclear fragmentation, blebbing of the plasma membrane with membrane process formation, and the formation of apoptotic bodies (**Fig. 1**). In contrast, necrotic cells are characterized by nuclear and cytoplasmic swelling, chromatin flocculation, and loss of cell membrane viability. These features are particularly apparent if the technique is combined with staining of the nucleus and cytoplasm of the cells with a combination of acidic and basic dyes.

1. Culture cells on coverslips or on chamber slides. Remove the culture medium and air-dry for 5 min.
2. Fix in methanol for 10 s. Allow to drain.
3. Add acid dye mix for 10 s.
4. Add basic dye mix for 10 s.
5. Rinse off dyes and air-dry.
6. Mount slides and cover slip. Examine under 40× objective.

3.1.2. Propidium Iodide and Hoechst 332589 (HO258) or 33342 (HO342) Staining

Propidium iodide or Hoechst staining without prior fixation identify intense fluorescence in apoptotic cells, predominantly due to altered membrane uptake and staining of condensed chromatin in apoptotic cells. Live cells stain faintly with either dye.

1. Culture cells on chamber slides, coverslips or dishes.
2. Wash in PBS.
3. Add 10 μL of HO258 or HO342/mL of PBS.
   OR
   Add 10 μg/mL PI.
4. Fix in 4% paraformaldehyde for 10 min.
5. Examine with a fluorescence microscope. Excitation wavelength for HO258 or HO342 is 340 nm, and for PI is 488 nm.

3.1.3. Electron Microscopy

Electron microscopy is the definitive method for identifying that the mode of cell death is apoptotic. Electron microscopy identifies the chromatin condensation, lack of cytoplasmic disruption (except some swelling of the endoplasmic reticulum), membrane blebbing, vacuolization, and even the presence

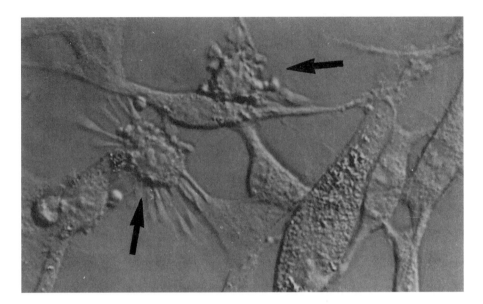

Fig. 1. Phase contrast microscope appearance of apoptotic vascular smooth muscle cells. Arrowed cells show evidence of cell shrinkage, retraction from adjacent cells, and membrane bleb formation.

of internalized apoptotic bodies, seen in apoptosis (**Fig. 2**). However, owing to the extensive preparation required, this is not a good method for quantification of apoptosis.

1. Culture cells in dishes, on coverslips or in chamber slides.
2. Wash cells in PBS.
3. Fix cells in glutaraldehyde/paraformaldehyde at 4°C overnight.
4. Rinse with three changes of 0.1 M sodium cacodylate buffer, pH 7.4, and post fix in 1% osmium tetroxide in 0.1 M sodium cacodylate buffer, pH 7.4, for 2 h at room temperature.
5. Rinse with two changes of 0.1 M sodium cacodylate buffer, pH 7.4, and two changes of 0.1 M maleate buffer, pH 5.2.
6. Stain cells with 2% uranyl acetate in 0.1 M maleate buffer, pH 5.2 for 1 h at room temperature (in the dark), and rinse in three changes of 0.1 M maleate buffer, pH 6.0.
7. Dehydrate cells in increasing concentrations of ethanol.
8. Dry with propylene oxide.
9. Embed in EPON resin.
10. Cut ultrathin sections (60 nm) with an ultramicrotome and mount.
11. Stain ultrathin sections with 2% uranyl acetate in 70% ethanol, followed by Reynold's lead citrate stain for 10 min.
12. Examine using a transmission electron microscope.

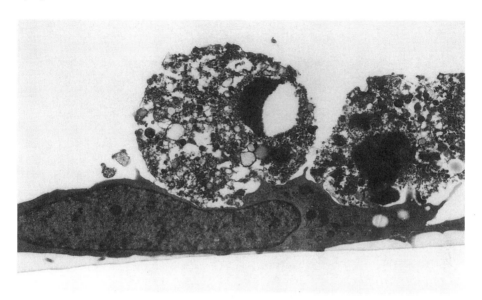

Fig. 2. Transmission electron microscopic appearance of apoptotic vascular smooth muscle cells. Two apoptotic cells lie adjacent to a cell monolayer of cells showing a normal appearance. The apoptotic cells demonstrate chromatin condensation, cell shrinkage, vacuolisation, and breakdown of plasma membrane continuity.

3.2. DNA Degradation

One of the final events of apoptosis is DNA degradation during which the DNA strands are broken by endonucleases releasing oligonucleosomal DNA pieces of 180–200 bp multiples (**Fig. 3**) *(6,7)*. This can be detected by agarose gel electrophoresis as DNA ladders. Alternatively, DNA degradation can be detected by TUNEL assay, which labels nicked DNA ends with fluorescein-dUTP in an end tailing reaction using terminal transferase (*see also* Chapter 19).

3.2.1. Agarose Gel Electrophoresis

1. Spin down apoptotic bodies in the supernatant of the cell culture.
2. Lyse the remaining adherent cells in 0.4 mL of DNA lysis buffer. Use a cell scraper to scrape off cells and transfer to an Eppendorf tube with a 1-mL pipet tip.
3. Add 1 μL of 50 mg/mL proteinase K and incubate for 1 h at 37°C.
4. Add 8 μL of 500 μg/mL RNase A and incubate for 1 h at 37°C.
5. Extract by mixing with 0.4 mL of phenol/chloroform (1X) and chloroform (1X) (*see* **Note 2**).
6. Microfuge at 13,000*g* for 5 min at room temperature and collect the upper aqueous phase containing the DNA.

M   A   A

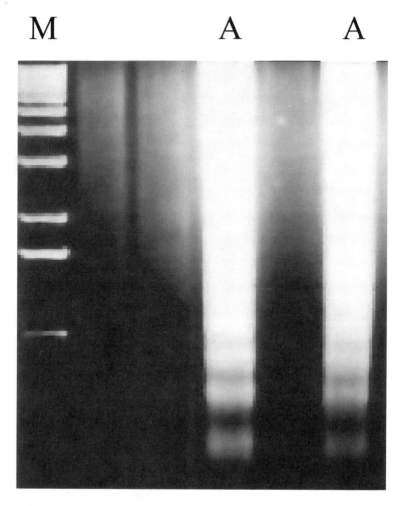

Fig. 3. DNA fragmentation due to apoptosis. Lanes marked A show evidence of internucleosomal DNA fragmentation with size fragments of multiples of 180 bp, in comparison with DNA markers (M).

7. Precipitate the DNA with 1 mL of ethanol and 40 μL of 3 *M* sodium acetate, pH 5.2. Leave at –20°C overnight.
8. Microfuge at 13,000*g* for 15 min. Dry the pellet and resuspend in 20 μL of TE.
9. Add 4 μL of 6X DNA sample loading buffer. Load onto a 1.5% agarose 1X TAE gel. Run the gel at 15 V for 16 h or until the blue dye has reached the last few centimetes of the gel.
10. Stain the gel with 0.5 μg/mL ethidium bromide in 1X TAE buffer or water for several hours or until the DNA bands are visible under a UV transilluminator (*see* **Note 3**).

3.2.2. Incorporation of Labeled Nucleotides (TUNEL)
(see also Chapter 19)

Here we describe a method based on that of *In Situ* Cell Death Detection Kit (Boehringer Mannheim), which offers the flexibility of detection by fluorescent or light microscopy.

1. Grow cells in eight-well chamber slides and leave overnight (*see* **Note 4**).
2. Treat the cells to induce apoptosis.
3. Air-dry cells, fix in 4% paraformaldehyde in PBS, pH 7.4 for 30 min at room temperature.
4. Rinse the slides with PBS. Block endogenous peroxidase activity with 0.3% H_2O_2 in methanol for 30 min at room temperature.
5. Rinse the slides with PBS and permeabilize cells with 0.1% Triton X-100 in 0.1% sodium citrate for 2 min on ice.
6. Rinse the slides twice with PBS. Dry the slides slightly.
7. Dilute solution 1 1:10 in solution 2. Add 10 μL to each chamber making sure that it covers all of the area. Cut a piece of parafilm to the exact size of the chamber and carefully lay it on top of the reaction mixture. Incubate in a humidified chamber for 60 min at 37°C.
8. Rinse the slides three times with PBS. Dry the slides slightly. Add 10 μL of Converter-POD to each chamber, cover with a parafilm. Incubate in a humidified chamber for 30 min at 37°C.
9. Rinse the slides three times with PBS. Add 100 μL of DAB for 10 min at room temperature.
10. Rinse slides three times with PBS. Counterstain the nuclei with Harris Haematoxylin Solution for 10 min at room temperature.
11. Immerse once in 0.25% HCl, 50% MeOH. Rinse with PBS.
12. Mount the slides in mounting medium.
13. Observe under a light microscope (*see* **Note 5**). Count the number of dead cells (brown staining) against the total number of cells (blue staining).

3.3. Flow Cytometry

Flow cytometry is usually used to detect cell membrane surface receptors such as Fas or tumor necrosis factor receptor (TNFR). It can also be used to detect cytoplasmic proteins after the cells are permeabilized by a reagent such as alcohol. This method has been adapted to detect apoptotic cells by ANNEXIN V binding to externalized PS. The differential permeability of live and dead cells to Hoechst and PI, respectively, serves as a useful parameter for distinguishing between live and dead cells. This is achieved by collecting the Hoechst and PI signals in different channels by flow cytometry. Here we describe an example of the method for detection of surface and cytoplasmic Fas (**Fig. 4**).

1. Trypsinize the cells with 2 mL of trypsin-EDTA per 75 cm² tissue culture flask for just long enough to dislodge the cells (*see* **Note 6**).

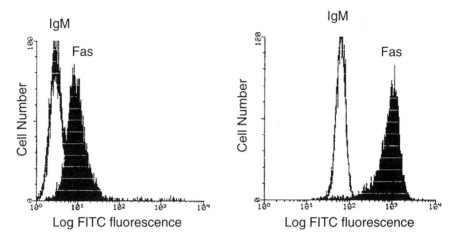

Fig. 4. Flow cytometry of (A) surface Fas and (B) cytoplasmic Fas in coronary vascular smooth muscle cells. The cells were permeablized with 70% ethanol for the detection of cytoplasmic Fas. The blank histograms (IgM) represent the log FITC fluorescence of isotypic IgM controls. The solid histograms (Fas) represents the log FITC fluorescence of Fas.

2. Pool cells together. Add 10 mL of 1 mg/mL soybean trypsin inhibitor. Spin at 95g for 5 min at 4°C.
3. Resuspend in 2% FCS in PBS at 10^7cells/mL. Aliquot 100 μL (=10^6 cells) into each Eppendorf (×8).
4a. To detect cytoplasmic proteins, permeabilize cells with 1 mL of 70% ice-cold ethanol and leave for 30 min on ice (*see* **Note 7**). Spin at 95g at 4°C.
4b. To detect surface proteins, proceed to **step 5**.
5. Wash once with 1 mL of 2% FCS in PBS. Spin at 95g at 4°C.
6. Resuspend the pellet in 50 μL of 2% FCS in PBS. Add to the cells:
   a. Nothing (untreated control).
   b. 20 μg/mL first antibody, e.g., mouse monoclonal antiFas IgM clone CH-11 (Upstate) (experimental).
   c. 20 μg/mL isotypic immunoglobulin, e.g., mouse IgM (Sigma) (isotypic control).
   d. Nothing until **step 8** (background staining).
   Leave for 30 min on ice.
7. Wash with 1 mL of 2% FCS in PBS. Spin at 95g at 4°C.
8. Resuspend in 50 mL of 2% FCS in PBS.
9. Add 0.5 μL (1:100) of FITC-conjugated secondary antibody, e.g., FITC-conjugated antimouse antibody (Sigma) to tubes b, c, and d, respectively. Incubate for 30 min on ice.
10. Wash once with 1 mL of 2% FCS in PBS. Spin at 95g at 4°C.
11. Resuspend in 0.5 mL of 2% FCS in PBS.
12. Analyze with FACS.

3.4. Cell Membrane Changes

3.4.1. PS/Annexin V Binding

In living cells, PS resides on the cytoplasmic face of the cell membrane. Externalization of PS is an early event in apoptosis *(8)*, which can be detected by Annexin V binding to PS (*see* **Note 8**). Fluorescein-conjugated Annexin V is commercially available, which offers direct detection of externalized PS by flow cytometry or fluorescent microscopy.

1. Wash cells once in PBS. Resuspend 10^5 cells in 100 µL of 1X binding buffer.
2. Add 10 µL of 10 µg/mL Annexin V-FITC and 10 µL of 50 µg/mL PI (*see* **Note 9**). Mix gently. Incubate at room temperature in the dark for 5–15 min.
3a. Add 0.4 mL of 1X binding buffer. Analyze immediately by flow cytometry with laser emitting excitation wavelength at 488 nm. Collect the FITC signal with FL1 detector and the PI signal with FL2.
3b. Alternatively, count the cells under a fluorescent microscope using a dual filter set for FITC (green fluorescence for Annexin V) and rhodamine (red fluorescence for PI).

3.4.2. Trypan Blue Exclusion

Trypan blue has been used as a dye to differentiate between live and dead cells based on the fact that live cells do not take up the dye, whereas dead cells do.

1. Trypsinize cells and resuspend in a suitable dilution in 0.5 mL EBSS (*see* **Note 10**).
2. Add 0.5 mL of 0.4% Trypan blue solution. Stand for 5–15 min.
3. Count the number of stained (blue) and unstained cells with a haemocytometer. The percentage viability is the number of unstained cells/total number of cells x100%.

3.5. Cleavage of Apoptosis-Associated Substrates

The process of apoptosis involves sequential cleavage and activation of caspases from inactive proforms into active mature forms. These caspases subsequently activate the cleavage of a number of death substrates such as PARP and nuclear lamins, resulting in the eventual death of the cells. Cleavage of caspases and the death substrates can easily be detected by Western blot. An example is given here concerning the detection of PARP cleavage. PARP is frequently used as a marker of apoptosis. Cleavage of PARP (116 kD) generates a signature fragment of 85 kD.

1. Seed cells in 75 cm^2 tissue culture flask overnight to subconfluence (*see* **Note 11**).
2. Treat the cells to induce apoptosis.
3. Add 100 µL of preheated 2X protein sample buffer to each flask.
4. Scrape off the cells with a cell scraper.
5. Transfer the sample into an Eppendorf tube.
6. Heat at 100°C for 10 min.

7. Pass three times through a 25G needle.
8. Microfuge at 13,000g for 10 min at room temperature. Collect the supernatant.
9. Determine the protein concentrations using Bradford Reagent.
10. Load an equal quantity of protein onto an 8% SDS-PAGE gel (Bio-Rad Mini-Protean II Electrophoresis Cell). Alternatively, load protein equivalent to an equal number of cells into each lane.
11. Run at 100 V for 2 h.
12. Transfer proteins onto Immobilon-P membrane at 25 V for 1 h using transfer buffer.
13. Block the membrane in blocking buffer for 1 h at room temperature with gentle agitation.
14. Seal the membrane in a plastic bag. Incubate with mouse monoclonal antiPARP antibody clone C-2-10 (1:10,000) in incubation buffer overnight in the cold room with gentle agitation.
15. Wash the membrane in 4X wash buffer, each of 200 mL for 5 min at room temperature, with vigorous shaking.
16. Seal membrane in a plastic bag. Incubate with peroxidase conjugated antimouse antibody (1:1000) in incubation buffer for 2 h at room temperature with gentle agitation.
17. Wash the membrane in 4X wash buffer, each of 200 mL for 5 min at room temperature, with vigorous shaking. Wash the membrane in a final wash of 1X TBS for 5 min.
18. Develop the signal with a suitable ECL kit (e.g., from Amersham) (*see* **Note 12**). Drip the membrane to remove excess TBS but do not let dry. Place on Saran Wrap.
19. Mix 0.5 mL of each of solutions 1 and 2 from the kit.
20. Pipet onto the membrane and stand for 1 min.
21. Drain off excess fluid by soaking onto a tissue paper.
22. Cover the membrane with the Saran Wrap.
23. Put a film on in the dark room. Develop the film after an appropriate length of exposure (*see* **Note 13**).

3.6. Cell Free Apoptosis Assay

Cell free assays provide useful tools to dissect individual components involved in apoptosis. Indicator nuclei are usually taken from HeLa cells, although autologous nuclei can be used. Cytosolic extract is then added to induce apoptotic changes in the HeLa nuclei, which in turn can be detected by microscopy, DNA laddering, and/or PARP cleavage.

3.6.1. Preparation of HeLa Nuclei

1. Trypsinise the cells. Stop the trypsin reaction with complete medium.
2. Wash the cells 2X PBS and once with buffer A.
3. Lyse the cells with cell lysis buffer for 10 min on ice. Spin at 110g for 10 min at 4°C.
4. Wash the nuclei in 3X with buffer A, with spinning at 110g for 10 min at 4°C.
5. Use immediately.

3.6.2. Preparation of Cytosolic Extract

1. Treat the cells to induce apoptosis.
2. Same as **Subheading 3.6.1, steps 1–3**.
3. Take off the supernatant as cytosolic extract. Determine the protein concentration by Bio-Rad DC Protein Assay (*see* **Note 14**).

3.6.3. Cell Free Assay (see **Notes 15** and **16**)

1. Incubate 10^6 nuclei with 300 mg of protein (from **Subheading 3.6.2., step 3**) in a final volume of 25 µL. Incubate at 37°C for 1 h.
2. Remove 3.5 µL of the cell-free mixture to mix with 1.5 µL of 10 µ *M* Hoechst in formalin on a slide. Observe under a fluorescent microscope for nuclei morphological changes.
3. Spin down the nuclei. Wash three times with buffer A.
4. Extract half of the nuclei for DNA analysis (proceed as in **Subheading 3.2.1.**). Extract the other half of the nuclei for PARP cleavage detection (proceed as in **Subheading 3.5.**).

4. Notes

1. Uranyl acetate in 0.1 *M* maleate buffer, pH 5.2 should be stored in the dark.
2. Repeat phenol/chloroform extraction if the aqueous phase becomes too viscous.
3. Sometimes, a prolonged staining is required to visualize the smaller bands. However, it is usually not necessary to destain the gel. In case the background is too high, the gel can be destained by soaking in water or 1 m*M* $MgSO_4$ for 20 min at room temperature.
4. Negative and positive controls should be included with each run. For negative controls, incubate cells with solution 2 only. For positive controls, incubate cells with 1 mg/mL to 1 µg/mL of DNase I for 10 min at room temperature to induce DNA strand breaks.
5. Alternatively, the cells can be detected by fluorescent microscopy after **step 7**. Rinse slides three times with PBS, counterstain with 10 µg/mL of PI for 1 min at room temperature. Rinse slides three times with PBS. Mount slides in Fluorescent Mounting Medium (Dako). Count the number of dead cells (green fluorescence) against the total number of cells (red fluorescence). In this case, omit **step 4**.
6. Trypsin changes some surface proteins. In this case, one can replace trypsin with other cell dislodging agents such as the nonenzymatic cell dissociation solution (Sigma) and 0.02% EDTA solution or the Accutase Cell Dispersal Preparation (TCS).
7. Other permeabilizing agents include ice-cold or –20°C methanol, 4% paraformaldehyde in PBS, etc.
8. Live cells will not stain with either Annexin-V FITC or PI. Early apoptotic cells will stain with Annexin-V FITC only. Necrotic cells and late apoptotic cells will stain with both FITC and PI.
9. Controls include unstained cells, cells stained with FITC only and cells stained with PI only.

10. EBSS can be replaced by other balanced salt solution such as Hank's balanced salt solution (HBSS).
11. Positive controls for PARP Western blot include noninduced HL60 cells and HL60 cells induced with etoposide, both available as whole cell extracts from BIOMOL.
12. There is no fixed conditions for Western blotting detection. A useful guide is to use 5% Marvel in the blocking medium. Add 0.05% or 0.1% Tween-20 or NP40 to the incubation and/or blocking buffers in case of high background. The optimal concentrations for each antibodies also differ depending on the antibodies. The starting point is to try using dilutions of 1:1000 for both the primary and secondary antibodies. If sensitivity is too low or the background is too high, the dilutions can then be adjusted accordingly. A 1:1000 dilution is usually sufficient for most monoclonal antibodies, whereas dilutions as high as 1:5000 are sometimes necessary to eliminate high background when using polyclonal antibodies.
13. It usually requires multiple exposures to obtain the best picture. Exposure time varies depending on the abundance of the protein in the whole cell lysate and the sensitivity of the antibodies. Usually a 1 min exposure is carried out as a test and subsequent exposure time varies according to the intensity of the bands.
14. It is very important to use the correct protein assay since different protein assays are compatible with different detergents and/or reducing agents used in the extraction of proteins.
15. The apoptotic effect of individual component can be tested by this method by adding the corresponding recombinant protein to the nuclei in the presence of naive cytosolic extract from uninduced cells.
16. The specificity of the apoptotic effect can be assessed by preincubating the cytosolic extract with nM to µM range of peptide inhibitors such as Ac-YVAD-CHO, Ac-DEVD-CHO or zVAD-fmk for 2 h at 37°C before the nuclei are added.

Acknowledgments

Dr. Chan is supported by a British Heart Foundation project grant. Dr. Bennett is a British Heart Foundation Senior Research Fellow.

References

1. Kerr, J. F., Wyllie, A. H., and Currie, A. R. (1972) Apoptosis: a basic biological phenomenon with wide-ranging implications in tissue kinetics. *Br. J. Cancer* **26,** 239–257.
2. Martin, S., Reutelingsperger, C., Mcgahon, A., et al. (1995) Early redistribution of plasma-membrane phosphatidylserine is a general feature of apoptosis regardless of the initiating stimulus - inhibition by overexpression of bcl-2 and abl. *J. Exp. Med.* **182,** 1545–1556.
3. Bennett, M., Gibson, D., Schwartz, S., and Tait, J. (1995) Binding and phagocytosis of apoptotic rat vascular smooth muscle cells is mediated in part by exposure to phosphatidylserine. *Circ. Res.* **77,** 1136–1142.

4. Mashima, T., Naito, M., Fujita, N., Noguchi, K., and Tsuruo, T. (1995) Identification of actin as a substrate of ICE and an ICE-like protease and involvement of an ICE-like protease but not ICE in VP-16-induced U937 apoptosis. *Biochem. Biophys. Res. Comm.* **217,** 1185–1192.

5. Kayalar, C., Ord, T., Testa, M. P., Zhong, L. T., and Bredesen, D. E. (1996) Cleavage Of Actin By Interleukin 1-Beta-Converting Enzyme to Reverse Dnase-I Inhibition. *Proc. Natl. Acad. Sci. USA* **93,** 2234–2238.

6. Enari, M., Sakahira, H., Yokoyama, H., Okawa, K., Iwamatsu, A., and Nagata, S. (1998) A caspase-activated DNase that degrades DNA during apoptosis and its inhibitor ICAD. *Nature* **391,** 43–50.

7. Sakahira, H., Enari, M., and Nagata, S. (1998) Cleavage of CAD inhibitor in CAD activation and DNA degradation during apoptosis. *Nature* **391,** 96–99.

8. Martin, S., Finucane, D., Amarantemendes, G., O'Brien, G., and Green, D. (1996) Phosphatidylserine externalization during cd95-induced apoptosis of cells and cytoplasts requires ice/ced-3 protease activity. *J. Biol.Chem.* **271,** 28,753–28,756.

9. Darmon, A., Ley, T., Nicholson, D., and Bleackley, R. (1996) Cleavage of CPP32 by Granzyme-B represents a critical role for Granzyme-B in the induction of target cell DNA fragmentation. *J. Biol. Chem.* **271,** 21,709–21,712.

10. Tewari, M., Quan, L., O' Rourke, K., et al. (1995) Yama/cpp32-beta, a mammalian homolog of ced-3, is a crma-inhibitable protease that cleaves the death substrate poly(adp-ribose) polymerase. *Cell* **81,** 801–809.

11. Casciola-Rosen, L., Miller, D., Anhalt, G., and Rosen, A. (1994) Specific cleavage of the 70-KDa protein component of the U1 small nuclear ribonucleoprotein is a charcateristic biochemical feature of apoptotic cell death. *J. Biol. Chem.* **269,** 30,57–30,760.

12. Tewari, M., Beidler, D., and Dixit, V. (1995) crmA-inhibitable cleavage of the 70-kda protein-component of the u1 small nuclear ribonucleoprotein during fas-induced and tumor necrosis factor-induced apoptosis. *J. Biol. Chem.* **270,** 18,738–18,741.

13. Casciola-Rosen, L., Anhalt, G., and Rosen, A. (1995) DNA-dependent protein kinase is one of a subset of autoantigens specifically cleaved early during apoptosis. *J. Exp. Med.* **182,** 1625–1634.

14. Cryns, V. L., Bergeron, L., Zhu, H., Li, H. L., and Yuan, J. Y. (1996) Specific cleavage of alpha-fodrin during Fas-induced and tumor necrosis factor-induced apoptosis is mediated by an interleukin-1-beta-converting rnzyme/Ced-3 protease distinct from the poly(Adp-ribose) rolymerase protease. *J. Biol.Chem.* **271,** 31,277–31,282.

15. Orth, K., Chinnaiyan, A., Garg, M., Froelich, C., and Dixit, V. (1996) The ced-3/ice-like protease mch2 is activated during apoptosis and cleaves the death substrate lamina. *J. Biol. Chem.* **271,** 16,443–16,446.

16. Lazebnik, Y A., Cole, S., Cooke, C. A., Nelson, W. G., and Earnshaw. W-C. (1993) Nuclear events of apoptosis in vitro in cell-free mitotic extracts a model system for analysis of the active phase of apoptosis. *J. Cell. Biol.* **123,** 7–22.

21

Molecular Assessment of the Phenotypic Changes Associated with Smooth Muscle Cells Using Two-Dimension Electrophoresis and Microsequence Analysis

Rachel Johnatty, Giulio Gabbiani, and Pascal Neuville

1. Introduction

Phenotypic modulation of arterial smooth muscle cells (SMC) is essential for the evolution of atheromatosis and restenosis after angioplasty *(1)*. During these pathological phenomena, SMC express numerous genes such as those responsible for cell migration and proliferation *(2)*. The identification of genes differentially expressed is obviously important for the understanding of the mechanisms leading to restenosis and atheromatous plaque development and may be a key step in the planning of new therapeutic approaches. Among the different techniques available for the identification of differentially expressed genes, in this chapter we describe the two-dimensional analytical gel electrophoresis (2-D PAGE) protein expression analysis *(3)*. This method offers the advantage of producing protein maps of defined SMC phenotypes, which can be used as references for such applications as SMC phenotype comparison and drug effect analysis *(4,5)*. In the last decade, this classical biochemical technique has benefited from modifications improving the reproducibility and the quality of 2-D gels. One of the most important contributions was the introduction of immobilized pH gradients (IPGs) as the first dimension *(3)*. In comparison to the conventional carrier ampholyte, they ensure reproducible gradients that are insensitive to disturbances from sample components. Moreover, recent developments concerning protein databases as well as computer systems facilitate spot detection and protein identification *(6)*. In this chapter, we describe a detailed protocol, developed in the Geneva laboratory of Professor

From: *Methods in Molecular Medicine, Vascular Disease: Molecular Biology and Gene Therapy Protocols*
Edited by: A. H. Baker © Humana Press Inc., Totowa, NJ

D. Hochstrasser, for sample preparation and 2-D PAGE. Solutions to the problems most frequently encountered are given. The procedure for 2-D PAGE image analysis and protein identification is also approached. Finally, using an example, we show how to link 2-D PAGE images to protein databases.

2. Materials

2.1. Reagents (see Notes 1 and 2)

1. Resolyte 3.5–10 (BDH, London, UK).
2. Resolyte 4–8 (BDH).
3. 2-D SDS PAGE Std (Bio-Rad, Hercules, CA).
4. Acrylamide.
5. Extra thick blotting paper (Bio-Rad).
6. Piperazine diacrylyl (PDA) (Bio-Rad).
7. PVDF membrane (Bio-Rad).
8. Sodium dodecyl sulfate (SDS).
9. BSA fraction V (Boerhinger Mannheim, Germany).
10. Acetic acid.
11. Amido black (Fluka, Buchs, Switzerland).
12. Ammonium hydroxide solution (25%).
13. Bromophenol blue.
14. CHAPS (Fluka).
15. Ethanol (Et-OH).
16. Glutaraldehyde solution.
17. Glycerol 87% (Fluka).
18. Glycine.
19. Hydrochloric acid (HCl).
20. Iodoacetamide.
21. Isopropanol.
22. Kerosene.
23. Methanol (Met-OH).
24. Met-OH (HPLC).
25. Silicone oil DC 200 (Fluka).
26. Silver nitrate.
27. Sodium acetate.3H$_2$O.
28. Sodium azide.
29. Sodium hydroxide.
30. N,N,N',N'-tetramethylethylenediamine (TEMED).
31. Ammonium persulfate.
32. Dithioerytheritol (DTE).
33. TRIS ultra pure.
34. 2,7-Napthalene disulfonic acid (NDS, Kodak, Rochester, NY): 0.05% (w/v). Make up just before use.
35. Citric acid.
36. Formaldehyde solution (35%).

37. Sodium thiosulfate.5H$_2$O.
38. Urea.
39. Immobiline dry plate pH 3.0–10.0 NL/L (17-1221-05) (Pharmacia Biotech, Uppsala, Sweden).
40. Repel-Silane ES (Pharmacia Biotech).
41. Agarose.
42. CAPS (Sigma, St. Louis, MO).
43. EGTA (100 mM). Store at room temperature.
44. PMSF (35 mg/mL). Store at –20°C.
45. TAME (76 mg/mL). Store at –20°C.
46. Aprotinin (2.8 mg/mL). Store at 4°C.
47. Benzamidine.
48. Tween 20.
49. IPG gel strips (Immobiline, Pharmacia).
50. Electrofocusing Electrode Paper (Pharmacia).
51. 10 M NaOH.

2.2. Buffers

All water used throughout this technique should be ultra-pure grade. Glassware should have a final rinse in deionized water.

2.2.1. Buffers for Sample Preparation

1. Wash buffer: 10 mL 100 mM EGTA, 1 mL PMSF 35 mg/ mL, 1 mL 76 mg/mL TAME, 1.43 mL 2.8 mg/mL aprotinin, 7.8 mg benzamidine (make up fresh before use). Make up to 100 mL with saline (0.8% NaCl). Do not use PBS; physiological saline is preferable.
2. Lysis buffer: 162 mM DTE, 1% (v/v) TWEEN 20, 9 M urea, 40 mM Tris-HCl. Prepare 10 mL in water. Store at –20°C in 0.5-mL aliquots. Thaw once only.

2.2.2. Buffers for Rehydration

1. Rehydration buffer: 8 M urea, 32.5 mM CHAPS, 10 mM DTE, 40 μL bromophenol blue solution (0.5% w/v). Prepare 20 mL in water. Add just prior to use: 200 μL of Resolyte pH 4.0–8.0 and 200 μL of Resolyte pH 3.5–10.0. The quality of ampholytes is crucial to the effective isoelectric focusing of the proteins and hence to the quality of 2-D gels. Use a syringe and needle to dispense.

2.2.3. Buffers for Equilibration

1. Equilibration buffer: 20 mL of 0.5 M Tris-HCl, pH 6.8, 6 M urea, 65 mL glycerol (stock solution 87%), 2% (w/v) SDS. Prepare 200 mL in water. Divide into two parts of 100 mL to make Buffers A and B (*see* **steps 2** and **3**). Add only just before use.
2. Buffer A: 2 g DTE (2%) facilitates the resolubilization of proteins and the reduction of S-S bonding.

3. Buffer B: 2.5 g iodoacetamide (2.5%). Blocks the formation of -SH groups.

Do not reuse these solutions.

2.2.4. Solutions for the Second Dimension

1. Upper chamber buffer: 50 mM Tris-HCl, 380 mM glycine, 0.1% (w/v) SDS. Dissolve in water.
2. Lower chamber buffer: 50 mM Tris-HCl, 380 mM glycine, 3.1 mM sodium azide, 0.1% (w/v) SDS. Dissolve in water.
3. Agarose Solution: 0.4% (w/v) agarose, 25 mM Tris-HCl, 0.1% (w/v) SDS, 0.19 M glycine, 0.5% bromophenol blue solution (enough to visualize). Dissolve in water with gentle warming.

2.2.5. Solutions for Silver Staining

1. Fixative A: 40% (v/v) Et-OH, 10% (v/v) acetic acid. Stable for many months at room temperature in a dark bottle.
2. Fixative B: 5% (v/v) Et-OH, 5% (v/v) acetic acid. Stable for many months at room temperature in a dark bottle.
3. Glutaraldehyde solution: 0.5 M sodium acetate, 1% glutaraldehyde solution (prepare a 50% stock solution). Store sodium acetate stock (0.5 M) at 4°C. Add glutaraldehyde (also store at 4°C) when needed.
4. Silver nitrate solution: mix in the following order: 160 mL water, 1.5 mL 10 M NaOH solution, 10 ml 25% NH_4OH solution, silver nitrate solution (6 g/ 30 mL water). Dissolve the silver nitrate separately, do not expose to light for long periods before use. Add to the main mixture slowly while stirring; a transient brown precipitate will appear. Make up with water up to 750 mL (enough for four gels). Do not prepare the solution too far in advance or expose to light for long periods. NB: Care must be taken when disposing of the used solution as it is potentially explosive.
5. Developer: 2.38 mM citric acid, 0.1% (v/v) formaldehyde. Prepare in water (2 L/ four gels) just prior to use.
6. Stop solution: 5% (v/v) acetic acid. Stable for many months at room temperature in a dark bottle.
7. Gel storage solution: 0.5 M Tris-HCl, 3% (v/v) acetic acid. Stable for many months at room temperature in a dark bottle.

2.2.6. Reagents for Electrophoretic Transfer to PVDF Membranes

1. Towbin transfer buffer: 25 mM Tris-HCl, 0.19 M glycine, 20% (v/v) Met-OH. Prepare in water.
2. CAPS buffer: 10 mM CAPS + 10% (v/v) Met-OH, pH 11.0 (adjust with NaOH). Prepare in water.
3. Amido black stain: 0.2% (w/v) naphthol blue black B, 20% (v/v) Met-OH (HPLC). Prepare in water.

2.2.7. Solutions for Determining Amino Acid Composition

1. Denaturation buffer A: 10% (w/v) SDS, 150 mM DTE. Prepare in water. Heat the sample 5 min at 100°C. Use: 20 mL BSA solution, 10 mL Buffer A, and 50 mL lysis buffer.
2. CAPS buffer: 10 mM CAPS. Prepare in water. Adjust to pH 11.0 with 1 M NaOH.
3. Amido black stain: 0.1% (w/v) naphthol blue black B, 25% (w/v) isopropanol, 10% (v/v) acetic acid. Prepare in water.

2.3. List of Equipment for 2-D PAGE

2.3.1. For Isoelectric Focusing

1. Reswelling Cassette (Pharmacia Biotech).
2. Multiphor II Electrophoresis Unit (Pharmacia Biotech).
3. Immobiline DryStrip Kit (Pharmacia Biotech).
4. Microcomputer Electrophoresis E752 (Consort, Turnhout, Belgium).
5. MultiTemp Thermostatic Circulator (Pharmacia Biotech).

2.3.2. For Vertical Second Dimension Gels

1. Protean II xi Multi-Cell Casting Chamber (Bio-Rad).
2. Protean II Multi-Cell (Bio-Rad).
3. Gradient Gel Pourer (LargeScaleBiology/Bio-Rad).

2.3.3. For Electrophoretic Transfer

1. Trans-Blot Cell (Bio-Rad).

2.3.4. For Scanning and Image Analysis

1. Laser Densitometer (Molecular Dynamics).
2. GS-700 Imaging Densitometer (with appropriate image acquisition software) (Bio-Rad).
3. Melanie II 2-D PAGE software for PC/UNIX/Macintosh (Bio-Rad).
4. Computer and data storage facilities (according to requirements for software to be used).

3. Methods

3.1. Sample Preparation

It is crucial that a high level of care is maintained during SMC culture, sample preparation, and solubilization, if samples are to be used for comparative 2-D PAGE analysis. Small variations at this stage can result in differences in the final 2-D PAGE result, which may not be associated with the phenotypes being compared. Incomplete solubilization can leave protein aggregates and complexes, which may cause the appearance of artifactual spots.

If the samples are from freshly dissociated vessels, differences in the length of time and the holding conditions postexcision could also introduce unnecessary variation. It is important that all blood is washed off using physiological saline, and fat and connective tissue are carefully removed to avoid contamination and masking the proteins of interest.

1. Harvest cultured SMC preferably without the use of enzymes or with a trypsin-EDTA mixture. If fresh tissue is to be used, ensure that all lumps are dissociated and that any enzymes used are carefully removed—mechanical dissociation in liquid nitrogen is advisable.
2. Wash SMC three times in wash buffer. The addition of proteinase inhibitors helps to reduce protein damage by autolysis.
3. After the final wash, centrifuge to pellet the SMC and remove as much of the wash buffer as possible.
4. Add 75 µL of lysis buffer/1×10^7 cells and store immediately at –70°C, until ready for use. Do not boil the sample. If sonication is needed, use ice.

3.2. First Dimension

The first dimension migration is probably the step that has the greatest influence on the final outcome of the procedure. It is important that the greatest care is taken to ensure the best result.

3.2.1. Nonlinear Immobilized pH Gradient (IPG) Gel Strips

The use of IPG gel strips as the first dimension matrix greatly improves resolution, and reproducibility, is much easier to use, and allows greater amounts of proteins to be loaded, compared to conventional tube gels. For an unknown protein use pI 3.5–10.0 to determine where the pI is. For a known protein use a more specific pH range. For analytical gels use 3 mm widths 18 cm length.

The preparative gels used in this protocol are specifically adapted for loading quantities (1–3 mg) of sample. This produces a 2-D gel with spots containing the picomolar quantities of protein required for microsequencing. IPG strips with a width of 5 mm and adapted to 15 mm at the sample end are used (*see* **Fig. 1**).

1. Rehydrate the strips overnight in a Pharmacia Reswelling Cassette.

The sample can also be introduced into the gel during the IPG strip rehydration step using modified rehydration chambers. This avoids the use of sample cups and reduces the risk of sample precipitation at the application site *(7,8)*.

3.2.2. Rehydration

Rehydrate the Immobiline gel strips the night before, for a minimum of 6 h.

1. Using Repel-Silane (dimethyl-dichloro-silane), silanize the glass plate that will be in contact with the gel side of the strip, to prevent sticking (resilanize after every four uses).

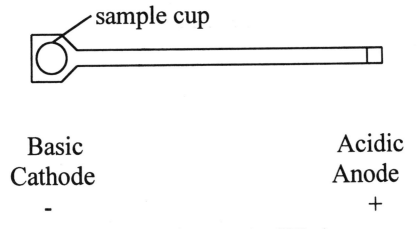

Fig. 1. Diagrammatic representation of IPG strips.

2. Remove the plastic backing of the gel strips and lay gel side up on the unsilanized plate.
3. Squirt buffer liberally over the strips and lay the silanized plate on top.
4. Clamp and fill vertically using a syringe, ensuring that no bubbles are trapped in the cassette.

Leave overnight at room temperature with the syringe still in place.

3.2.3. Mounting the First-Dimension Gel Strips for Electrophoresis

1. Connect the Multiphor II Electrophoresis Chamber to a refrigerated circulating water bath at 15°C (*see* **Note 3**).
2. Wet the electrode wicks (Electrofocusing Electrode Paper) with water.
3. Blot well with tissue paper, as excess water will cause lateral streaking of the spots on the gel. For preparative gels, put a ring of agarose outside the edge of the preparative well to prevent spreading of sample and cut out two electrode wicks from extra-thick blotting paper.
4. Cover the white base-plate with kerosene (about 10–20 mL) and lay the glass plate carefully on top, avoiding bubbles.
5. Cover the bottom of the glass plate with silicone oil (about 10–15 mL) and carefully lay the plastic strip tray, avoiding bubbles and without allowing oil to escape to the top surface.

For preparative gels, do not use strip tray and put the IPG strip directly onto the glass.

6. Withdraw the rehydration buffer using the attached syringe and carefully dismantle the Reswelling Cassette. Work quickly to avoid crystallization of the urea in the strips.
7. Wipe off excess buffer from the base of each gel strip and position carefully onto the strip tray, gel side uppermost with the basic end orientated to the cathode.

8. Lay the humidified electrode wicks onto the both ends of the IPG strips.
9. Slot in the electrodes onto the wicks and position the sample application wells at the cathode end.
10. Cover entirely with silicone oil just over the level of the wells (checking that they do not leak).
11. Adjust the protein concentration of the sample to be loaded with lysis buffer. The total volume of the wells is 60 µL; you may use a maximum of 200 µg protein for analytical gels (*see* **Note 4**). For preparative gels, load 1–3 mg of protein.
12. Cover and attach to a power supply which adjusts the variable voltage required automatically. The voltage must be increased linearly from 300 to 3500 V during the first 3 h, followed by 3 h at 3500 V, and the remaining time at 5000 V.

The total voltage hours should be 100 kVh for analytical gels (and 400 kVh for preparative gels). The number of milliamperes must be between 0.1–0.2; if not, it indicates a problem with the strip (*see* **Table 1**).

3.3. Equilibration

1. Check the total number of hours that the first dimension gel has run.
2. When completed, disconnect the power supply and the water bath.
3. Remove the plastic wells and lift off the glass assembly from the base plate.
4. Pour off as much of the silicone oil as possible and wipe off residual kerosene from the base (*see* **Note 5**).
5. Strips must be equilibrated before loading onto the second-dimension gel. Remove the sample wells (but not the electrodes) and incubate the strips in the assembly first in Equilibration Buffer A for 10 min, then Equilibration Buffer B for 5 min.

3.4. The Second Dimension

This is a vertical gradient (9–16%) slab gel about 1.5-mm thick (*see* **Table 2**). A multigel electrophoretic system allowing four to eight gels to be run at a time, is used. This improves reproducibility and speed.

This protocol developed by Professor Hochstrasser's group *(3,9)* uses piperazine diacrylyl (PDA) with acrylamide instead of the more conventionally used bisacrylamide. It is thought that this reduces N-terminal protein blockage and gives better protein resolution. The addition of thiosulfate reduces backgrounds during silver staining. The gels are not polymerized in the presence of SDS, but the SDS in the running buffer is sufficient to maintain the necessary negative charge. They have found that this prevents the formation of micelles containing acrylamide monomer, thereby increasing the homogeneity of pore size and reducing the concentration of unpolymerized monomer in the polyacrylamide.

Because multigel systems use a great deal of lower chamber buffer, it is recommended to reuse only up to 3 wk. The inclusion of azide prevents the growth of bacteria and other contaminants.

Table 1
First-Dimension Gel Electrophoresis

	Analytical gels		Preparative gels	
Program	Volts	Hours	Volts	Hours
1	350	0.5	350	0.5
2	450	0.5	450	0.5
3	800	0.5	800	0.5
4	1250	0.5	1250	0.5
5	1700	0.5	1700	0.5
6	2150	0.5	2150	0.5
7	2600	0.5	2600	0.5
8	3050	0.5	3050	0.5
9	3500	0.5	3500	0.5
10	5000	19	5000	80
	Vh: 100,000		Vh: 400,000	

Table 2
For Four 8–16% Gradient Gels[a]

	9%	16%
1.5 M Tris-HCl, pH 8.8 (mL)	31.34	31.34
Acryl/PDA 30%/0.8% (mL)	35.82	69.66
Water (mL)	56.63	22.79
Sodium thiosulfate 5% (mL)	0.66	0.66
TEMED (µL)	50	50
APS 10% (µL)	500	500

[a]These are for single (not double) gels made in the PROTEAN II XI Multigel Casting Chamber, (Bio-Rad). Double gels are also possible but resolution is often not as good.

1. Assemble the second-dimension tank. Cast gradient gels carefully to about 1.5 cm from the top, using the appropriate equipment and being careful to avoid disruption of the gradient by bubbles.
2. Overlay with sec-butanol and leave for about 2–3 h before washing off with deionized water.
3. Disassemble the remainder of the first-dimension apparatus.
4. Remove the electrodes and the wicks carefully, and gently draw the base of each strip over absorbent tissue to remove excess buffer.
5. Trim the ends off the gel strip, about 7 mm from the anode end and 15 mm from the cathode end. For preparative gels, trim off the extra width from the sample end also.
6. Fill the top of the gel with warmed agarose solution (at about 75°C), and load the strip so it makes contact with the interface (preferably with the gel side facing out).

Remove bubbles. Contact with the interface will not be exact but the proteins will migrate through the agarose.

7. Allow to migrate: 40 mA/gel for about 4.5 h (or until the dye front reaches the end) at 15°C.
8. Upon completion gels may be silver stained.

3.5. Ammoniacal Silver Staining for Analytical 2-D Gels

Always use gloves and rinse off powder whenever touching gels. All staining is done with constant gentle agitation, preferably inside a fume cabinet. Ethanol used throughout is absolute ethanol. Preparative gels are NOT silver stained if they are to be used for microsequencing.

1. After migration of the second dimension, disassemble plates and cut off the top 5 mm of the resolving gel—ensuring all agarose is removed.
2. Wash the gels in water for about 5–10 min to remove SDS.
3. In a plastic tray (four gels/tray) with cover, incubate the gels in Fixative A for 1 h.
4. Incubate the gels (four gels/tray) covered, for 1 h (or maximum overnight) in Fixative B.
5. Rinse in water for about 5 min.

After this point it is essential to use glass trays. Agarose left on the gel at this stage will stick to the glass and tear the gel.

6. Incubate the gels for 30 min in the glutaraldehyde solution (700 mL/four gels).
7. Rinse the gels with water three times for 10 min each rinse.
8. Incubate the gels two times for 30 min each in NDS solution (700 mL/four gels).
9. Rinse the gels in wate four times for 15 min each.
10. Incubate for 30 min in the silver solution.
11. Rinse the gels in water five times for 5 min each.
12. Develop in fresh glass trays: one gel at a time. 500 mL of developer solution is sufficient for two gels. Any acetic acid that gets into the developer will stop the reaction.
13. When the spots are clearly visible, remove to the stop solution. This will cause the spots to darken somewhat. The stop solution may need to be changed if it begins to change color.
14. To maintain stability, store gels in the storage solution and scan or photograph as soon as possible. For long-term storage, seal wet in plastic bags or dry between acetate sheets.

3.6. Scanning

The gels must be scanned as soon as possible after staining to avoid possible deterioration of the quality of the stain, loss of resolution, or the appearance of artifactual spots. It is best to use a laser densitometer for scanning. Two devices that have been shown to be adequate are Molecular Dynamics Laser Densitometer (4000 × 5000 pixels, 12 bits/ pixel) and the GS-700 from Bio-Rad. The size of the gels and the high resolution required for imaging means that the resulting scanned images maybe quite large, up to 10–15 MB and adequate data storage facilities are therefore essential.

3.7. Image Analysis

There are several programs now commercially available for the computerized analysis of 2-D PAGE images. The Melanie II program developed in Geneva by Hochstrasser's group is now marketed by Bio-Rad and supports UNIX, Macintosh, and PC platforms. The main features of this program are that it combines algorithms, which facilitate spot detection, gel alignment, and matching, and differential and statistical analyses. Unlike some other commercially available programs, it is also capable of interfacing and utilizing information available on compatible internet-linked 2-D databases.

3.8. Limitations of the Study

The ability of the 2-D technique to analyze complicated or highly variable samples is limited. This would restrict its use, for example, in epidemiological studies using human vascular samples, but is likely to be of more use in studies using animal models or established transformed SMC lines. In these situations the variability between samples is potentially smaller, conditions for preparation of samples are more controllable, and large amounts of sample needed for generating high quality reproducible 2-D maps are possible.

3.9. Preparative Gels

Preparative gels are used to facilitate identification and characterization of the proteins of interest by generating enough protein material to transfer onto PVDF membrane and to microsequence. The same sample as for analytical analysis is used, and the first and second dimensions are essentially identical as those described above with the slight modifications indicated. After proteins have been separated on the two dimensions, the preparative gel is blotted onto PVDF membrane. This can be carried out using any of the conventional methods available *(10)*. The most widely used methods use either semidry or (wet) vertical tank electrophoretic transfer systems with either Towbin's transfer buffer or CAPS transfer buffer, which contains no glycine. For highly expressed proteins, spots stained with Coomassie blue may be excised directly from the gel for microsequencing.

3.9.1. Electrophoretic Transfer to PVDF Membrane (for Protein Microsequencing)

1. Wet the membrane (PVDF) in Met-OH HPLC for 1 min.
2. Equilibrate in transfer buffer (dilute Towbin 1:2 in water or full strength CAPS buffer), for 30 min (minimum*).*

3. After the migration of the second dimension, wash the gel in water for 5 min and equilibrate in the Transfer buffer (Towbin diluted 1:2 in water or full strength CAPS buffer) for 20 min. It is useful to rinse all the filter paper to be used in transfer buffer also.
4. Assemble blot and transfer at 90 V for about 1 h, then 35 V overnight, at 8°C.
5. Incubate in amido black stain for about 2–5 min.
6. Wash twice for 5 min each in water.

3.9.2. Electrophoretic Transfer to PVDF Membrane (for Determining the Amino Acid Composition).

A standard reference must be included: BSA fraction V without lipid dissolved in water. Load 20 mg.

1. Wash the membrane (PVDF) in a 30% (w/v) SDS solution for 5 min and equilibrate in the CAPS transfer buffer.
2. After the migration of the second dimension, wash the gel in water for 5 min.
3. Equilibrate the gel in CAPS transfer buffer for 20 min. It is useful to rinse all the filter paper to be used in transfer buffer also.
4. Assemble blot and transfer at 90 V for about 1 h, then 35 V overnight, at 8°C.
5. Stain for 2–5 min.
6. Wash (twice for 5 min each) in deionized water.

3.10. Protein Identification

After selecting differentially-expressed spots by image analysis, the proteins of interest can be identified. Protein spots obtained by preparative gel electophoresis and blotting that are visible after amido black staining (indicating sufficient protein content [approx 1–2 pmol]) are excised. N-terminal sequence determination can be achieved by the Edman degradation technique *(11)*. For proteins that are N-terminally-blocked other methods can be used. First, proteins can be cleaved by proteolytic enzymes to produce internal peptides that can be subjected to the Edman degradation *(12)*. Second, proteins can be identified by their amino acid composition in conjunction with their pI and molecular mass estimated from 2-D gels *(13)*. These data are then matched with the corresponding theoretical values of proteins present in databases. Finally, a rapid protein identification method was recently presented. A three to four amino acid N-terminal "sequence tag" is generated by Edman degradation, and the same sample is then subjected to amino acid composition analysis *(14)*. The combination of these two methods increases the accuracy of protein identification. Another technique that uses peptide mass fingerprinting has recently been described *(15,16)*.

3.11. Internet Tools

Many proteins have been identified by the 2-D PAGE technique in different tissues, cell lines, and species. Access to these data is available on the ExPASy

World Wide Web (WWW) molecular biology server from the Swiss Institute of Bioinformatics (SIB, *17*). The database called SWISS-2-DPAGE (http://expasy.hcuge.ch/ch2d/) provides 2-D PAGE maps as well as links to other related databases. Despite the fact that no SMC 2-D PAGE maps are available on these databases, there are others that can help to identify SMC proteins (such as fibroblast and muscle maps) or that are of interest in the field of cardiovascular disease (such as platelet, heart, macrophage, and endothelial cell maps). Some internet sites containing 2-D PAGE maps of these cells are listed below.

- Rat and human heart 2-D PAGE (http://gelmatching.inf.fu-berlin.de/~pleiss/2d/ *and* http://gelmatching.inf.fu-berlin.de/~pleiss/dhzb.html).
- MRC-5 Fibroblasts, Adult human fibroblasts and endothelial cells, lymphocytes, muscle (http://biosun.biobase.dk/~pdi/2Dgallery/2Dgallery_java.html#i_h_cult).
- Kidney, liver, platelet, macrophage-like-cell line (http://expasy.hcuge.ch/cgi-bin/map1).

3.12. Examples

Finally, we give examples of two SMC proteins, the cellular retinol binding protein-1 (CRBP-1) and the cytokeratin 8 (CK8), that were recently identified in particular rat SMC phenotypes *(4,5)*. Two representative analytical 2-D gels of aged and newborn rat SMC isolated from the aorta are given in **Fig. 2** (the figure captions are those of the publication of Cremona et al.—courtesy of Experimental Cell Research, Academic Press, 6277 Sea Harbor Drive, Orlando, FL 32887). The spots no. 859 and no. 394 have been microsequenced and identified as the CRBP-1 and the CK8. The entries in the SWISS-PROT database are presented in **Figs. 3A** and **B**. The CRBP-1 was not previously identified in the mouse and human 2-D PAGE maps available, but an estimated location of the protein obtained according to the computed protein's pI and molecular mass can be visualized (**Fig. 4A**). In contrast, the CK8 was identified in the mouse liver 2-D PAGE map and the location of the spot is indicated as well as a region likely to contain CK8 from other species according to the variation in molecular mass and pI (**Fig. 4B**).

3.13. Troubleshooting Guide

1. Horizontal Streaks. This may be due to incomplete isoelectric focusing (IEF)—either the migration time was not sufficient or there was protein precipitation prior to or during the IEF run. Check that samples are loaded at the cathode end, that sample solubilization is complete (centrifuge to pellet any remaining particulates) and ensure that the voltage increments are accurate.
2. Vertical Streaks. Often caused by excess water left in the electrode wicks—blot well between absorbent tissue before use. This may also be caused by continuous solubilization of protein aggregates during the second dimension migration.

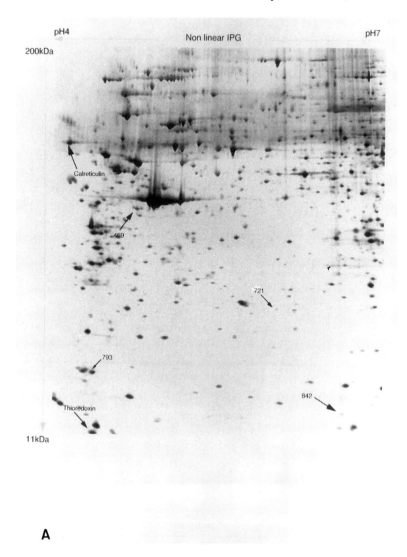

A

Fig. 2. Silver-stained 2-D PAGE map of newborn (**A**) and aged (**B**) rat aortic SMC. Differentially expressed spots are highlighted together with calreticulin and thioredoxin.

3. Horizontal Spot Elongation. Generally due to poor contact of the IPG strips with the second-dimension gel interface. Ensure that the IPG gel strips are cut in a straight line and that the SDS-PAGE interface has polymerized horizontally.

4. Vertical Spot Elongation. This could be due to oxidation of DTE during the first dimension migration.

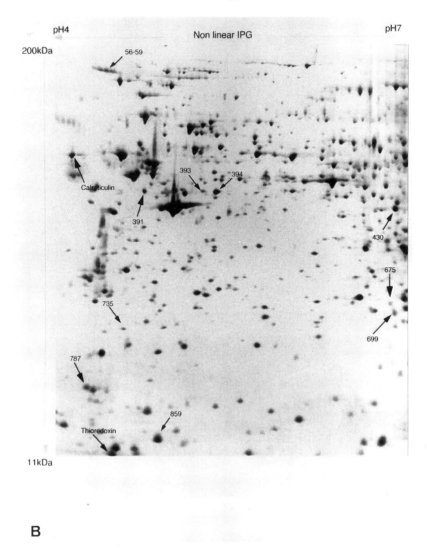

B

Fig. 2B.

5. Highly Diffuse Spots. This could be caused by a number of different reasons, such as sample overloading in the first dimension. In the second dimension, placing a magnetic flea at the bottom of the electrophoresis tank, improving buffer recirculation may reduce insufficient heat exchange causing a temperature gradient through the gel. If you are running "double gels," switch to "single" gels. Do not apply more than 40 mA per gel. Check that the gel cassettes are assembled correctly as the upper chamber buffer may leak, disrupting the flow of current. This increases the current to the other gels in the tank.

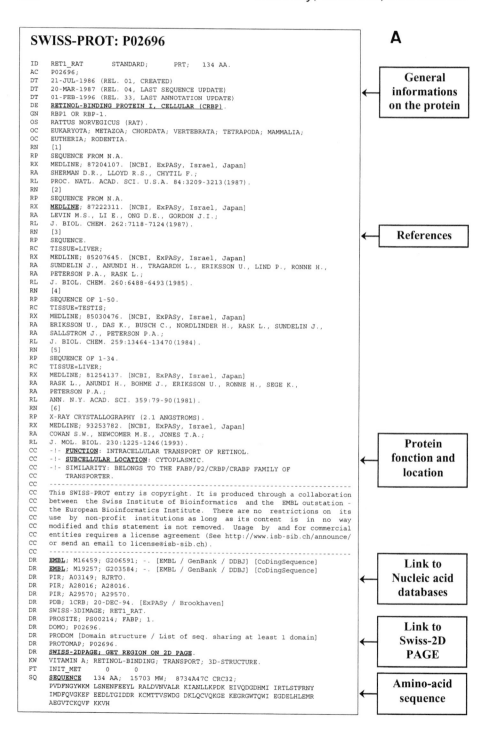

SWISS-PROT: P02696   **A**

```
ID   RET1_RAT        STANDARD;     PRT;    134 AA.
AC   P02696;
DT   21-JUL-1986 (REL. 01, CREATED)
DT   20-MAR-1987 (REL. 04, LAST SEQUENCE UPDATE)
DT   01-FEB-1996 (REL. 33, LAST ANNOTATION UPDATE)
DE   RETINOL-BINDING PROTEIN I, CELLULAR (CRBP).
GN   RBP1 OR RBP-1.
OS   RATTUS NORVEGICUS (RAT).
OC   EUKARYOTA; METAZOA; CHORDATA; VERTEBRATA; TETRAPODA; MAMMALIA;
OC   EUTHERIA; RODENTIA.
RN   [1]
RP   SEQUENCE FROM N.A.
RX   MEDLINE; 87204107. [NCBI, ExPASy, Israel, Japan]
RA   SHERMAN D.R., LLOYD R.S., CHYTIL F.;
RL   PROC. NATL. ACAD. SCI. U.S.A. 84:3209-3213(1987).
RN   [2]
RP   SEQUENCE FROM N.A.
RX   MEDLINE; 87222311. [NCBI, ExPASy, Israel, Japan]
RA   LEVIN M.S., LI E., ONG D.E., GORDON J.I.;
RL   J. BIOL. CHEM. 262:7118-7124(1987).
RN   [3]
RP   SEQUENCE.
RC   TISSUE=LIVER;
RX   MEDLINE; 85207645. [NCBI, ExPASy, Israel, Japan]
RA   SUNDELIN J., ANUNDI H., TRAGARDH L., ERIKSSON U., LIND P., RONNE H.,
RA   PETERSON P.A., RASK L.;
RL   J. BIOL. CHEM. 260:6488-6493(1985).
RN   [4]
RP   SEQUENCE OF 1-50.
RC   TISSUE=TESTIS;
RX   MEDLINE; 85030476. [NCBI, ExPASy, Israel, Japan]
RA   ERIKSSON U., DAS K., BUSCH C., NORDLINDER H., RASK L., SUNDELIN J.,
RA   SALLSTROM J., PETERSON P.A.;
RL   J. BIOL. CHEM. 259:13464-13470(1984).
RN   [5]
RP   SEQUENCE OF 1-34.
RC   TISSUE=LIVER;
RX   MEDLINE; 81254137. [NCBI, ExPASy, Israel, Japan]
RA   RASK L., ANUNDI H., BOHME J., ERIKSSON U., RONNE H., SEGE K.,
RA   PETERSON P.A.;
RL   ANN. N.Y. ACAD. SCI. 359:79-90(1981).
RN   [6]
RP   X-RAY CRYSTALLOGRAPHY (2.1 ANGSTROMS).
RX   MEDLINE; 93253782. [NCBI, ExPASy, Israel, Japan]
RA   COWAN S.W., NEWCOMER M.E., JONES T.A.;
RL   J. MOL. BIOL. 230:1225-1246(1993).
CC   -!- FUNCTION: INTRACELLULAR TRANSPORT OF RETINOL.
CC   -!- SUBCELLULAR LOCATION: CYTOPLASMIC.
CC   -!- SIMILARITY: BELONGS TO THE FABP/P2/CRBP/CRABP FAMILY OF
CC       TRANSPORTER.
CC
CC   ------------------------------------------------------------------------
CC   This SWISS-PROT entry is copyright. It is produced through a collaboration
CC   between  the Swiss Institute of Bioinformatics  and the  EMBL outstation -
CC   the European Bioinformatics Institute.  There are no  restrictions on  its
CC   use  by  non-profit  institutions as long  as its content  is  in  no  way
CC   modified and this statement is not removed.  Usage  by and for commercial
CC   entities requires a license agreement (See http://www.isb-sib.ch/announce/
CC   or send an email to license@isb-sib.ch).
CC   ------------------------------------------------------------------------
DR   EMBL; M16459; G206591; -. [EMBL / GenBank / DDBJ] [CoDingSequence]
DR   EMBL; M19257; G203584; -. [EMBL / GenBank / DDBJ] [CoDingSequence]
DR   PIR; A03149; RJRTO.
DR   PIR; A28016; A28016.
DR   PIR; A29570; A29570.
DR   PDB; 1CRB; 20-DEC-94. [ExPASy / Brookhaven]
DR   SWISS-3DIMAGE; RET1_RAT.
DR   PROSITE; PS00214; FABP; 1.
DR   DOMO; P02696.
DR   PRODOM [Domain structure / List of seq. sharing at least 1 domain]
DR   PROTOMAP; P02696.
DR   SWISS-2DPAGE; GET REGION ON 2D PAGE.
KW   VITAMIN A; RETINOL-BINDING; TRANSPORT; 3D-STRUCTURE.
FT   INIT_MET       0       0
SQ   SEQUENCE   134 AA;  15703 MW;  8734A47C CRC32;
     PVDFNGYWKM LSNENFEEYL RALDVNVALR KIANLLKPDK EIVQDGDHMI IRTLSTFRNY
     IMDFQVGKEF EEDLTGIDDR KCMTTVSWDG DKLQCVQKGE KEGRGWTQWI EGDELHLEMR
     AEGVTCKQVF KKVH
```

General
informations
on the protein

References

Protein
fonction and
location

Link to
Nucleic acid
databases

Link to
Swiss-2D
PAGE

Amino-acid
sequence

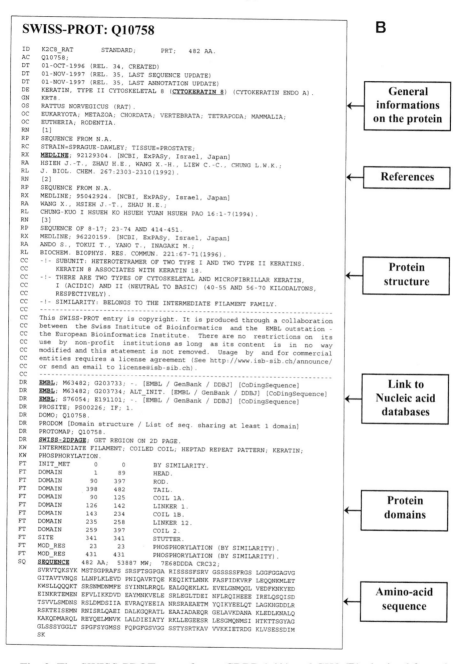

B

SWISS-PROT: Q10758

```
ID   K2C8_RAT        STANDARD;      PRT;    482 AA.
AC   Q10758;
DT   01-OCT-1996 (REL. 34, CREATED)
DT   01-NOV-1997 (REL. 35, LAST SEQUENCE UPDATE)
DT   01-NOV-1997 (REL. 35, LAST ANNOTATION UPDATE)
DE   KERATIN, TYPE II CYTOSKELETAL 8 (CYTOKERATIN 8) (CYTOKERATIN ENDO A).
GN   KRT8.
OS   RATTUS NORVEGICUS (RAT).
OC   EUKARYOTA; METAZOA; CHORDATA; VERTEBRATA; TETRAPODA; MAMMALIA;
OC   EUTHERIA; RODENTIA.
RN   [1]
RP   SEQUENCE FROM N.A.
RC   STRAIN=SPRAGUE-DAWLEY; TISSUE=PROSTATE;
RX   MEDLINE; 92129304. [NCBI, ExPASy, Israel, Japan]
RA   HSIEH J.-T., ZHAU H.E., WANG X.-H., LIEW C.-C., CHUNG L.W.K.;
RL   J. BIOL. CHEM. 267:2303-2310(1992).
RN   [2]
RP   SEQUENCE FROM N.A.
RX   MEDLINE; 95042924. [NCBI, ExPASy, Israel, Japan]
RA   WANG X., HSIEH J.-T., ZHAU H.E.;
RL   CHUNG-KUO I HSUEH KO HSUEH YUAN HSUEH PAO 16:1-7(1994).
RN   [3]
RP   SEQUENCE OF 8-17; 23-74 AND 414-451.
RX   MEDLINE; 96220159. [NCBI, ExPASy, Israel, Japan]
RA   ANDO S., TOKUI T., YANO T., INAGAKI M.;
RL   BIOCHEM. BIOPHYS. RES. COMMUN. 221:67-71(1996).
CC   -!- SUBUNIT: HETEROTETRAMER OF TWO TYPE I AND TWO TYPE II KERATINS.
CC       KERATIN 8 ASSOCIATES WITH KERATIN 18.
CC   -!- THERE ARE TWO TYPES OF CYTOSKELETAL AND MICROFIBRILLAR KERATIN,
CC       I (ACIDIC) AND II (NEUTRAL TO BASIC) (40-55 AND 56-70 KILODALTONS,
CC       RESPECTIVELY).
CC   -!- SIMILARITY: BELONGS TO THE INTERMEDIATE FILAMENT FAMILY.
CC   ---------------------------------------------------------------------
CC   This SWISS-PROT entry is copyright. It is produced through a collaboration
CC   between the Swiss Institute of Bioinformatics and the EMBL outstation -
CC   the European Bioinformatics Institute. There are no restrictions on its
CC   use by non-profit institutions as long as its content is in no way
CC   modified and this statement is not removed. Usage by and for commercial
CC   entities requires a license agreement (See http://www.isb-sib.ch/announce/
CC   or send an email to license@isb-sib.ch).
CC   ---------------------------------------------------------------------
DR   EMBL; M63482; G203733; -. [EMBL / GenBank / DDBJ] [CoDingSequence]
DR   EMBL; M63482; G203734; ALT_INIT. [EMBL / GenBank / DDBJ] [CoDingSequence]
DR   EMBL; S76054; E191101; -. [EMBL / GenBank / DDBJ] [CoDingSequence]
DR   PROSITE; PS00226; IF; 1.
DR   DOMO; Q10758.
DR   PRODOM [Domain structure / List of seq. sharing at least 1 domain]
DR   PROTOMAP; Q10758.
DR   SWISS-2DPAGE; GET REGION ON 2D PAGE.
KW   INTERMEDIATE FILAMENT; COILED COIL; HEPTAD REPEAT PATTERN; KERATIN;
KW   PHOSPHORYLATION.
FT   INIT_MET      0      0
FT   DOMAIN        1     89       HEAD.
FT   DOMAIN       90    397       ROD.
FT   DOMAIN      398    482       TAIL.
FT   DOMAIN       90    125       COIL 1A.
FT   DOMAIN      126    142       LINKER 1.
FT   DOMAIN      143    234       COIL 1B.
FT   DOMAIN      235    258       LINKER 12.
FT   DOMAIN      259    397       COIL 2.
FT   SITE        341    341       STUTTER.
FT   MOD_RES      23     23       PHOSPHORYLATION (BY SIMILARITY).
FT   MOD_RES     431    431       PHOSPHORYLATION (BY SIMILARITY).
SQ   SEQUENCE   482 AA;  53887 MW;  7E68DDDA CRC32;
     SVRVTQKSYK MSTSGPRAFS SRSFTSGPGA RISSSSFSRV GSSSSSFRGS LGGFGGAGVG
     GITAVTVNQS LLNPLKLEVD PNIQAVRTQE KEQIKTLNNK FASFIDKVRF LEQQNKMLET
     KWSLLQQQKT SRSNMDNMFE SYINNLRRQL EALGQEKLKL EVELGNMQGL VEDFKNKYED
     EINKRTEMEN EFVLIKKDVD EAYMNKVELE SRLEGLTDEI NFLRQIHEEE IRELQSQISD
     TSVVLSMDNS RSLDMDSIIA EVRAQYEEIA NRSRAEAETM YQIKYEELQT LAGKHGDDLR
     RSKTEISEMN RNISRLQAEI DALKGQRATL EAAIADAEQR GELAVKDANA KLEDLKNALQ
     KAKQDMARQL REYQELMNVK LALDIEIATY RKLLEGEESR LESGMQNMSI HTKTTSGYAG
     GLSSSYGGLT SPGFSYGMSS FQPGFGSVGG SSTYSRTKAV VVKKIETRDG KLVSESSDIM
     SK
```

General informations on the protein ←

References ←

Protein structure ←

Link to Nucleic acid databases ←

Protein domains ←

Amino-acid sequence ←

Fig. 3. The SWISS-PROT entry for rat CRBP-1 (**A**) and CK8 (**B**) obtained from the ExPASy WWW server. References and the amino-acid sequence are provided as well as links to other databases such as EMBL and GenBank for nucleic acid sequences. A link to the SWISS-2-D PAGE allows the visualisation of the spot region in other 2-D gels.

P02696:

```
Compute the theoretical pI/Mw

This protein does not exist in the current release of SWISS-2DPAGE.
```

2D PAGE maps for unidentified proteins:

```
You may obtain an estimated location of the protein on various 2D PAGE maps, provided the whole
amino acid sequence is known. The estimation is obtained
according to the computed protein's pI and Mw.

Warning 1: the displayed region reflects an area around the theoretical pI and molecular weight of
the protein and is only provided for the user's
information. It should be used with caution, as the experimental and theoretical positions of a
protein may differ significantly.
```

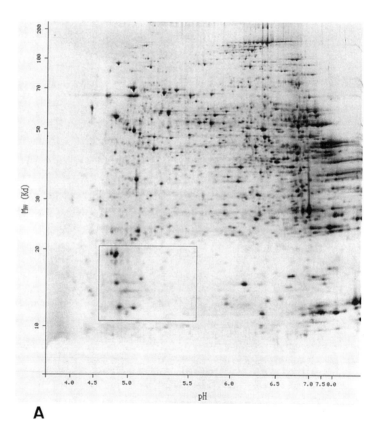

A

Fig. 4. 2-D PAGE map of mouse liver showing the estimated location of the CRBP-1 (**A**, rectangular box) and the CK8 (**B**, rectangular box). The precise position of the CK8 spot is also indicated (B, arrow).

6. Contaminants. Spurious spots ranging from 50 to 70 kD may be due to keratin proteins from skin. Ensure that gloves are worn and all powder is rinsed off when touching gels.

Q10758:

Compute the theoretical pI/Mw

This protein does not exist in the current release of SWISS-2DPAGE.

(SWISS-2D PAGE does not contain rat 2-D maps but the CK8 protein was identified in the mouse liver)

P11679:

Compute the theoretical pI/Mw

2D PAGE maps for identified proteins:

The following 2D PAGE maps are available for this protein (see how to interpret a protein map):

Mouse liver

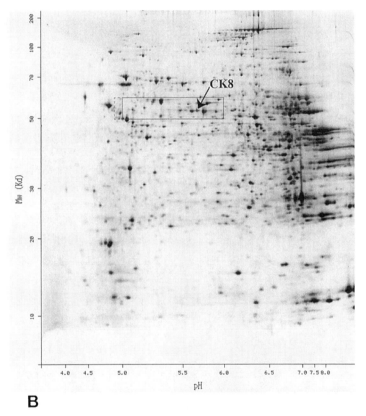

B

Fig. 4B.

7. High or Irregular Background. Poor quality water or old reagents used during the silver staining procedure.

4. Notes

1. Water. Contaminating ions and other organic substances will interfere with the IEF, the polymerization and migration of the second dimension and the subse-

quent silver staining, or electrophoretic transfer. Adequate water purification must remove as much contaminants as possible. This 2-D PAGE procedure uses large quantities of buffers and other solutions. All glassware and gel running/ preparation equipment also requires a final rinse in deionized water before use. Another consideration therefore is sufficient output without the need for long-term storage in plastic bottles, which are susceptible to bacterial and other contamination. Water quality varies widely from region to region, and it may be necessary to test various systems to determine which gives best results.

2. Chemicals. Ensure that all reagents used are "electrophoresis grade," as contaminants will reduce the quality and reproducibility of the end. Ampholytes may vary depending on supplier and batches.
3. Temperature is a critical parameter in the reproducibility of this IEF step.
4. It is advisable to do a protein titration as overloading may cause a spot to decrease rather than increase.
5. Silicone oil may be reused several times.

Acknowledgments

We are grateful to The Laboratory of Professor D Hochstrasser and Dr. RD Appel for expert advice. We thank Dr. J. C. Sanchez for critically reading this manuscript. We thank Antoine Geinoz for technical assistance, Mr. J. C. Rumbeli and Mr. E. Denkinger for photographic work, and Mrs. M. Vitali for typing the manuscript. This work was supported in part by the Swiss National Science Foundation, Grant No. 3100-50568.97. Dr. R. Johnatty is funded by a British Heart Foundation Grant (No. 96052) held jointly by Professor G. Gabbiani (Geneva) and Dr. P. Chan, Senior Clinical Lecturer, Department of Surgical Sciences, University of Sheffield Medical School, Sheffield, S5 7AU, UK.

References

1. Ross, R. (1995) Cell biology of atherosclerosis. *Annu. Rev. Physiol.* **57,** 791–804.
2. Shanahan, C. M. and Weissberg, P. L. (1998) Smooth Muscle Cell Heterogeneity. Patterns of gene expression in vascular smooth muscle cells in vitro and in vivo. *Arterioscler. Thromb. Vasc. Biol.* **18,** 333–338.
3. Bjellqvist, B., Pasquali, C., Ravier, F., Sanchez, J. C., and Hochstrasser, D. F. (1993) A nonlinear wide range immobilized pH gradient for two-dimensional electrophoresis and its definition in a relevant pH scale. *Electrophoresis* **14,** 1357–1365.
4. Cremona, O., Muda, M., Appel, R.D., Frutiger, S., Hughes, G. J., Hochstrasser, D. F., Geinoz, A., and Gabbiani, G. (1995) Differential protein expression in aortic smooth muscle cells cultured from newborn and aged rats. *Exp. Cell Res.* **217,** 280–287.
5. Neuville, P., Geinoz, A., Benzonana, G., Redard, M., Gabbiani, F., Ropraz, P., and Gabbiani, G. (1997) Cellular Retinol-Binding Protein I is expressed by distinct subsets of rat arterial smooth muscle cells in vitro and in vivo. *Am. J. Pathol.* **150,** 509–521.

6. Hoogland, C., Sanchez, J. C., Tonella, L., Bairoch, A., Hochstrasser, D. F., and Appel, R. D. (1998) Current status of the SWISS-2DPAGE database. *Nucleic Acids Res.* **26**, 332,333.

7. Rabilloud, T., Valette, C., and Lawrence, J. J. (1994) Sample application by in-gel rehydration improves the resolution of two-dimensional electrophoresis with immobilized pH gradient in the first dimension. *Electrophoresis* **15**, 1552–1558.

8. Sanchez, J. C., Rouge, V., Pisteur, M., Ravier, F., Tonella, L., Moosmayer, M., Wilkins, M. R., and Hochstrasser, D. F. (1997) Improved and simplified in-gel sample application using reswelling of dry immobilized pH gradients. *Electrophoresis* **18**, 324–327.

9. Hochstrasser, D. F., Harrington, M. G., Hochstrasser, A. C., Miller, M. J., and Merril, C .R. (1988) Methods for increasing the resolution of two-dimensional protein electrophoresis. *Anal. Biochem.* **173**, 424–435.

10. Sanchez, J. C., Ravier, F., Pasquali, C., Frutiger, S., Paquet, N., Bjellqvist, B., Hochstrasser, D. F., and Hughes, G. J. (1992) Improving the detection of proteins after transfer to polyvinylidene difluoride membranes. *Electrophoresis* **13**, 715–717.

11. Allen, G., ed. (1981) *Sequencing of Proteins and Peptides,* Elseiver Press, Amsterdam, The Netherlands.

12. Matsudaira, P. (1987) Sequence from picomole quantities of proteins electroblotted onto polyvinylidene difluoride membranes. *J. Biol. Chem.* **262**, 10,035–10,038.

13. Golaz, O., Wilkins, M. R., Sanchez, J. C., Appel, R. D., Hochstrasser, D. F., and Williams, K. L. (1996) Identification of proteins by their amino acid composition: an evaluation of the method. *Electrophoresis* **17**, 573–579.

14. Wilkins, M. R., Ou, K., Appel, R. D., Sanchez, J.C., Yan, J. X., Golaz, O., et al. (1996) Rapid protein identification using N-terminal «sequence tag» and amino acid analysis. *Biochem. Biophys. Res. Commun.* **221**, 609–613.

15. Cottrell, J. S. (1994) Protein identification by peptide mass fingerprinting. *Pept. Res.* **7**, 115–124.

16. Wilkins, M. R. and Williams, K. L. (1997) Cross-species protein identification using amino acid composition, peptide mass fingerprinting, isoelectric point and molecular mass: a theoretical evaluation. *J. Theor. Biol.* **186**, 7-15.

17. Appel, R. D., Bairoch, A., and Hochstrasser, D. F. A. (1994) New generation of information retrieval tools for biologists: the example of the ExPASy WWW server. *Trends Biochem. Sci.* **19**, 258–260.

VI

IN VITRO METHODS TO EXPRESS FOREIGN GENES IN VASCULAR CELLS

22

Simple Methods for Preparing Recombinant Adenoviruses for High-Efficiency Transduction of Vascular Cells

Stuart A. Nicklin and Andrew H. Baker

1. Introduction

Adenoviruses are icosahedral viruses 70–90 nm in diameter with a double-stranded, linear DNA genome of approx 36 kb. They are widely utilized in gene transfer protocols owing to their relative ease of genetic manipulation, ability to grow to high titres (10^9–10^{12} plaque forming units [pfu]/mL), and their ability to infect both dividing and nondividing cells efficiently. The latter reason makes them extremely suitable for investigations in vascular systems where the low proliferative indices of cells is a limiting factor for retroviral gene transfer.

In 1977 Frank Graham et al. developed the 293 cell line, a human embryonic kidney cell line transformed with the entire left-hand end of the adenovirus serotype 5 genome (1). Subsequently, a simple method was developed for derivation of recombinant adenoviruses by cotransfection of two plasmids into 293 cells (2) (**Fig. 1**).

This chapter describes simple techniques relevant to the the derivation, purification, propagation, and titration of recombinant adenoviruses, including transfection of low passage 293 cells, recombination, plaque purification, generation of pure high-titer stocks, cesium chloride (CsCl) purification, and titration by end-point dilution. The chapter will also detail characterization of recombinant adenoviruses, including immunofluorescence for E1a and infections of nonpermissive cell lines to test for contaminating replication competent adenoviruses (RCA).

From: *Methods in Molecular Medicine, Vascular Disease: Molecular Biology and Gene Therapy Protocols*
Edited by: A. H. Baker © Humana Press Inc., Totowa, NJ

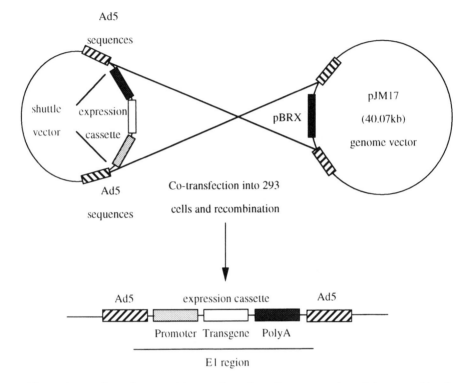

Fig. 1. Generation of a recombinant adenovirus. Representation of the recombination event which takes place in order to generate recombinant adenoviruses in low passage 293 cells. The insertion of pBRX (4.3 kB) in pJM17 exceeds the packaging limits of the adenovirus. Homologous recombination between adenoviral sequences flanking both pBRX in the genome vector and the expression cassette in the shuttle vector generates an E1 deleted, replication-deficient, recombinant adenovirus expressing the transgene.

2. Materials

2.1. Preparation of Recombinant Adenoviruses

2.1.1. Calcium-Phosphate-Mediated Transfection into Low Passage 293 Cells for Derivation of Adenoviruses

1. 10X citric saline: dissolve 100 g of potassium chloride and 44 g of sodium citrate in 100 mL of deionized water (dH$_2$O). Sterilize by autoclaving. Stable for up to 1 yr at room temperature. For a working solution, dilute the stock 10X in sterile phosphate-buffered saline (PBS). Make fresh as required.
2. 2 M CaCl$_2$: dissolve 54 g of CaCl$_2$.6H$_2$O in 100 mL of dH$_2$O. Sterilize by passage through a 0.22-mm filter and store in 1-mL aliquots at 4°C for up to 6 mo.
3. 2 X HEPES-buffered saline (2X HBS), final concentrations in parentheses: dissolve 1.6 g of NaCl (280 mM), 0.074 g of KCl (10 mM), 0.027 g of

$Na_2HPO_4.2H_2O$ (1.5 mM), 0.20 g of dextrose (12 mM) and 1 g of HEPES (50 mM) in 100 mL of dH_2O. Adjust the pH to 7.05 with 0.5 N NaOH. Store in 5-mL aliquots. Stable at 4°C for up to 6 mo.

4. T-25 cm² tissue culture flasks.
5. Tissue culture grade PBS.
6. Low passage human kidney embryonic 293 cells (Microbix, Toronto, Canada).
7. 293 cell growth media: minimal essential medium (MEM) containing 10% fetal calf serum (FCS), 2 mM L-glutamine, 100 international units (IU)/mL penicillin and 100 µg/mL streptomycin. Stable at 4°C for up to 1 mo.

2.1.2. Generation of Crude Adenovirus Stocks

1. ArkloneP (trichlorotrifluoroethane) (ICI Ltd., Cheshire, UK).

2.1.3. Plaque Purification by End-Point Dilution

1. 96-well plates.

2.1.4. Generation of Pure High Titer Stocks of Recombinant Adenoviruses

1. T-150 cm² tissue culture flasks.
2. Quick-Seal tubes (16 × 76 mm) (Beckman, CA).
3. Cordless Tube Topper (Beckman).
4. TD solution: 750 mM NaCl, 50 mM KCl, 250 mM Tris-HCl, 10 mM Na_2HPO_4, pH 7.4.
5. CsCl (density 1.34) in TD solution. Stable at room temperature for up to 6 mo.
6. CsCl (density 1.4) in TD solution. Stable at room temperature for up to 6 mo.
7. Collodion dialysis bags (Sartorius, Gottingen, Germany).
8. Dialysis buffer, final concentrations in parentheses: dissolve 27 mL of 5 M NaCl (135 mM), 10 mL of 1 M Tris-HCl, pH 7.5 (10 mM), and 0.5 mL of 2 M $MgCl_2$ (1 mM) in 1000 mL dH_2O. Sterilize all reagents separately by autoclaving. Make fresh as required.
9. Dialysis buffer with 10% glycerol: as dialysis buffer (900 mL) above plus 100 mL of sterile autoclaved glycerol. Make fresh as required.

2.2. Assays for Replication Competent Adenoviruses

2.2.1. Infections in Nonpermissive Cells

1. HeLa cells (European Collection of Animal Cell Cultures, Salisbury, UK).
2. Growth media for HeLa cells: MEM containing 10% FCS, 2 mM L-glutamine, 100 IU/mL penicillin, and 100 µg/mL streptomycin. Stable at 4°C for up to 1 mo.

2.2.2. Immunofluorescent Cytochemistry for Adenovirus Type 5 E1a

1. Anti-E1a antibody: clone M73 (Calbiochem-Novabiochem, Nottingham, UK). Stable at 4°C for up to 1 yr.
2. Fluorescein-isothiocyanate (FITC)-conjugated F(ab')₂ fragment of goat-anti-mouse immunoglobulins (IgG): clone F 0479 (Dako, UK). Stable at 4°C for up to 1 yr.

3. Vectashield (Vector Laboratories, Inc., Burlingame, CA). Stable at 4°C for up to 1 yr.
4. 1% formalin: add 2.5 mL of 40% formaldehyde to 97.5 mL of PBS. Stable at room temperature for up to 1 yr.
5. 0.1% Triton-X-100 (Sigma, Dorset, UK): add 0.1 mL of Triton-X-100 to 99.9 mL of PBS. Stable at room temperature for up to 1 yr.

3. Methods

3.1. Preparation of Recombinant Adenoviruses

3.1.1. Calcium-Phosphate-Mediated Transfection into Low Passage 293 Cells for Derivation of Adenoviruses

The first stage in the production of a recombinant adenovirus is the recombination event itself, in low passage 293 cells. We have generated a number of novel recombinant adenoviruses following calcium-phosphate-mediated transfection into 293 cells *(3,4)*. This method produces a transfection efficiency of approx 40%. In our experience this produces lower cytotoxicity in comparison to liposome mediated transfection.

1. Subculture low passage 293 cells (<P40) into T-25 tissue culture flasks, three per proposed recombination (*see* **Note 1**). Seed each flask with 2×10^6 cells so that they reach approx 70–80% confluence the following day. It is important that the cells are in mid-log phase for optimum transfection efficiency.
2. Premix 5 µg of genome vector DNA and 5 µg shuttle vector DNA (*see* **Notes 2** and **3**) in a sterile polypropylene tube and add deionized water to 180 µL.
3. Slowly add 30 µL of 2 M CaCl$_2$ to the DNA solution drop-wise whilst vortexing vigorously.
4. Add this mixture drop-wise to another tube containing 240 µL 2X HBS while vortexing at medium speed (*see* **Notes 4** and **5**).
5. Allow the precipitate to form over 30 min. Immediately prior to the addition of the precipitate, wash the cells in complete media and add 4.55 mL of fresh, prewarmed media.
6. Add the precipitate drop-wise to the cells. Swirl the media gently around the flask every few drops in order to disperse the precipitate evenly. Incubate the cells at 37°C in 5% CO_2 for 4–24 h (*see* **Note 6**).
7. Gently wash the cells twice with prewarmed PBS and then add 5 mL of fresh, prewarmed media. Replace the media every 2–3 d or when acidity is evident (*see* **Note 7**).

3.1.2. Generation of Crude Adenovirus Stocks

Once a recombination has taken place and a plaque has been observed (*see* **Fig. 2**), allow the cytopathic effect to spread throughout the monolayer of 293 cells. Because adenovirus has no release mechanism from infected cells, approx 90% will remain within the cell. Therefore, a simple extraction with a

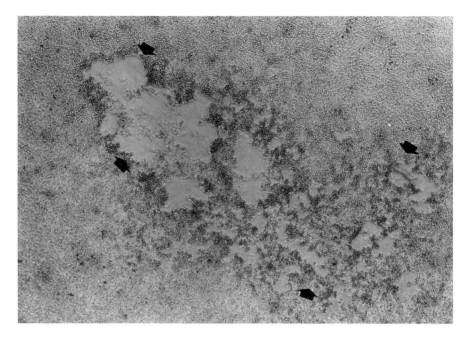

Fig. 2. Recombinant adenoviral plaque. Arrows indicate the boundaries of the plaque generated within a monolayer of 293 cells.

commercial solvent such as ArkloneP, or three cycles of freeze/thawing at –80°C will release the adenovirus.

1. Collect the media containing the cells into a Falcon tube. Wash the flask with 5 mL of media and pool. Pellet the cells in a sealed container at 250*g* for 10 min at room temperature.
2. Decant the media and resuspend the pellet in 1 mL of sterile PBS. Add an equal volume of ArkloneP, then invert the tube for 10 s followed by shaking (not too vigorously) for 5 s. Repeat the mixing step (*see* **Note 8**).
3. Centrifuge the tube at 750*g* for 15 min at room temperature. The tube will now contain three layers, the lower layer is solvent, the middle darker layer contains cellular debris, and the top layer is an aqueous solution containing the adenovirus.
4. Remove the adenovirus with a pipet, taking care not to disturb the layer of cellular debris, and store in sterile Eppendorfs in 50-µL aliquots at –80°C (*see* **Note 9**). This crude preparation of adenovirus is suitable for initial investigations to determine whether the transgene is expressed and for the extraction of DNA for polymerase chain reaction analysis and Southern blot analysis.

3.1.3. Plaque Purification by End-Point Dilution

During calcium-phosphate-mediated transfection into 293 cells, plaques may arise as a result of multiple recombination events. It is important to have pure

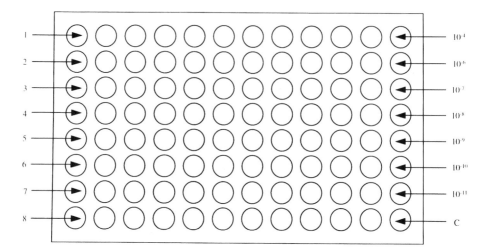

Fig. 3. Layout of a 96 well plate for plaque purification and titering by end point dilution. The left-hand column represents row numbers as per **Table 1** and the numbers in the right-hand column represent adenoviral dilutions. Cells are subcultured into the middle 80 wells, and adenovirus is added to 10 wells on each row at the appropriate dilutions. C = control (media only).

stocks of adenovirus, i.e., stocks which have been generated by the multiplication of a single adenovirus. We utilize a simple method of plaque purification by serial dilution of the crude stock onto 293 cells. This method is an alternative method to that described by Graham et al. and the cells do not require an agarose overlay *(5)*.

1. Subculture low passage 293 cells into a 96-well plate (80 wells in 8 rows of 10) (see **Fig. 3**) in order to achieve 50–60 % confluence the following day (*see* **Note 10**).
2. Prepare serial dilutions of adenovirus from the crude stock as per **Table 1**.
3. Beginning at row 8, replace the media with 100 μL of fresh media. Next replace the media in row 7 with the correct adenoviral dilution, followed by row 6 and so on. Under aseptic conditions and starting with the control wells and working through to the higher concentrations of adenovirus, the same tip can be used for all wells.
4. Incubate the plate in a humidified chamber for 16–18 h at 37°C in 5% CO_2.
5. Replace the media with 200 μL of fresh complete media (*see* **Note 11**).
6. Replace the media every 2–3 d for 8 d. Once the cytopathic effect is apparent in a well, mark it and stop replacing the media in that well. On the seventh day, prepare another 96-well plate as previously described, for a second round of plaque purification. Once the assay is complete collect the cells and media from three positive wells at the highest dilution for which the cytopathic effect is apparent. Collect them by pipeting up and down three times and then store them in sterile Eppendorfs. These plaques will have arisen from a single adenovirus,

Table 1
Preparation of Serial Dilutions of Adenovirus for Plaque Purification and End-Point Dilution[a]

Row on plate	Final dilution of virus	Volume of virus (μL)	Volume of media (μL)
—	10^{-2}	50 stock	4950
1	10^{-4}	50 @ 10^{-2}	4950
2	10^{-6}	50 @ 10^{-4}	4950
3	10^{-7}	500 @ 10^{-6}	4500
4	10^{-8}	500 @ 10^{-7}	4500
5	10^{-9}	500 @ 10^{-8}	4500
6	10^{-10}	500 @ 10^{-9}	4500
7	10^{-11}	500 @ 10^{-10}	4500

[a]Adenovirus at appropriate dilution is added to 10 wells on the appropriate row as per **Fig. 3.**

therefore freeze two of the samples and extract the other by either two cycles of freeze/thawing or with an equal volume of ArkloneP.

7. Take 50 μL of this adenovirus stock and repeat the plaque purification assay with the plate prepared on d 7. At this point plaques taken from the highest dilutions on the next plate can be considered plaque pure.

3.1.4. Generation of Pure High-Titer Stocks of Recombinant Adenoviruses

High-titer stocks of recombinant adenoviruses are generated by large scale multiplication of the initial pure recombinant in 293 cells. The cytopathic effect of the adenovirus in these permissive cells causes them to detach from the tissue culture flask allowing them to be collected easily.

1. Subculture low passage 293 cells into 30X T-150 tissue culture flasks. As a rule of thumb, one confluent T-150 flask can be split into 20 T-150 flasks for infection after approx 1 wk.
2. Once cells have reached 80–90% confluence, they can be infected with a multiplicity of infection (MOI) of 0.1–10 per flask (*see* **Notes 12** and **13**).
3. Change the media every 3 d until the cytopathic effect begins and the cells start to detach from the flask. After this if the cells need to be fed before the cytopathic effect is complete, then add an additional 10–15 mL complete media to each flask.
4. Once the cytopathic effect is complete, collect the cells immediately as prolonged incubation of detached cells will result in a decrease in titer of the adenovirus. Centrifuge in sterile Falcon tubes at 250*g* for 10 min at room temperature.
5. Decant the supernatant to waste and resuspend cells in a total volume of 12–15 mL of PBS. Add an equal volume of ArkloneP, then invert the tube for 10 s followed by shaking (not to vigorously) for 5 s. Repeat the mixing step (*see* **Note 8**). Centrifuge the tube at 750*g* for 15 min at room temperature.

6. Remove the top layer containing the adenovirus to a fresh tube, taking care not to disturb the lower layers.

7. Add a further 10 mL of PBS to the remaining solvent and cell debris and repeat the extraction. Add the upper layer to the adenovirus already extracted. The adenoviral stocks can be immediately purified on a CsCl gradient or stored at –80°C.

Freeze/thawing and ArkloneP extraction are crude methods for adenovirus extraction and preparations are contaminated with cellular proteins which may be cytotoxic in vitro and in vivo. Centrifugation on CsCl density gradients provides an efficient and simple method for both concentrating and purifying stocks of recombinant adenoviruses.

8. Sterilize ultracentrifuge tubes by rinsing with 70% ethanol followed by sterile water.

9. Pipet 3 mL of CsCl (density 1.34) into a sterile ultracentrifuge tube. Underlay this with 1.6 mL of CsCl (density 1.4) using a sterile glass pipet (*see* **Note 14**). Put the pipette to the bottom of the tube and release the CsCl gently with even pressure so that the layers do not mix.

10. Lay the crude adenovirus preparation on top of the gradient drop-wise using a sterile glass pipet. If necessary, top the tubes up with either PBS or dialysis buffer depending upon the constitution of the viral solution.

11. Centrifuge at 90,000*g* for 2 h at 18°C with zero deceleration.

12. At the end of the centrifugation step, the recombinant adenovirus presents as a discrete white layer between the two CsCl layers (see **Fig. 4**) (*see* **Note 15**). Using a 21-gauge needle pierce the top of the tube several times. Take a fresh needle and a 1.5-mL syringe and gently pierce the side of the tube just underneath the adenovirus band, with a gentle side to side sweeping motion collect the adeno-virus into the syringe without collecting to much of the solution (*see* **Note 16**).

13. Dilute the virus solution in two volumes of PBS and layer onto a preformed gradient (1.5 mL of CsCl [density 1.34] underlayed with 1 mL of CsCl [density 1.4]).

14. Centrifuge at 100,000*g* for 18 h.

15. Remove the adenovirus band (**step 12**) formed at density 1.34–1.35.

16. Dialyze the adenovirus in the Collodion dialysis bag for 2 h against 1000 mL dialysis buffer in a sterile beaker on a magnetic stirrer.

17. Repeat **step 16** with fresh dialysis buffer.

18. Dialyze the adenovirus for at least a further 2 h (or preferably overnight) against 1000 mL of fresh dialysis buffer containing 10% glycerol. Aliquot the adenoviral stocks and store them at –80°C.

3.1.5. Titration of Adenovirus by End-Point Dilution

Once recombinant adenovirus has been purified on a CsCl gradient it can be titered by serial dilution on 293 cells as per **Subheading 3.1.3.**

1. Subculture low passage 293 cells into 80 wells of a 96-well plate as laid out in **Fig. 2** for approx 50–60% confluence after 24 h (*see* **Note 10**).

2. Make serial dilutions of the adenovirus in complete media as per **Table 1**.

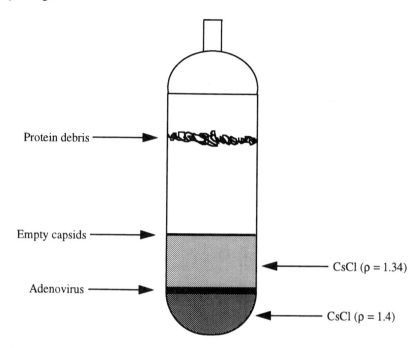

Protein debris

Empty capsids

CsCl (ρ = 1.34)

Adenovirus

CsCl (ρ = 1.4)

Fig. 4. CsCl gradient for purifying recombinant adenoviruses. Schematic representation of a CsCl gradient after centrifugation. The two shaded areas represent the different densities of CsCl. The recombinant adenovirus lies as a layer between them. The band above this represents empty capsids. The cellular protein debris (which sometimes smears down the side of the tube) sits above the other two bands.

3. Add 100 μL of each adenovirus dilution to the appropriate wells and incubate for 16–18 h at 37°C in 5% CO_2.
4. After 18 h, replace the media containing the adenovirus with 200 μL fresh complete media and incubate at 37°C in 5% CO_2 (*see* **Note 11**). Change the media every 2–3 d or when acidity shows. Once the cytopathic effect is apparent in a well mark it and stop replacing the media in that well.
5. After 8 d incubation, count the number of wells containing plaques and fit the results into the equation below in order to obtain the titer of the adenoviral stocks in pfu/mL (**6**).
6. The proportionate distance equals

$$\frac{\% \text{ positive above } 50 - 50\%}{\% \text{ positive above } 50\% - \text{ positive below } 50\%}$$

$\log ID_{50}$ (infectivity dose) = log dilution above 50% + (proportionate distance $\times$ dilution factor)

For example: titration gives

@ 10^{-4} all wells positive 10/10

@ 10^{-6} 10/10

@ 10^{-7} 10/10

@ 10^{-8} 9/10

@ 10^{-9} 3/10

@ 10^{-10} 0/10

@ 10^{-11} 0/10

$$\text{The proportionate distance} = \frac{90 - 50}{90 - 30} = 0.67$$

$$\log \text{ID}_{50} = -8 + (0.67 \times -1) = -8.67$$

$$\text{ID}_{50} = 10^{-8.67}$$

$$\text{TCID}_{50} \text{ (tissue culture infectivity dose 50)} = \frac{1}{10^{-8.67}}$$

$\text{TCID}_{50} / 100\ \mu L = 10^{8.67} \times$ dilution factor [Multiply by 10 to account for initial dilution of viral stock]

$\text{TCID}_{50} / \text{mL} = 10^{9.67}$ which is equivalent to $6.7 \times 10^{9}\ \text{TCID}_{50}/\text{mL}$

but

$1\ \text{TCID}_{50} \simeq 0.7\ \text{pfu},$

therefore,

Final titer $= 4.7 \times 10^{9}\ \text{pfu/mL}$

3.2. Assays for Replication Competent Adenoviruses

3.2.1. Infection in Nonpermissive Cells

The 293 cell line contains adenovirus type 5 sequences that are homologous with sequences in pJM17; therefore it is possible that RCA may contaminate stocks of recombinant adenoviruses. Stocks of recombinant adenoviruses can be tested in nonpermissive cell lines such as HeLa.

1. Subculture HeLa cells into 80 wells of a 96-well plate as per **Fig. 3**. Aim for 50–60% confluence the following day.
2. Prepare serial dilutions of the adenoviral stocks as per **Table 1**. Replace the media in row 8 with fresh media. Replace the media in rows 1–7 with 100 µL of the appropriate adenoviral dilution (starting at the highest dilution and working through to the lowest using the same tip) and incubate overnight at 37°C in 5% CO_2.
3. The following day replace the media in all the wells with 200 µL of fresh media. Change the media every 2–3 d or when acidity is apparent (*see* **Note 11**).
4. Incubate the plate for 8 d at 37°C in 5% CO_2 and observe any cytopathic effect that occurs. If after 8 d no cytopathology is apparent, recombinant adenoviral stocks can be assumed to be free of RCA.

3.2.2. Immunofluorescent Cytochemistry for Adenovirus Type 5 E1a

1. Prepare Hela cells and 293 cells the day before infection. Subculture 2×10^5 cells/well onto sterile coverslips in 6-well plates (*see* **Note 17**)
2. The following day infect the HeLa cells with 80 pfu/cell of recombinant adenoviruses for 16–18 h (*see* **Note 18**). The following steps are for both the HeLa cells and the 293 cells.
3. Wash the cells twice gently with PBS, for 5 min per wash at room temperature using a plastic Pasteur pipet.
4. Fix the cells in 1% formalin in PBS for 10 min at room temperature.
5. Wash the cells twice with PBS, for 5 minutes per wash.
6. Permeabilize the cells in 0.1% Triton-X-100 for 30 min at room temperature.
7. Wash the cells three times in PBS, for 5 min per wash at room temperature.
8. All antibodies are diluted in PBS and blocked in 20% goat serum. Make a 1/25 dilution of anti-E1a. Incubate the cells for 60 min with the primary antibody, or the appropriate isotype matched control (mouse IgG).
9. Wash the cells in PBS three times, for 5 minutes per wash at room temperature.
10. Make a 1/200 dilution of goat-anti-mouse IgG FITC-conjugate. Incubate the cells for 60 min with the secondary antibody.
11. Wash the cells in PBS three times, for 5 min per wash at room temperature (*see* **Note 19**).
12. Mount each cover slip in Vectashield. Seal the coverslip to the slide using clear nail varnish at each corner. The 293 cells will be E1a positive while HeLa cells infected with recombinant adenoviruses will be E1a negative, assuming no RCA are present.

4. Notes

1. Standard trypsinisation procedures for subculturing low passage 293 cells are too harsh. An alternative procedure is to subculture them in 1X citric saline. Briefly, for a T-150 flask make 50 mL of 1X citric saline (in PBS), wash the cells with 25 mL and decant to waste, wash the cells with a further 25 mL and leave approx 2 mL on the cells. Leave the flask at room temperature until the cells detach, add 10 mL of media and pipet the cells up and down to avoid clumping. Cells can be

counted and subcultured at this point, they do not require pelleting and resuspending in fresh media.

2. For assessing the transfection efficiency into 293 cells, a plasmid containing β-galactosidase can be substituted for the shuttle vector. Following 2–3 d of transfection, the cells can be X-gal-stained and the positive cells counted. The efficiency of transfection can be optimized by carrying out trial transfections in 6- or 12-well plates varying the conditions discussed in **Notes 4–6**, before scaling up to T-25 flasks for the recombination.

3. Only use high-quality DNA for transfections. Either CsCl banded DNA or DNA prepared using high-grade commercial kits is acceptable.

4. The efficiency of transfection can be optimized by carrying out transfections with 2X HBS solutions of different pH's, in the range of 6.97–7.10. Full details of various alternative methods for calcium-phosphate-mediated transfection can be found elsewhere.

5. Generally, the finer the precipitate is, the lower the cytotoxicity will be and therefore the higher the transfection efficiency. Experiment with the speed of the vortexer to determine the effect on precipitate density.

6. Adjusting the time scale of the transfection period within a range of 4–24 h can influence the transfection efficiency and the level of cytotoxicity observed.

7. Generally, plaques begin to arise after approx 7 d, but if after 10–12 d there is no evidence of a cytopathic effect, discard the flasks and repeat the transfection. Prolonged incubation of the cells increases the likelihood of RCA production.

8. Too vigorous mixing of ArkloneP and the cell suspension will result in the loss of adenoviral fibers and therefore a decrease in infectivity.

9. Avoid freeze/thawing the adenoviral stocks more than twice as it will result in a loss of titer. Aliquot all adenoviral stocks into suitable volumes for experiments.

10. Subculturing the cells at higher densities in 96-well plates will mean that after 5–7 d the monolayer will begin to peel off from the edges of the well; this will make observation of any cytopathic effect difficult. As a rule of thumb, subculture a confluent T-150 flask into 15 mL of media, take 3 mL of the media containing the cells and add 10 mL of fresh media to this. Add 100 μL of cell suspension per well.

11. In order to avoid cross-contaminating the wells when changing the media on plaque assays, but still change the media quickly and efficiently we use a simple strategy. Rest the plate edge on its upturned lid and then the media will automatically collect at one side, this leaves one hand free in order to hold a tube for the collection of waste media. The media must be removed with one pipet tip per well completing one row at a time. When adding fresh media, use a single tip per row and ensure that you do not touch the wells with the tip.

12. Typically, infection can be performed at the time of a media change. Mix 50–100 μL of crude adenovirus stock with 750 ml of complete media and then feed 25 mL to each flask.

13. Avoid multiply passaging recombinant adenoviruses in 293 cells as rearrangements are more likely *(7)*. Try to always use an original plaque pure stock for infecting the cells when generating new stocks.

14. When setting up CsCl gradients, a simple way to test that the layers are forming correctly is to mix a dye (e.g., trypan blue) with the density 1.4 CsCl. Discrete separation between the two layers can then be easily observed.
15. To avoid confusion between the bands place 1.6 mL water into a centrifuge tube and line it up with the tube containing the banded adenovirus. If there are no clear, separate bands repeat the CsCl purification.
16. Take adenovirus in a minimum of 500 µL of solution per 10 T-150 flasks to avoid aggregation during dialysis.
17. Take care when washing and fixing 293 cells on coverslips as they do not adhere very tightly. We have found that plating the cells at higher densities, i.e., more cells are touching each other, usually means more cells are lost during the washing stages of the experiment; therefore, 50–60% confluence gives the best results.
18. Infecting HeLa cells at 80 pfu/cell gives an infection efficiency of approx 80–90%.
19. We have found that a nuclear counter stain with propidium iodide at 1 µM does not mask the fluorescence for E1a and allows differentiation between positive and negative cells on the same slide.

References

1. Graham, F. L., Smiley, J., Russel, W. C., and Nairu, R. (1977) Characteristics of a human cell line transformed by DNA from human adenovirus type 5. *J. Gen. Virol.* **36,** 59–72.
2. McGrory, W. J., Bautista, D. S., and Graham, F. L. (1988) A simple technique for the rescue of early region I mutations into infectious human adenovirus type 5. *Virology* **163,** 614–617.
3. Baker, A. H., Wilkinson, G. W. G., Hembury, R. M., Murphy, G., and Newby, A. C. (1996) Development of recombinant adenoviruses that drive high level expression of the human metalloproteinase-9 and tissue inhibitor of metalloproteinase-1 and -2 genes: characterisation of their infection into rabbit smooth muscle cells and human MCF-7 adenocarcinoma cells. *Matrix Biol.* **15,** 383–395.
4. Baker, A. H., Zaltsman, A. B., George, S. J., Newby, A. C. (1998) Divergent effects of tissue inhibitor of metalloproteinase-1,-2 or -3 overexpression on rat vascular smooth muscle cell invasion, proliferation and death in vitro. *J. Clin. Invest.* **101,** 1478–1487.
5. Graham, F. L. and Prevec, L. (1991) Manipulation of adenovirus vectors, in *Methods in Molecular Biology, Vol. 7: Gene Transfer and Expression Protocols* (Murray, E. J., ed.), The Humana Press, Totowa, NJ, pp. 109–127.
6. Lowenstein, P. R., Shering, I. A. F., Bain, D., Castro, M. G., and Wilkinson, G. W. G. (1996) How to examine the interactions between adenoviral mediated gene transfer and different identified target brain cell types *in vitro* in, *Towards Gene Therapy for Neurological Disorders* (Lowenstein, P. R. and Enquist, L. W., eds.), Wiley, Chichester, UK, pp. 93–114.
7. Lochmuller, H., Jani, A., Huard, J., et al. (1994) Emergency of early region 1-containing replication-competent adenovirus in stocks of replication-defective adenovirus recombinants (E1+E3) during multiple passages in 293 cells. *Human Gene Ther.* 5, 1485–1491.

23

Generation of Recombinant Adeno-Associated Viruses for Delivery of Genes into Vascular Cells

Carmel M. Lynch

1. Introduction

A variety of delivery systems, both viral and nonviral, have been employed to genetically modify vascular endothelial cells and smooth muscle cells (SMC) in vitro and by direct in vivo gene transfer into the vessel wall. The most recent addition to gene delivery technology for the vasculature has been the use of adeno-associated virus (AAV) vectors *(1–5)*.

1.1. AAV

AAV is a human parvovirus with a single-stranded linear DNA genome of 4680 nucleotides (**Fig. 1A**). The genome is comprised of two open reading frames *rep* and *cap* flanked by a 145 nucleotide inverted terminal repeat (ITR). The *rep* and *cap* genes encode the Rep proteins and viral capsid proteins necessary for replication and encapsidation of the viral genome, respectively. The ITRs contain the viral origin of replication and the signals necessary for packaging of the genome. The ITRs are required *in cis* for viral replication and encapsidation, while the *rep* and *cap* gene products can function *in trans* to promote DNA replication and form nonenveloped icosahedral particles, respectively. The single-stranded viral DNA progeny of replication are packaged into preformed capsids.

1.2. AAV Life Cycle

AAV requires a helper virus, such as adenovirus, for viral DNA replication. As a result the AAV life cycle can be divided into two states, lytic and latent, distinguished by the presence and absence of the helper virus, respectively (**Fig. 2**). In the presence of Ad helper virus AAV undergoes DNA replication

From: *Methods in Molecular Medicine, Vascular Disease: Molecular Biology and Gene Therapy Protocols*
Edited by: A. H. Baker © Humana Press Inc., Totowa, NJ

A Wild-type AAV

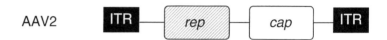

B Recombinant AAV

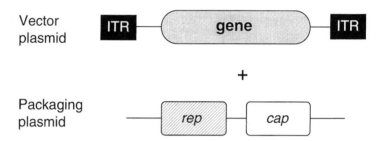

Fig. 1. rAAV vector construction. (**A**) The wild-type AAV genome is presented schematically as the *rep* and *cap* genes flanked by inverted terminal repeat (ITR) sequences (filled boxes). The *rep* and *cap* gene expression cassette is comprised of the native AAV promoters and polyadenylation signal in addition to the coding sequences (promoters and polyadenylation signal are not indicated in the diagram for simplicity). (**B**) A recombinant AAV vector plasmid is constructed from the wtAAV genome by removing the *rep* and *cap* gene cassette and inserting a gene of interest between the ITRs. The *rep* and *cap* gene cassette removed from the wtAAV genome is cloned into a second plasmid to generate a packaging plasmid. The packaging plasmid provides the *rep* and *cap* gene products *in trans* for vector production. The signals required *in cis* for vector replication and encapsidation are provided by the ITRs in the vector plasmid. The packaging plasmid will not be replicated and encapsidated since it lacks ITRs. Together the rAAV vector and packaging plasmids are functionally equivalent to the wild-type AAV genome.

resulting in the production of progeny virus (**Fig. 2A**). The host cell undergoes lysis due to adenovirus allowing for release of the newly produced AAV virions.

   In the absence of Ad helper virus, AAV persists in an episomal or integrated state in the host cell (**Fig. 2B**). While the latent AAV genome cannot undergo DNA replication in the absence of Ad helper virus, AAV gene expression can occur using the host cell machinery. The ability of AAV to establish latency allows the use of AAV vectors for transduction (i.e., gene transfer and expression, reviewed in *[6]*).

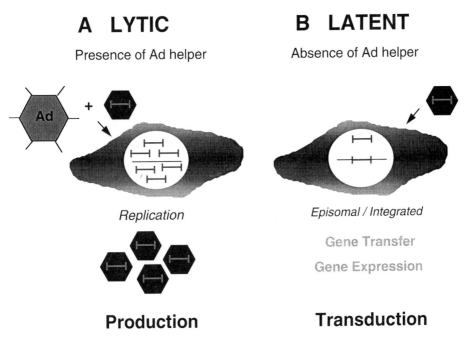

Fig. 2. Aspects of the AAV life cycle related to rAAV vector production and transduction. **(A)** In the presence of a helper adenovirus (Ad) the AAV genome undergoes DNA replication resulting in amplification of the genome and production of progeny virions. Concomitant production of adenovirus (not shown) results in cell lysis, and as a result, is referred to as the lytic phase of the AAV life cycle. Production of rAAV vectors requires Ad helper and is analogous to the lytic phase of the life cycle. **(B)** In the absence of Ad helper the AAV genome persists in the host cell in an episomal state or integrated into the host cell genome and is known as latency. Thus, genes carried in the AAV genome are transferred to the host cell. The latent AAV genome cannot undergo replication and production of progeny virions in the absence of Ad helper. However, gene expression can occur. The process of gene transfer and gene expression that occur during the latent phase of the AAV life cycle are utilized for the purpose of AAV-vector mediated transduction.

1.3. Principles of rAAV Vector Development

The overall principle of AAV vector development is simply to remove all of the viral sequences except for the ITRs and substitute them with a heterologous gene expression cassette comprised minimally of a promoter, gene, and polyadenlyation signal. The AAV *rep* and *cap* genes that have been removed must then be provided *in trans* to support replication and packaging of the recombinant AAV genome (**Fig. 1B**). One advantage of this system is that the recombinant AAV genome is devoid of any viral coding sequences and will not illicit immune responses related to viral gene expression, which have limited the in vivo utility of other viral vectors.

1.4. General Considerations in rAAV Vector Construction

AAV vector construction begins with a duplex copy of the AAV genome inserted in a bacterial plasmid. A number of AAV serotypes have been cloned, the most commonly used for vector construction is AAV serotype two (AAV-2). AAV-2 was originally cloned by two groups and is available as plasmids pAV2 *(7)* and psub201 *(8)*. AAV vectors are constructed in AAV plasmids by substituting a gene of interest for the AAV *rep* and *cap* genes using standard molecular biology subcloning techniques. The primary consideration is the size of the DNA insert, which ideally should not exceed 4.4 kb so that together with the ITR sequences the total size of the recombinant AAV genome is similar to that of wild-type AAV. The packaging limit is 110% of the wtAAV genome and the efficiency of packaging declines sharply after 105% of the wtAAV genome size *(9)*. A recombinant vector typically contains: flanking ITR sequences, promoter, gene of interest, and polyadenylation signal. Tissue specific promoters or common viral promoters such as, the human cytomegalovirus (CMV) immediate early promoter or Simain Virus 40 (SV40) promoter, can be inserted upstream of the gene of interest. The ITR has not been shown to effect transcription from downstream promoters. Additional gene expression regulatory elements such as introns may be included as permitted by the packaging constraints.

2. Materials

1. 225 cm² cell culture flask, preferably with vent caps (Costar Corporation, Cambridge, MA).
2. Dulbecco's modified Eagle's medium (BioWhitaker, Wakersville, MD).
3. Fetal bovine serum (HyClone Laboratories, Inc., Logan, UT).
4. HeLa cells (American Type Culture Collection, Rockville, MD).
5. Trypsin-EDTA solution: 0.05% trypsin, 0.02% EDTA (JRH Biosciences, Lenexa, KS).
6. 0.4% trypan blue solution (Sigma Chemical Company, St. Louis, MO).
7. Adenovirus 5 (American Type Culture Collection).
8. Chloroquine (Sigma Chemical Company): Make a stock solution at 10 m*M* in phosphate-buffered saline (PBS). Single use aliquots can be stored at –20°C for up to 1 yr. Chloroquine is light sensitive, and aliquots should be wrapped in aluminum foil.
9. Diethylaminoethyl-Dextran, DEAE-Dextran (Sigma Chemical Company): make a stock solution at 4 mg/mL in Tris-buffered saline. Single use aliquots can be stored at –20°C for up to 1 yr.
10. Dimethyl sulfoxide (DMSO) (Sigma Chemical Company).

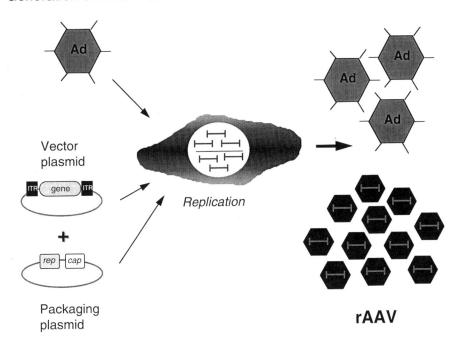

Fig. 3. rAAV vector production. Cells are cotransfected with a rAAV vector plasmid containing the gene of interest flanked by AAV inverted terminal repeat (ITR) sequences and with a packaging plasmid which provides the *rep* and *cap* gene functions. Cells are also infected with adenovirus (Ad) to provide helper function. The AAV vector is excised from the vector plasmid and undergoes DNA replication with the aid of the *rep* gene products provided by the packaging plasmid. Capsid proteins are also provided *in trans* by the packaging plasmid and encapsidate the newly replicated vector genomes to produce new progeny rAAV virions. The helper Ad virus also undergoes replication and generates new Ad virus. The resulting rAAV vector preparation is thus a mixture of the desired progeny rAAV virions and contaminating Ad virus. The rAAV vector preparation is subsequently purified to remove and/or inactivate the contaminating Ad virus.

11. 50 mM Tris-HCl, pH 8.0, 5 mM MgCl$_2$, 1 mM EDTA, and 5% glycerol (TMEG solution). Store at 4°C.
12. Benzonase, ultra-pure, 250 U/μL (American International Chemical Inc., Natick, MA): dilute 1:10 in TMEG for a concentration of 25 U/μL immediately prior to use.
13. Ringer's balanced salt solution (BioWhitaker).

3. Methods

The following vector production (**Fig. 3**) and purification procedures should be performed in a biosafety cabinet under BL-2 conditions.

3.1. Vector Production by Transient Transfection of Vector and Packaging Plasmids

1. Seed 21 225 cm^2 vented cap flasks with HeLa cells (*see* **Note 1**) at a density of 5×10^6 cells per flask.
2. Culture the cells in 10% FBS DMEM in a humidified 10% CO_2 atmosphere at 37°C for 16–24 h.
3. Note the confluence of the cells (*see* **Note 2**). Count one flask of cells to determine the cell number (*see* **Note 3**).
4. Prepare a batch of Ad 5 at $1 \times x10^8$ pfu/mL in complete medium.
5. Aspirate medium from cells and replace with 28 mL of fresh medium per flask.
6. Add 1 mL (1×10^8 pfu) of Ad 5 to each flask (*see* **Note 3**) for a multiplicity of infection (MOI) of 10.
7. Incubate the cells for 1 h @37°C in 10% CO_2.
8. During the 1 h incubation prepare the DNA for transfection. Prepare a batch of DNA/DEAE-dextran sufficient for 20 flasks plus 1 extra. Add the following in order to a centrifuge tube:

DMEM (no serum)	7,612.5 µL
Packaging plasmid (1 µg/µL)	787.5 µL
Vector plasmid (1 µg/µL)	787.5 µL
<Vortex>	
10 m*M* chloroquine	7,875.0 µL
<Vortex>	
4 mg/mL DEAE-Dextran	3,937.5 µL

9. Add 1 mL of the DNA/DEAE-dextran mixture per flask to a final volume of 30 mL/ flask containing 37.5 µg each of the packaging and vector plasmid, 125 µ*M* chloroquine, and 25 µg/mL DEAE-dextran. Distribute evenly over the cells.
10. Incubate for 4 h @37°C in 10% CO_2.
11. Prepare a solution of 10% DMSO in complete medium (10 mL/flask). Carefully aspirate the Ad-containing supernatant from the cells (*see* **Note 4**). Cover the cell monolayer with 10 mL of the 10% DMSO solution. Incubate at room temperature for 5 min.
12. Aspirate the DMSO solution. Wash the cells with 10 mL of DMEM per flask.
13. Add 30 mL of complete medium per flask and incubate for 48–72 h @ 37°C in 10% CO_2.
14. Examine the cells microscopically for cytopathic effect (CPE) due to Ad (*see* **Note 5**).
15. If maximal CPE is evident, scrape the cells into the supernatant and harvest.
16. Pellet the cells by centrifugation at 2700*g* for 10 min.
17. Resuspend the cells at a concentration of 5×10^6 cell/mL in TMEG.
18. Freeze the cells at –70°C until ready to purify the rAAV particles.

3.2. Vector Purification by CsCl Isopycnic Gradient Centrifugation

1. Remove cells from –70°C freezer and allow to thaw at room temperature.
2. Lyse the cells by sonication, 4×15 s bursts (*see* **Notes 6** and **7**).

3. Add 25 U of benzonase/mL of lysate and incubate at 37°C for 1 h.
4. Add CsCl to a final density of 1.387 g/mL. Remove 10 µL and read the refractive index at room temperature. A refractive index of 1.3710 ± 0.0005, which is equal to a density of 1.387 g/mL ± 0.005 is required. Add CsCl or TMEG as necessary to adjust the density.
5. Transfer sample to a 12.5-mL polyallomer ultracentrifuge tube (10.0–10.5 mL) and overlay with 0.5 mL of mineral oil to a final volume of 10.5–11 mL/tube.
6. Centrifuge at 151,000g at 15°C for 48 h.
7. Visually inspect the gradient, the Ad virus band should be visible in the top half of the gradient. The rAAV band should be present in the bottom half of the gradient but will not be visible.
8. Attach a stop cock to an 18-gage needle.
9. Puncture one side of the centrifuge tube with the needle (stop cock in the OFF position) approximately one third to one quarter distance from the bottom of the tube.
10. Collect 0.5-mL fractions by turning the stop cock to the ON position and allowing the gradient to drip by gravity flow. Store the fractions at 4°C.
11. Read the refractive index and determine the density of each fraction (*see* **Note 8**).
12. Assay the fractions to determine those that contain rAAV. Fractions may be assayed for biological titer and/or particle number (*see* **Note 9**).
13. Pool fractions containing rAAV and exclude fractions which contain Ad virus based on visual inspection of the gradient (*see* **Note 10**).
14. Repeat **steps 4–13**.
15. Heat the pooled fractions at 56°C for 30 min to inactivate any residual Ad virus.
16. Dialyze the pooled fractions against three changes of Ringer's balanced salt solution containing 5% glycerol (*see* **Note 11**).
17. Aliquot rAAV and store at –70°C (*see* **Note 12**).

4. Notes

1. 293-1 cells and Cos-7 cells can also be used for rAAV production. DEAE-Dextran is not suitable for use with 293-1 cells as it causes cells to round-up and become displaced from tissue culture ware. If 293-1 cells are used, the CaPO$_4$ precipitation method of transfection should be used instead of DEAE-dextran. A subclone of 293-1 cells selected for their adherent properties called 293-A are recommended for ease of handling and can be purchased from Quantum BioTechnologies, Montreal, Quebec, Canada.
2. It is best to use cells that are in the exponential growth phase for vector production. Cell cultures should be approx 50–70 % confluent.
3. Each 225 cm^2 flask should contain approx 1×10^7 cells per flask at the time of transfection. Variations of two- to threefold in cell number do not require adjustment of the amount of Ad 5 virus or plasmid DNA used for transfection.
4. The Ad 5 virus-containing medium can be inactivated by addition of bleach to a final concentration of 10% by volume. The medium should be left in contact with the bleach for a minimum of 15 min prior to disposal.

5. Cytopathic effects of adenovirus are evident when cells round-up and detach from the bottom of the tissue culture flask. The majority of cells can be displaced by gently tapping the side of the culture flask against the palm of one hand. The remaining adherent cells can be removed using a disposable cell scraper (e.g., Costar Corporation, Cambridge, MA).

6. Check that the cells have been lysed by addition of trypan blue in a 1:1 ratio to an aliquot of cells. Examine the cells in a hemacytometer under a microscope. Cells that have not been lysed will exclude the trypan blue. If unlysed cells are present perform an additional round of sonication. Examine the cells again for lysis as described above. Lysis of 80–90% of the cells is desirable.

7. Alternatively, if a sonicator is not available cell lysis can be achieved by three cycles of freeze/thaw on dry ice/ethanol and 37°C. We have found vector yield to be reduced 10-fold after freeze/thaw lysis compared with cell lysis by sonication.

8. AAV has a buoyant density of 1.41 g/cm^3 in CsCl, and rAAV vectors of similar genome length to wild-type AAV should band at densities close to 1.41 g/cm^3. Ad 5 virus has a buoyant density of 1.35 g/cm^3 in CsCl. CsCl equilibrium density gradient centrifugation of rAAV vector preparations is aimed primarily at achieving separation of the rAAV vector particles from Ad used as a helper virus during production.

9. Biological titer should be assayed based on expression of the gene present in the vector. Particle number is commonly determined by measuring encapsidated vector genomes resistant to DNase treatment by DNA hybridization methodology (a protocol can be found in *[6]*). It is particularly important to adequately treat rAAV preparations generated by DNA transfection with DNase. Unencapsidated DNA that is not removed by inadequate DNase treatment could result in an overestimate of the particle number.

10. Usually only the peak fractions (3–5 fractions) are pooled in order to obtain a high titer vector preparation and minimize the amount of Ad virus contamination.

11. Glycerol is added as a stabilizing agent to permit long-term storage of the vector. Ringer's balanced salt solution without glycerol or phosphate buffered saline may be used for dialysis if long-term preservation of vector is not required.

12. This procedure should yield 1–2 mL of purified vector with a titer of 1×10^{10} DNase resistant particles (DRP) per mL. The use of 1000 DRP per cell is recommended for transduction of vascular cells in culture. This results in transduction efficiencies of 5–31% *(3)*. For in vitro transductions, retroviruses may provide a better tool, especially if derivation of stable cell lines is required (*see* Chapter 27). It is not possible to derive stable drug-resistant cell lines following rAAV transduction in actively proliferating cells. (The episomal vector is lost and formation of concatemeric structures that mediate long-term persistence only occurs in quiescent cells.)

References

1. Kaplitt, M. G., Xiao, X., Samulski, R. J., Li, J., Ojamaa, K., Klein, I. L., Makimura, H., Kaplitt, M. J., Strumpf, R. K., and Diethrich, E. B. (1996) Long-

term gene transfer in porcine myocardium after coronary infusion of an adeno-associated virus vector. *Ann. Thorac. Surg.* **62(6),** 1669–1676.

2. Gnatenko, D., Arnold, T. E., Zolotukhin, S., Nuovo, G. J., Muzyczka, N., and Bahou, W. F. (1997) Characterization of recombinant adeno-associated virus-2 as a vehicle for gene delivery and expression into vascular cells. *J. Investig. Med.* **45(2),** 87–98.

3. Lynch, C. M., Hara, P. S., Leonard, J. C., Williams, J. K., Dean, R. H., and Geary, L. G. (1997) Adeno-associated virus vectors for vascular gene deliver. *Circ. Res.* **80.**

4. Arnold, T. E., Gnatenko, D., and Bahou, W. F. (1997) In vivo gene transfer into rat arterial walls with novel adeno-associated virus vectors. *J. Vasc. Surg.* **25(2),** 347–355.

5. Rolling, F., Nong, Z., Pisvin, S., and Collen, D. (1997) Adeno-associated virus-mediated gene transfer into rat carotid arteries. *Gene. Ther.* **4(8),** 757–761.

6. Muzyczka, N. (1992) Use of adeno-associated virus as a general transduction vector for mammalian cells. *Curr. Top. Microbiol. Immunol.* **158,** 97–129.

7. Laughlin, C. A., Tratschin, J. D., Coon, H., and Carter, B. J. (1983) Cloning of infectious adeno-associated virus genomes in bacterial plasmids *Gene* **23(1),** 65–73.

8. Samulski, R. J., Berns, K. I., Tan, M., and Muzyczka, N. (1982) Cloning of adeno-associated virus into pBR322: rescue of intact virus from the recombinant plasmid in human cells *Proc Natl Acad Sci U S A* **79(6),** 2077-81

9. Dong, J. Y., Fan, P. D., and Frizzell, R. A. (1996) Quantitative analysis of the packaging capacity of recombinant adeno- associated virus. *Hum. Gene. Ther.* **7(17),** 2101–2112.

24

Hemagglutinating Virus of Japan Liposome-Mediated Gene Delivery to Vascular Cells

Yoshikazu Yonemitsu and Yasufumi Kaneda

1. Introduction

Since the first report of in vivo direct gene transfer to the vessel wall in 1990 *(1)* several vectors, such as adenovirus, liposomes, and adeno-associated virus have been employed to introduce foreign genes to the vascular tissue in vivo. Hemagglutinating virus of Japan (HVJ, Sendai virus), a member of the mouse paramyxovirus family, has been combined with liposomes to produce a novel gene transfer system, namely, HVJ liposomes *(2,3)*. This vector system is constructed with inactivated viral particles and nonviral lamellar liposomes, and is defined as a "viral, nonviral hybrid vector." We and others have shown that this vector system can introduce foreign genes into the vascular tissue efficiently *(4–9)*, and have also demonstrated that these genes and synthetic oligodeoxynucleotides (ODNs) transferred by this system could add some functions to the vessel wall *(4–6)* or prevent the vascular proliferative diseases *(7–9)*.

HVJ liposomes are able to encapsulate gene expression cassettes into their inner lumen, as opposed to cationic liposomes, which complex with the negatively charged DNA, the so-called lipofection method *(10,11)*. DNA entrapped in the HVJ liposomes is directly introduced into cellular cytoplasm by means of the fusion activity of HVJ. Also, incorporation of nuclear protein, HMG-1, with DNA facilitates its nuclear localization, and this results in enhanced gene expression, especially in vivo *(3)*. HVJ liposomes are applicable for gene transfer to almost all mammalian cells with the ganglioside (sialic acid, receptor for HVJ), except for lymphocytes.

From: *Methods in Molecular Medicine, Vascular Disease: Molecular Biology and Gene Therapy Protocols*
Edited by: A. H. Baker © Humana Press Inc., Totowa, NJ

In this article, we describe the preparation of HVJ liposomes and procedures of gene transfer into the vascular cells and tissue. Also, we include details of cationic lipid-complexed HVJ liposome, HVJ cationic liposome *(12)*, which has proved to be a powerful technique especially for in vitro gene transfer *(13,14)*. Anionic HVJ liposomes achieve highly efficient gene transfer to the vessel walls of some animals, including carotid arteries of rat *(5,7,8)* and rabbit *(4,6,9)* or vein grafts of rabbits and dogs *(15)* and, in particular, more than 80% of vascular smooth muscle cells of rabbit carotid arteries under appropriate conditions *(4)*. However, it should be noted that;

1. Complements inactivate HVJ liposomes rapidly.
2. Red blood cells easily fuse to HVJ liposomes.
3. HN protein on the surface of HVJ liposomes makes red blood cells aggregate.

HVJ cationic liposomes are not suitable for direct gene transfer to vessel wall, because of reduced gene expression by cell damage due to concentrated cationic lipid.

2. Materials

2.1. Preparation of Virus

2.1.1. Culture of HVJ in Eggs

1. HVJ seed: Store 100-µL aliquots of chorioallantonic fluid with the best seed of HVJ (Z strain) in 10% dimethylsulfoxide in liquid nitrogen. This strain shows the highest fusion activity. This strain can be obtained from the authors.
2. Polypepton solution: 1% polypepton (pancreatic digest of casein, Wako Pure Chemicals, Osaka, Japan), 0.2% NaCl, pH 7.2. To make a 500 mL solution, dissolve 5 g of polypepton and 1 g NaCl in distilled water, adjust the pH to 7.2 with 1 N NaOH solution, and make up to 500 mL volume with distilled water. Sterilize by autoclaving at 121°C for 20 min and store at 4°C.
3. Balanced salt solution (BSS): 137 mM NaCl, 5.4 mM KCl, 10 mM Tris-HCl, pH 7.6. Dissolve 8 g of NaCl, 0.4 g of KCl, and 1.21 g of Tris base in distilled water, adjust the pH to 7.6 with 1 N HCl, and fill up to a liter with distilled water. Sterilize by autoclaving at 121°C for 20 min and store at 4°C.
4. Light illuminator.
5. Iodine for sterilization.
6. Needle to puncture the egg shell.
7. 1-mL disposable syringes with a 26-gage needle.
8. Incubator.
9. 10-mL disposable syringe with 18-gage needle.

2.1.2. Viral Titer

1. SSC: Dissolve 8.5 g of NaCl and 4.4 g of tri-sodium citrate·2H$_2$O in 1 L of distilled water.

2. Chicken red blood cells (cRBC): Prepare cRBC (Sigma, Dorset, UK) and dilute to 0.5% with SSC just before use (*see* **Note 1**).
3. Hemmagglutination plate (Merck, UK).
4. Spectrophotometer.

2.1.3. Purification of HVJ from Chrioallantoic Fluid

1. 30-mL disposable conical tubes.
2. Low-speed centrifuge.
3. 30-mL ultracentrifuge tubes.
4. Ultracentrifuge.

2.2. Preparation of Lipid Mixture

The lipid composition of the HVJ liposomes is a key determinant of optimal gene transfer efficiency. The preparation of two types of liposomes is now available, negatively charged and positively charged liposomes (HVJ cationic liposomes). The former contains anionic lipid (PS: phosphatidylserine), and the latter contains cationic lipid (TMAG: *N*-(trimethylammonioacetyl)-didodecyl-*D*-glutamate chloride or DC-Chol: DC-Cholesterol), with phosphatidylcoline (PC) and cholesterol (Chol). The positively charged HVJ liposomes (HVJ cationic liposomes) are especially effective for in vitro gene transfer *(13,14)*. Lipid oxidation seriously affects cell viability and reduces gene transfer efficiency. To avoid this, purge tubes with nitrogen gas at all steps of procedures except during incubation step during conjugation with HVJ.

2.2.1. Lipid Mixture for Negatively Charged Liposomes

1. Chromatographically pure bovine brain phosphatidylserine-sodium salt (PS) (*see* **Note 2**).
2. Egg yolk phosphatidylcholine (PC); dissolved in chloroform and divided into 48-mg aliquots in sterilized glass tubes. Stored at –20°C.
3. Cholesterol (Chol).
4. Chloroform (molecular biology grade).
5. Custom made glass tubes (24-mm caliber and 12 cm long): The new tubes should be immersed in saturated KOH-ethanol solutions for 24 h, rinsed with distilled water, and heated at 180°C for 2 h before use.
6. Rotary evaporator.
7. Vacuum pump with a pressure gauge.
8. Water bath.
9. Water bath shaker.

2.2.2. Lipid Mixture for Positively Charged Liposomes

1. TMAG (Sogo Yakuko Chemicals, Tokyo, Japan) or DC-Chol (Sigma, Dorset, UK).

2.3. Preparation of DNA Encapsulated Liposomes

2.3.1. Preparation of Negatively Charged Liposomes

1. Plasmid DNA: Dissolve in 10 mM Tris-HCl, pH 8.0, 0.1 mM EDTA or BSS (final concentration; 200 μg/136 μL). Store at –20 °C (*see* **Note 3**).
2. High mobility group-1, 2 protein (HMG-1, 2, 1 mg/mL) for plasmid DNA transfer (Wako Pure Chemicals, Inc., Osaka, Japan).
3. Oligodeoxynucleotide (ODN) solutions: Nuclease-resistant phosphorothioate ODN (15-25 bases long) can be made by a number of suppliers. Dissolve ODN with BSS at 100–350 μM and divide into 200-μL aliquots in autoclaved tubes. Store at –20°C.
4. Vortex mixer.
5. Water bath shaker.
6. Bath type sonicator.

2.3.2. Preparation of Positively Charged Liposomes

Complexes of HVJ liposomes with positively charged cationic lipid has several advantages, namely, a higher amount of negatively charged DNA entrapment, higher interaction between the negatively charged virion and positively charged liposomes, and enhanced interaction to negatively charged cellular membrane. In particular, HVJ cationic liposomes are effective for in vitro gene transfer *(13)*, whereas in vivo direct injection may result in decreased gene expression due to relatively high concentration of cationic lipid. Unlike with anionic HVJ liposome system, use of HMG-1 and 2 sometimes reduces gene expression efficiency due to inhibiting DNA entrapment.

1. Solutions and equipment as for **Subheading 2.3.1.**

2.4. Preparation of Anionic and Cationic HVJ Liposomes

1. Sucrose solutions: To prepare a 30% (w/v) and a 50 % (w/v) sucrose solutions, dissolve 150 and 250 g of sucrose in BSS, respectively. Adjust the volume to 500 mL, sterilize by autoclaving, and store at 4°C.
2. Ultraviolet spectrolinker.

2.5. Gene Transfer to Cultured Vascular Cells

Suitable conditions for in vitro gene transfection by HVJ liposomes are variable and depend on cell type or animal species. For example, we recommend the use of collagen-coated plates for culture of endothelial cells undergoing HVJ liposome-mediated gene transfer. Transfection of subconfluent cultured cells may result in formation of multinuclear giant cells due to cell-to-cell fusion. Pilot studies are needed to establish suitable concentrations of HVJ liposomes for good gene expression by using reporter genes assays.

1. BSS containing 2 mM $CaCl_2$.
2. 1 M $CaCl_2$: Dissolve 11.1 g of $CaCl_2$ in 100 mL of diluted water, and sterilize by autoclaving.

3. Methods

3.1. Preparation of Virus

3.1.1. Culture of HVJ in Eggs

1. Rapidly thaw the seed and dilute 1000 times with the polypepton solution. The diluted seed should be kept on ice.
2. Observe embryonated eggs (9–10 d after fertilization) under a light illuminator in a dark room and mark an injection point about 5 mm above the chrioallantonic membrane (*see* **Fig. 1**).
3. Inject 0.1 mL of diluted seed into each egg using a 1-mL disposable syringe with a 26-gage needle. The needle should be inserted vertically to reach the chrioallantonic membrane (**Fig. 1**).
4. Cover the injected site on the egg shell with melted paraffin. Then incubate the eggs for 4 d at 35.5°C in sufficient moisture (*see* **Note 4**).
5. Chill the eggs at 4°C for more than 6 h before harvesting the chrioallantonic fluid containing the amplified virus (*see* **Note 5**).
6. Partially remove the egg shell with forceps, and transfer the chrioallantoic fluid to a sterilized bottle using a 10-mL syringe with an 18-gage needle. The chrioallantoic fluid should be cloudy. The fluid should be kept at 4°C to avoid freezing. The virus is stable in the fluid for at least 3 mo (*see* **Note 6**).

3.1.2. Viral Titer

1. Purify the HVJ (*see* **Subheading 3.1.3.**), check the absorbance at 540 nm (1 OD_{540} should be approx 15,000 hemagglutinating activity units (HAU)/mL), and dilute to 2000–4000 HAU/mL with SSC.
2. Apply 0.5 mL of SSC in each well of the hemagglutination plate.
3. Add 0.5 mL of virus solution on the left well, remove 0.5 mL of mixture, and add it to next right well. Repeat this procedure to make a 2X dilution series.
4. Add 0.5% of cRBC and gently mix in each well. Incubate the plate for 1 h at 4°C.
5. Read hemagglutination pattern, and calculate HAU. Make sure the HAU measurement by titer is almost equivalent to the value by spectrophotometrical measurement.

3.1.3. Purification of HVJ from Chrioallantoic Fluid

1. Transfer 20 mL of the chrioallantoic fluid into a 30-mL disposable conical tube and centrifuge at 1000g for 10 min at 4 C in a low-speed centrifuge.
2. Collect the supernatant, transfer into a 30-mL ultracentrifuge tube, and centrifuge at 27,000g for 30 min at 4°C.
3. Add 2 mL of BSS to the pellet and leave at 4°C overnight (*see* **Note 7**).
4. Gently resuspend the pellets, and centrifuge again as above. Add 1 mL of BSS and leave at 4°C for more than 8 h.

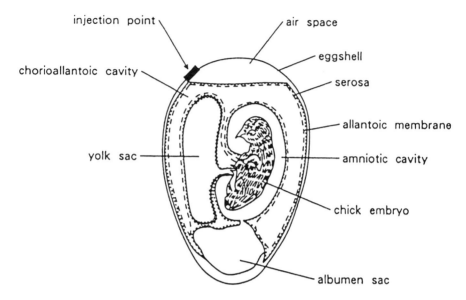

Fig. 1. Injection site of HVJ seed marked at approx 5 mm above the chrioallantoic membrane.

5. Gently resuspend the pellet and centrifuge at 1000*g* for 10 min at 4°C.
6. Transfer the supernatant to an aseptic tube and store at 4°C.
7. Measure the virus titer by the absorbance at 540 nm of 10- to 100-times-diluted supernatant using spectrophotometer. An optical density at 540 nm corresponds to 15,000 HAU, which correlates with optimal fusion activity. Adjust the concentration to 30,000 HAU with BSS. Aseptically prepared virus in BSS maintains fusion activity for 3 wk. The virus should not be frozen.

3.2. Preparation of Lipid Mixture

3.2.1. Lipid mixture for Negatively Charged Liposomes

1. Dissolve PC (48 mg), Chol (20 mg), and PS (10 mg) in 3.9 mL of chloroform, and mix gently.
2. Divide the lipid solution into 0.5-mL aliquots in to seven glass tubes (10 mg of lipid/tube). Keep the tubes at –20°C under nitrogen gas before evaporation. The lipid solution should be evaporated as soon as possible.
3. Connect the tube to a rotary evaporator. The tube should be kept at 40°C in a water bath.
4. Evaporate the chloroform in a rotary evaporator under very slow infusion of nitrogen gas (less than 1 L/min) at a pressure of less than 20 mmHg for few minutes. Then, increase the pressure to 700 mmHg for more than 5 min (**Fig. 2** and *see* **Note 8**).
5. The dried lipid mixture can be stored at –20°C in nitrogen gas for at least 2 wk.

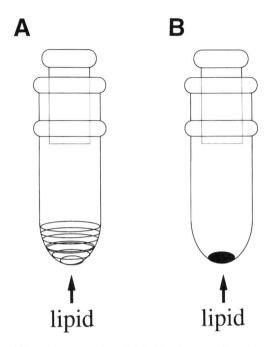

A   **B**

lipid   lipid

Fig. 2. Appropriate (**A**) and inappropriate (**B**) lipid mixtures after chloroform evaporation.

3.2.2. Lipid Mixture for Positively Charged Liposomes

1. Dissolve PC, Chol, and TMAG in 4.0 mL of chloroform, respectively, and mix gently (*see* **Note 9**).
2. Divide the lipid solution into 0.5-mL aliquots in seven glass tubes. Keep the lipid at –20°C under nitrogen before evaporation. The lipid solution should be evaporated as soon as possible.
3. Following procedures are same as above (**Subheading 3.2.1., steps 3–5**).

3.3. Preparation of DNA Encapsulated Liposomes

3.3.1. Preparation of Negatively Charged Liposomes

1. Mix 136 µL plasmid DNA (1.47 mg/mL, total 200 µg) and 64 µL HMG-1 (1.0 mg/mL, 64 µg) in a 0.5 mL of nuclease-free Eppendorf tube. Incubate the mixture in a water bath at 20°C for 1 h.
2. Transfer 200 µL of the DNA-HMG-1, 2 complex (or 200 µL of ODN solution) to a glass tube with the required dried lipid mixture. Agitate vigorously by vortexing for 30 s, and allow the tube to stand in a 37°C water bath for 30 s. Repeat this vortex-incubation cycle more than eight times.
3. Briefly sonicate in a bath type sonicator (3–5 s), then vortex again for 45 s.
4. Add 300 µL of BSS, and stand in a water bath reciprocal shaker (120 strokes/min) for 30 min.

3.3.2. Preparation of Positively Charged Liposomes

1. Transfer 200 µg/200 µL of the DNA in BSS (or 200 µL of 100–350 µ *M* ODN solution) to a glass tube with dried lipid mixture. Agitate vigorously by vortexing for 30 s, and allow the tube to stand in a 37°C water bath for 30 s. Repeat this vortex-incubation cycle more than eight times to form fine small liposome particles.
2. Add BSS to the tube to a 1.0 mL final volume.
3. Using a 1-mL syringe, extrude the liposome suspension through a 0.45-µm pore nitrocellulose filter membrane filled with BSS. Then extrude 0.5 mL of BSS to collect the liposomes left in the membrane filter. The 1.5 mL of liposome solution is then excluded through a 0.20-µm filter to obtain sized-unilamellar liposomes using a 2.5-mL syringe. Again, apply 0.5 mL of BSS and collect the residual liposomes (*see* **Note 10**).
4. Stand in a water bath reciprocal shaker (120 strokes/min) for 30 min.

3.4. Preparation of Anionic and Cationic HVJ Liposomes

1. Place the purified HVJ (30,000 HAU/mL) solution in a Petri dish and inactivate with ultraviolet irradiation (198 mJ/cm^2) using an ultraviolet crosslinker. Inactivated virus should be kept on ice and be used as soon as possible (in 1 h).
2. Place 1 mL of inactivated HVJ to 2 mL of liposome solution (total 30,000 HAU/tube). Keep the tubes on ice for 10 min, and incubate the HVJ liposome mixture at 37°C for more than 1 h with shaking (120 strokes/min) in a water bath.
3. During the incubation, construct a sucrose density gradient. Pour 1 mL of the 50% sucrose solution into an autoclaved ultracentrifuge tube (12–13 mL in size). Then overlay with 6.5 mL of 30% sucrose solution.
4. Place the HVJ liposome mixture on the sucrose density gradient and ultracentrifuge for 2 h at 62,800g at 4°C.
5. After centrifugation, pure HVJ liposomes are visualized in a layer between BSS and the 30% sucrose solution (upper band), whereas free HVJ sediments between 30 and 50% sucrose solutions (lower band, *see* **Fig. 3** and **Note 11**).
6. Carefully collect the HVJ liposomes with a sterilized Pasteur pipet. We usually adjust the volume to 1 mL with BSS. They can be stored for at least 2–3 d (anionic) or a week (cationic), but it is strongly recommended the mixture be used as soon as possible.

3.5. Gene Transfer to Cultured Vascular Cells

3.5.1 Anionic Liposomes

1. One to two days before transfection, seed the cells sparsely on 100-mm Petri dishes.
2. Wash the cell monolayer (endothelial cells, SMC, or fibroblasts) three times with BSS containing 2 mM CaCl$_2$.
3. Add 3 mL of the HVJ liposome solution with 2 mM CaCl$_2$ to the Petri dish. Incubate the cells at 37°C for 30–120 min (prolonged incubation may result in cell damage).

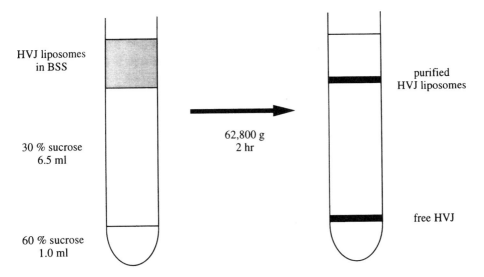

Fig. 3. Sucrose density gradient centrifugation for removal of unfused HVJ from HVJ liposome complex.

4. Observe the cells with a phase-contrast microscope every 30 min, and check cell integrity. Then remove the HVJ liposome solution, wash the cells with culture medium, and incubate in culture medium until assay. If cell damage is apparent using this protocol, try following the recipe for cationic liposomes.

3.5.2. Cationic Liposomes

1. Two days before transfection, seed the cells sparsely on 100-mm Petri dishes.
2. Add 1–100 µL of HVJ cationic liposome solution to the petri dish. Incubate the cells at 37°C for 30–120 min (prolonged incubation may result in cell damage).
3. Observe the cells in a phase-contrast microscope every 30 min, and check the condition of the cells. Then remove the medium with the HVJ cationic liposome, wash the cells with culture medium, and then incubate in culture medium until assay (*see* **Notes 12** and **13**).

3.6. Troubleshooting

If HVJ liposome system does not work, check the following;

1. Lipid peroxidation affects cell toxicity and gene transfer efficiency. To avoid this
   a. Use new batches of analytical biology grade chloroform and lipids.
   b. Fill tubes with nitrogen gas in all steps.
2. Purity of water. Calcium-, magnesium-, and nuclease-free conditions are critical in all steps of preparation except just prior to transfection. Use ultrapure and autoclaved distilled water.

4. Notes

1. Do not use cRBCs that have undergone hemolysis.
2. PS from Avanti Co. Ltd. (Alabaster, AL) is good for use in liposome preparation. The quality of lipids from other suppliers is varied and may affect gene transfer efficiency.
3. Equilibrium centrifugation in caesium chloride is recommended for DNA purification. Qiagen (Chatsworth, CA) column preparation is acceptable, and note that contamination of *Escherichia coli* genomic DNA or protein affects gene transfer efficiency.
4. HVJ is sensitive to culture temperature and passages grown at high temperature (e.g., 37°C) may result in mutated HVJ with a loss in fusion activity.
5. Chilling is necessary to make vessels spastic to avoid contamination of red blood cells.
6. Eggs and equipment should be sterilized by autoclaving before disposable.
7. Avoid vigorous pipeting. HVJ particles are extremely fragile.
8. After successful evaporation of a chloroform, there should be thin and layered lipid film inside the wall of glass tubes. Discard any tubes with lipid precipitation at the bottom of tube (**Fig. 2**).
9. In our experience, the following lipid formulation shows optimal transfection efficiency.

    TMAG : PC : Chol = 10 : 48 : 20 (mg) in 4.0 mL

    or

    DC-Chol : PC : Chol = 6 : 48 : 24 (mg) in 4.0 mL

10. Generally, cationic lipids make liposomes larger than anionic ones in the case of vigorous vortexing method (more than 1–2 μm). Before extrusion, you can see the colloidal liposome particles macroscopically. Sizing by membrane filter extrusion is recommended to reduce cytotoxicity and to enhance gene transfer efficiency *(13)*.
11. In the case of anionic HVJ liposomes, two bands are usually seen, and the BSS layer seems clear. A soft cushion-like upper band suggests good quality of HVJ liposomes. Lipid accumulation on the top of the tube or a cloudy BSS layer indicates failure of complexation of virus and liposomes. In the sucrose-density gradient centrifugation of cationic HVJ liposomes, the upper band shows a soft single layer and the lower layer is sometimes absent. A thick lower band indicates poor quality of virus.
12. Use 293 cells or HeLa cells as positive controls for transfection. These cells show minimal damage by HVJ liposomes, and express transgene efficiently.
13. To verify the transduction of macromolecules into cells by HVJ liposome system, we recommend trial transfections with FITC-labeled ODNs first. If successful, ODN is observed with the nuclear localizing fluorescence under a fluorescent microscopy in 30 min–6 h after transfection. Extracellular fluorescence with no nuclear signal means unsuccessful HVJ preparation.

References

1. Nabel, E. G., Plautz, G., and Nabel, G. J. (1990) Site-specific gene expression *in vivo* by direct gene transfer into the arterial wall. *Science* **249**, 1285–1288.
2. Kaneda, Y., Uchida, T., Kim, J., Ishiura, M., and Okada, Y. (1987) The improved efficient method for introducing macromolecules into cells using HVJ (Sendai virus) liposomes with gangliosides. *Exp. Cell Res.* **173**, 56-69.
3. Kaneda, Y., Iwai, K., and Uchida, T. (1989) Increased expression of DNA cointroduced with nuclear protein in adult rat liver. *Science* **243**, 375–378.
4. Yonemitsu, Y., Kaneda, Y., Morishita, R., Nakagawa, K., Nakashima, Y., and Sueishi, K. (1996) Characterization of *in vivo* gene transfer into the arterial wall mediated by the Sendai virus (HVJ)-liposomes: an effective tool for the *in vivo* study of arterial diseases. *Lab. Invest.* **75**, 313–323.
5. Von der Leyen, H. E., Gibbons, G. H., Morishita, R., Lewis, N. P., Zhang, L., Nakajima, M., Kaneda, Y., Cooke, J. P., and Dzau, V. J. (1995) Gene therapy inhibiting neointimal vascular lesion: *in vivo* transfer of endothelial cell nitric oxide synthase gene. *Proc. Natl. Acad. Sci. USA* **92**, 1137–1141.
6. Yonemitsu, Y., Kaneda, Y., Komori, K., Hirai, K., Sugimachi, K., and Sueishi, K. (1997) The immediate early gene of human cytomegalovirus stimulates vascular smooth muscle cell proliferation *in vitro* and *in vivo*. *Biochem. Biophys. Res. Commun.* **231**, 447–451.
7. Morishita, R., Gibbons, G. H., Ellison, K. E., Nakajima, M., Zhang, L., Kaneda, Y., et al. (1993) Single intraluminal delivery of antisense cdc2 kinase and proliferating-cell nuclear antigen oligonucleotides results in chronic inhibition of neointimal hyperplasia. *Proc. Natl. Acad. Sci. USA* **90**, 8474–8478.
8. Morishita, R., Gibbons, G. H., Horiuchi, M., Ellison, K. E., Nakajima, M., Zhang, L., et al. (1995) A gene therapy strategy using a transcription factor decoy of the E2F binding site inhibits smooth muscle proliferation *in vivo*. *Proc. Natl. Acad. Sci. USA* **92**, 5855–5859.
9. Yonemitsu, Y., Kaneda, Y., Tanaka, S., Nakashima, Y., Komori, K., Sugimachi, K., and Sueishi, K. (1998) Transfer of wild-Type p53 gene effectively inhibits vascular smooth muscle cell proliferation *in vitro* and *in vivo*. *Circ. Res.* **82**, 147–156.
10. Felgner, P. L., Gadek, T. R., Holm, M., Roman, R., Chan, H. W., Wenz, M., et al. (1987) Lipofection: a highly efficient, lipid-mediated DNA-transfection procedure. *Proc. Natl. Acad. Sci. USA* **84**, 7413–7417.
11. Yonemitsu, Y., Alton, E. W. F. W., Komori, K., Yoshizumi, T., Sugimachi, K., and Kaneda, Y. (1998) HVJ (Sendai virus) liposome-mediated gene transfer: current status and future perspectives. *Int. J. Oncol.* **12**, 1277–1285.
12. Yonemitsu, Y., Kaneda, Y., Muraishi, A., Yoshizumi, T., Sugimachi, K., and Sueishi, K. (1997) HVJ (Sendai virus)-cationic liposomes: a novel and potentially effective liposome-mediated technique for gene transfer to the airway epithelium. *Gene Ther.* **4**, 631–638.
13. Saeki, Y., Matsumoto, N., Nakano, Y., Mori, M., Awai, K., and Kaneda, Y. (1997) Development and characterization of cationic liposomes conjugated HVJ (Sendai

virus): reciprocal effect of cationic lipid for *in vitro* and *in vivo* gene transfer. *Hum. Gene Ther.* **8,** 2133–2141.

14. Namoto, M., Yonemitsu, Y., Nakagawa, K., Hashimoto, S., Kaneda, Y., Nawata, H., and Sueishi, K. (1998) Heterogeneous induction of apoptosis in colon cancer cells by wild-type p53 gene transfection. *Int. J. Oncol.* **12,** 777–784.

15. Matsumoto, T., Komori, K., Yonemitsu, Y., Morishita, R., Kaneda, Y., Sueishi, K., and Sugimachi, K. (1998) HVJ-liposome-mediated gene transfer of endothelial cell nitric oxide synthase inhibits intimal hyperplasia of canine vein grafts under conditions of poor runoff. *J. Vasc. Surg.* **27,** 135–144.

25

High-Efficiency and Low-Toxicity Adenovirus-Assisted Endothelial Transfection

Takamune Takahashi, Keiko Takahashi, and Thomas O. Daniel

1. Introduction

Cultured endothelial cells have provided a powerful tool for discovery of the molecular regulators of a range of vascular processes from angiogenesis to fibrinolysis *(1)*. Yet, the utility of genetic manipulation of endothelial culture systems to dissect critical intracellular signaling processes has been limited to date. Available methods such as retroviral transduction require endothelial proliferation, while cationic lipid mediated transfection is inefficient and evokes marked toxicity in cultured endothelial cells *(2–4)*. Adenoviral transduction of endothelial cells is efficient, but preparation of recombinant adenovirus vectors is cumbersome.

These experimental difficulties are enhanced by the challenge that endothelial cell heterogeneity imposes on the interpretation of results. Endothelial cells cultured from different vascular beds display marked differences in biochemical and phenotypic properties under identical culture conditions *(5–10)*, and immortalized endothelial lines display differences compared with microvascular and large-vessel-derived primary endothelial cells. For these reasons, methods for evaluating transient effects of gene expression in large populations of cultured primary and immortalized cell lines are needed. In order for such methods to be experimentally valuable for dissecting molecular roles for specific mediators of endothelial migration, attachment, proliferation, or apoptosis, they must be efficient and accompanied by low acute toxicity when applied to populations of endothelial cells. Under these conditions, transient high-level expression of dominant negative or antisense gene products offers a powerful method to dissect the molecular basis for endothelial cell behavior, including the basis for endothelial specialization that is retained in culture.

From: *Methods in Molecular Medicine, Vascular Disease: Molecular Biology and Gene Therapy Protocols*
Edited by: A. H. Baker © Humana Press Inc., Totowa, NJ

Here, we have identified critical variables that determine reproducible, efficient, and nontoxic transient transfection of cultured primary human renal microvascular endothelial cells (HRMEC), and of a human dermal microvascular endothelial cell line (HMEC-1). These experiments have significantly modified a less efficient and more toxic approach using replication-defective adenovirus as a "trojan horse" carrier of expression plasmid DNA that is adsorbed to viral particle surfaces in the presence of cationic lipid *(11–13)*.

2. Materials
2.1. Cells

1. Primary human renal microvascular endothelial cells (HRMEC cells, *14*). Cells from the third or fourth passage were used.
2. Human dermal microvascular endothelial cells (HMEC-1 cells).
3. HMEC-1 growth media: MCDB131 media (Sigma, St. Louis, MO) containing 15% calf serum (Hyclone Laboratories, Logan UT), 10 ng/ml epidermal growth factor (Collaborative Biomedical Products; Becton Dickinson, Bedford, MA), 1 mg/mL hydrocortisone (Sigma) 1 mM L-glutamine, 100 U/mL penicillin, and 100 mg/mL streptomycin (Gibco-BRL, Grand-Island, NY) *(15)*.

2.2. Propagation and Purification of Adenovirus

1. Ad5 transformed human embryonic kidney cells, HEK 293 (American Type Culture Collection, Rockville, MD, ATCC CRL 1583).
2. HEK 293 growth media: minimum essential media (MEM, Gibco-BRL), supplemented with 10% heat-inactivated fetal calf serum (Hyclone Laboratories), 2 mM L-glutamine, 100 U/mL penicillin, and 100 mg/mL streptomycin.
3. Serum free OPTIMEM media (Gibco-BRL).
4. 1 M Tris-HCl, pH 7.5.
5. BECKMAN SV40 rotor and ultracentrifuge (or equivalent).
6. Cesium chloride solutions (1.25 g/cm^3; 1.34 g/cm^3, and 1.43 g/cm^3).
7. Dialysis buffer: 10 mM Tris-HCl (pH 7.4), 1 mM MgCl$_2$.
8. Hydrate membrane: Molecular weight cut off 10,000 (Pierce, Rockford, IL).

2.3. Transfection

1. Plasmid DNA.
2. Lipofectamine (Gibco-BRL).
3. Polystyrene conical tubes (Falcon, Los Angeles, CA).

3. Methods
3.1. Propagation and Purification of Adenovirus
(see *also Chapter 22*)

1. Prior to adenoviral infection, discard HEK 293 culture medium and wash cells twice with serum-free medium OPTIMEM and discard.

2. Overlay 1.2 mL/p150 plate of stock cultures of adenovirus [Ad dl 312 (2×10^9 pfu/mL, kindly provided by Tom Shenk, Princeton University, and stored at $-80°C$ in serum-free medium] on cell monolayers and leave for 30 min at a multiplicity of infection (MOI) of 20.
3. Add 17 mL of growth medium to the cells and incubate for an additional 48–72 h, or until >90% of the cells showed a cytopathic effect.
4. Harvest cells by scraping, transferred to 50 mL polypropylene tubes and add 1 M Tris-HCl, pH 7.5 to 20 mM (final concentration).
5. Centrifuged for 8 min at 500g at 4°C.
6. Remove the supernatant and resuspend the pellet in 1.3 mL of serum free media/ 20 mM Tris-HCl.
7. Lyse the cell suspension by three freeze/thaw cycles ($-70°C/25°C$) to release intracellular adenoviral particles.
8. Centrifuge the lysate at 14,000g for 10 min at 4°C to remove the cellular debris.
9. Layer the supernatant fraction on top of a discontinuous CsCl step gradient (1.25 g/cm^3, 1.43 g/cm^3) and centrifuge at 150,000g (BECKMAN SV40 rotor) for 2 h at 20°C *(16,17)*.
10. Collect the visible adenovirus band by puncturing the lateral wall of the centrifuge tube using a 21-gage needle.
11. Increase the volume to 12.0 mL with 1.34 g/cm^3 CsCl solution.
12. Recover the adenovirus fraction after centrifugation at 150,000g for 16 h at 20°C *(18,19)*.
13. Dialyze 1 mL of adenovirus against 2.0 L of 10 mM Tris-HCl, pH 7.4, 1 mM MgCl$_2$ for 4 h at 4°C with three buffer changes.
14. Aliquot and freeze at $-70°C$ (*see* **Note 1**).

3.2. Preparation of Adenovirus/DNA/Cationic Lipid Complexes

1. Mix plasmid DNA (2.2 mg/p35 plate), lipofectamine (8.8 mg, reflecting a DNA:lipofectamine 1:4 ratio, *see* **Note 2**) and adenovirus (2×10^9 pfu/mL) in sequence by gentle tapping in 800 mL of serum free medium OPTIMEM in a polystyrene conical tube (Falcon) (*see* **Note 3**).
2. Incubate the mixture for 30 min at 37°C.

3.3. Transfection

1. Plate cells on p35 plates at a density of 7.2×10^5 cells 24 h prior to transfection to achieve a confluency of 90–100% (*see* **Note 4**).
2. Wash cells twice in serum free medium OPTIMEM.
3. Layer preformed DNA/Lipofectamine/adenovirus complexes (MOI = 42) on the cells, and incubate for 30 min at 37°C (*see* **Note 5**).
4. Add fetal bovine serum (FBS) 2% v/v final) to the medium and incubate cells for 30 min in the CO$_2$ incubator at 37°C (*see* **Note 6**).
5. Replace the medium with growth medium and culture cells overnight.

6. Forty-eight hours after transfection, change the medium again, and use cells for biological assays (*see* **Note 7**).

4. Notes

1. Extensive dialysis and freeze/thaw of virus dramatically reduces viral titer and the transfection efficiency.
2. The ratio of plasmid DNA to cationic liposome in the adenovirus complex is a critical independent variable that affects transfection efficiency, yet the amount of total DNA used is also quite important (**Fig. 1B**). Plasmid DNA used in these studies was prepared using an endotoxin-free DNA isolation kit (Qiagen, Chatsworth, CA). Other formulations of cationic lipid, including Lipofectamine plus™ (Gibco-BRL) did not improve results.
3. Polypropylene tubes reduce transfection efficiency.
4. Cell density at transfection is a critical determinant of cell recovery. When cells plated at low density are transfected, detachment of transfected cells appears to reduce apparent efficiency of transfection and viability at 48 h. Because it has been reported that $\alpha_v\beta_3$, $\alpha_v\beta_5$ promote adenovirus internalization *(20,21)*, adenovirus may competitively inhibit integrin-mediated attachment to the extracellular matrix. Optimal recoveries are obtained at 48 hours after transfection of plates containing cells at 90–100% confluency (**Fig. 1A**).
5. The high MOI (from 10 to 80) facilitates efficient transfection during abbreviated exposure times (**Fig. 1C**).
6. The duration of cell exposure to adenovirus/DNA/cationic lipid complexes in serum-free medium is an important factor affecting cell viability and subsequent function. Addition of 2% (v/v) FBS to the medium after 30 min exposure in serum-free conditions reduces toxicity, as it increases replating efficiency to greater than 90% and returns BrdU incorporation to levels comparable to those of nontransfected cells (**Fig. 2A**). Preserved function of endothelial cells transfected by this method was demonstrated in a wound closure assay, where we evaluated the rate at which confluent endothelial monolayers migrate to close a circular wound of 800 nm diameter (**Fig. 2B**). Transfected cells expressing β-galactosidase were as competent as cells not exposed to complexes, adenovirus, DNA, or lipofectamine alone to migrate in the wound closure assay.
7. With optimization of these variables, we consistently achieve transfection efficiencies of 40–45% in primary HRMEC and in the HMEC-1 line in over 20 independent experiments (**Fig. 1D**). Application of this improved method will make it possible to rapidly evaluate effects of transient expression of native or mutated forms of potential therapeutic targets in endothelial cells cultured from a range of different vascular sites. In conjunction with recent improvements in the capacity to culture endothelial cells from different tissue sources, we anticipate that any differences in molecular actions ascribed to endothelial heterogeneity may be rapidly and efficiently uncovered. Finally, this sort of analysis

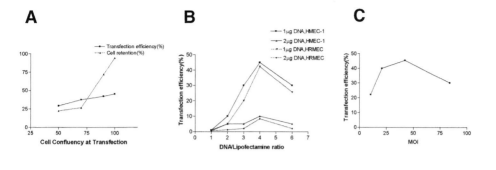

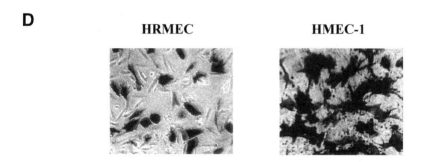

Fig. 1. Critical determinants for adenovirus assisted transfection. (**A**) High cell density preserve attachment of the transfected cells without reduction of transfection efficiency. HMEC-1 cells (3×10^5 cells) were plated at different cell densities to achieve the indicated cell confluency in 12-well plates, transfected with pSRα/βgal plasmid DNA and the detached cells were counted 48 h after transfection. The attached cells were stained for β-galactosidase activity *(22)*. (**B**) Expression plasmid DNA/Lipofectamine™ Ratio and DNA amount are critical transfection variables. HRMEC and HMEC-1 cells (3×10^5 cells) were plated in 12-well plates and transfected as described (MOI = 40) 48 h prior to staining for β-galactosidase activity. The mean ratio of β-galactosidase positive to total cells was determined in five independent fields representing over (400 cells) scored. (**C**) Optimization of MOI in endothelial transfection. HMEC-1 cells (3×10^5 cells) were plated in 12-well plates and transfected with plasmid DNA (1.0 mg)/Lipofectamine™ (4.0 mg) and varying MOI of adenovirus. (**D**) Adenovirus assisted lipofection showed high transfection efficiency in primary HRMEC cells as well as HMEC-1 cells. HRMEC or HMEC-1 (3×10^5 cells) were plated in 12-well plates, transfected and stained for β-galactosidase activity at 60 h after transfection, as described.

will permit evaluation of signaling molecules, transcription factors, and other gene products that play critical roles in endothelial proliferation, migration, assembly, and apoptosis.

A

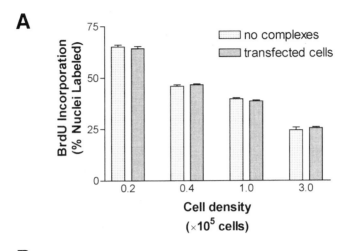

B

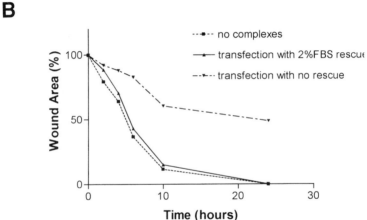

Fig. 2. Evaluation of cell viability (proliferation, migration) of transfected endothelial cells. (**A**) Bromodeoxyuridine incorporation in transfected cells. Transfected cells were replated 24 h after transfection. Effects of cell density on proliferation were examined by BrdU immunolabeling assay (Boeringer Mannheim, Indanapolis, IN) 48 h after transfection. Control cells were exposed to serum-free medium (no DNA, no Lipofectamine, no adenovirus) for 60 min. (**B**) Transfected HMEC-1 cells are competent to complete wound closure. HMEC-1 cells (7.2×10^5 cells) were plated in 35 mm culture dishes, transfected with pSRα/βgal plasmid DNA as described and allowed to grow to confluence for 36 h. A circular "wound" of approx 800 nm was created using a rotating silicon tipped bit mounted on a drill press. Visual images of the rate of wound closure were captured at the indicated time points and the wound area calculated using a computer image analysis system (Bioquant, Nashville, TN). Each data point represents the mean ratio of wound area to original area for three different wounds of similar size, at each indicated time. Control cells were prepared in the same manner without adenovirus/DNA/Lipofectamine complexes.

References

1. Bussolino, F., Mantovani, A., and Persico, G. (1997) Molecular mechanisms of blood vessel formation. *Trends Biochem. Sci.* **22,** 251–256.
2. Teifel, M., Heine, L. T., Milbredt, S., and Friedl, P. (1997) Optimization of transfection of human endothelial cells. *Endothelium* **5,** 21–35.
3. Dichek, D. A. (1991) Retroviral vector-mediated gene transfer into endothelial cells. *Mol. Biol. Med.* **8,** 257-266
4. Kahn, M. L., Lee, S. W., and Dichek, D. A. (1992) Optimization of retroviral vector-mediated gene transfer into endothelial cells in vitro. *Circ. Res.* **71,** 1508–1517.
5. Risau, W. (1995) Differentiation of endothelium. *FASEB J.* **9,** 926–933.
6. Craig, L. E., Spelman, J. P., Strandberg, J. D., and Zink, M. C. (1998) Endothelial cells from diverse tissues exhibit differences in growth and morphology. *Microvasc. Res.* **55,** 65–76.
7. Plendl, J., Sinowatz, F., and Auerbach, R. (1992) The heterogenicity of the vascular endothelium. *Anat. Histol. Embryol.* **21,** 256–262.
8. Mason, J. C., Yarwood, H., Sugars, K., and Haskard, D. O. (1997) Human umbilical vein and dermal microvascular endothelial cells show heterogeneity in response to PKC activation. *Am. J. Physiol.* **273,** C1233–C1240.
9. Wojta, J., Hoover, R. L., and Daniel, T. O. (1989) Vascular origin determines plasminogen activator expression in human endothelial cells. Renal endothelial cells produce large amounts of single chain urokinase type plasminogen activator. *J. Biol. Chem.* **264,** 2846–2852.
10. Obrig ,T. G., Louise, C. B., Lingwood, C. A., Boyd, B., Barley-Maloney, L., and Daniel, T. O. (1993) Endothelial heterogeneity in Shiga toxin receptors and responses. *J. Biol .Chem.* **268,** 15,484–15,488.
11. Yoshimura, K., Rosenfeld, M. A., Seth, P., and Crystal, R. G. (1993) Adenovirus-mediated augmentation of cell transfection with unmodified plasmid vectors. *J. Biol. Chem.* **268,** 2300–2303.
12. Raja-Walia, R., Webber, J., Naftilan, J., Chapman, G. D., and Naftilan, A. J. (1995) Enhancement of liposome-mediated gene transfer into vascular tissue by replication deficient adenovirus. *Gene Ther.* **2,** 521–530.
13. Kreuzer, J., Denger, S., Reifers, F., Beisel, C., Haack, K., Gebert, J., and Kubler, W. (1996) Adenovirus-assisted lipofection: efficient in vitro gene transfer of luciferase and cytosine deaminase to human smooth muscle cells. *Atherosclerosis* **124,** 49–60.
14. Martin, M., Schoecklmann, H., Foster, G., Barley-Maloney, L., McKanna, J., and Daniel, T. O. (1997) Identification of a subpopulation of human renal microvascular endothelial cells with capacity to form capillary-like cord and tube structures. *In Vitro Cell Dev. Biol.* **33,** 261–269.
15. Xu, Y., Swerlick, R. A., Sepp, N., Bosse, D., Ades, E. W., and Lawley, T. J. (1994) Characterization of expression and modulation of cell adhesion molecules on an immortalized human dermal microvascular endothelial cell line (HMEC-1). *J. Invest. Dermatol.* **102,** 833–837.

16. Kanegae, Y., Makimura, M., and Saito, I. (1994) A simple and efficient method for purification of infectious recombinant adenovirus. *Jpn. J. Med. Sci. Biol.* **47,** 157–166.
17. Kanegae, Y., Lee, G., Sato, Y., Tanaka, M., Nakai, M., Sakaki, T., Sugano, S., and Saito, I. (1995). Efficient gene activation in mammalian cells by using recombinant adenovirus expressing site-specific Cre recombinase. *Nucleic Acid Reserach* **23,** 3816–3821.
18. Graham, F. L., Van der, E. B. A. J. (1973) A new technique for the assay of infectivity of human adenovirus 5 DNA. *Virology* **52,** 456–467.
19. Graham, F. L. and Prevec, L.(1995) Methods for construction of adenovirus vectors. *Mol. Biotechnol.* **3,** 207–220.
20. Wickham, T. J., Mathias, P., Cheresh, D. A., and Nemerow, G. R. (1993) Integrins alpha v beta 3 and alpha v beta 5 promote adenovirus internalization but not virus attachment. *Cell* **73,** 309–319.
21. Wickham, T. J., Filardo, E. J., Cheresh, D. A., and Nemerow, G. R. (1994). Integrin alpha v beta 5 selectively promotes adenovirus mediated cell membrane permeabilization. *J. Cell. Biol.* 1994 **127,** 257–264.
22. Sanes, J. R., Rubenstein, J. L., and Nicolas, J. F. (1986) Use of a recombinant retrovirus to study post-implantation cell lineage in mouse embryos. *EMBO J.* **5,** 3133–3142.

26

Gene Transfer in Vascular Cells Using an Engineered Na-H Exchanger (NHE1) as a Selectable Marker

Jacques Pouysségur and Danièle Roux

1. Introduction

The techniques of gene transfer using transfection via electroporation, $CaPO_4$, or cationic lipids rely on selectable markers because of the low efficiency of this approach. Selectable markers range from fluorescent molecules to a variety of cytotoxic compounds, with the most commonly used in animal cells being neomycin, hygromycin, and gancyclovir. With fluorescent molecules or cell surface markers that can be visualized with fluorescent antibodies, one needs a cell sorting machine, whereas with cytotoxic drugs, the procedure is simpler, but requires several days to irradicate the majority of the cell population that has not received the gene of interest. In the case of vascular cells (smooth muscle or endothelial cells), the nontransfected population could easily exceed 90% of the total cell population.

The method we are proposing in this chapter is a simple technique of acid-loading that efficiently kills cells within 2 h. The principle of this approach exploits the high toxicity of cytoplasmic H^+ and the capacity of the Na-H exchanger (NHE) to extrude H^+ at the expense of the inwarded-directed Na^+ gradient.

The Na-H exchanger is a plasma membrane transporter expressed in all eukaryotic cells, whose major function is to regulate intracellular pH (for review *see* **ref. *1***). The first isoform cloned, NHE1 *(2)*, expressed in most mammalian cells including vascular smooth muscle cells and endothelial cells *(3–5)*, is sensitive to amiloride and its derivatives including commercially available ethyl isopropyl amiloride (EIPA). When cells are acutely acid-loaded,

From: *Methods in Molecular Medicine, Vascular Disease: Molecular Biology and Gene Therapy Protocols*
Edited by: A. H. Baker © Humana Press Inc., Totowa, NJ

Transfection   H⁺ Loading   pH Recovery
DAC-30

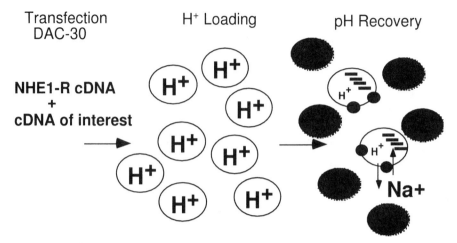

NHE1-R = Na-H Exchanger Amiloride-resistant (selective marker)

Fig. 1. Scheme of acid-load selection. Following the acidification, only cells that expresses NHE1-R are capable of regulating intracellular pH in presence of EIPA and therefore survive the selection. Note that these cells express the gene of interest (gene of interest denoted by thick black lines), whereas the rest of the cell population dies (black circles).

they recover this pHi insult within minutes, unless NHE1 is inhibited with EIPA. In this case all cells die by acidosis within 1 or 2 h. By appropriate mutations in the transmembrane segments of NHE1, we engineered a NHE1, referred to as NHE1-R, which represents an exchanger at least 1000-fold more resistant to EIPA than the parental form (*6*, Noël, J. and Pouysségur, J., unpublished results). When we transfect the plasmid encoding NHE1-R, only the cells expressing this marker survive an acid-load in the presence of EIPA. Because cell death occurs within 2 h of the acid load insult, this approach is efficient for "physically sorting" the transfected cells directly in the dish (**Fig. 1**). In our group we have extensively used this method for the selection of stable transfectants (*7,8*). However, owing to the rapid cell killing of nontransfected cells, its great advantage is in transient transfection experiments. With few variations, this technique has been successfully used to express constitutive active mutants of MAP kinase kinase (MEK1) (*9*), dominant-negative mutants of MEK1, p44MAPK (*9,10*), and SHC (*11*), as well as antisense cDNA for p44MAPK (*10*) or for the cell cycle inhibitors p27 (*12*).

2. Materials

1. Two incubators at 37°C, one regulated for CO_2 (tissue culture type), the other without CO_2 (bacterial type).

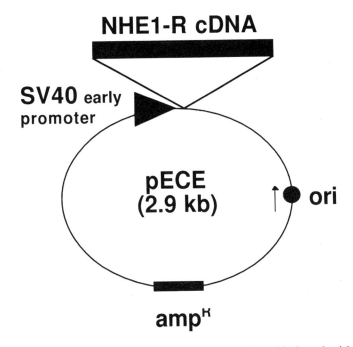

Fig. 2. Simplified map of the NHE1-R expression plasmid cloned within *Hind*III and *Xba* I sites in the polylinker of the pECE mammalian expression vector *(13)*. Digestion of this plasmid with *Bam*HI will generate three fragments of 0.9, 1.9, and 3.0 kb, respectively (there are two *Bam*H1 sites in the cDNA insert).

2. Ethyl isopropyl amiloride (EIPA) from (Sigma, St. Louis, MO, cat. no. A3085): make a 100X stock solution at 3 mM in DMSO and store at –20°C.
3. NHE1-R cDNA cloned in the mammalian expression vector pECE (*see* **Fig. 2**, *[13]*), this is provided by the authors upon request.
4. DAC-30™ cationic liposomes (Eurogentec, Liège, Belgium) (http:/ /www. eurogentec.be) with detailed transfection protocol.
5. Ammonium-loading buffer (ALB) (*[1], see* **Note 1**): 70 mM choline chloride, 50 mM ammonium chloride, 5 mM potassium chloride, 1 mM magnesium chloride, 2 mM calcium chloride, 5 mM glucose, and 15 mM HEPES (acid form). Adjust the pH to 7.5 with TRIS-base, add phenol red (optional), and steriliae through 0.22-µm filters. Store at 4°C.
6. Washing buffer (WB) (*see* **Note 1**): 130 mM choline chloride, 5 mM potassium chloride, 1 mM magnesium chloride, 2 mM calcium chloride, 5 mM glucose, and 15 mM MOPS (acid form). Adjust the pH to 7.0 with TRIS-base and sterilize through 0.22-µm filters. Store at 4°C. Before use, add EIPA to a final concentration of 30 µM.
7. PHi-recovery buffer (RB): 120 mM sodium chloride, 5 mM potassium chloride, 1 mM magnesium chloride, 2 mM calcium chloride, 5 mM glucose, and 15 mM

MOPS (acid form). Adjust the pH to 7.0 with TRIS-base, add phenol red (optional), and sterilize through 0.22-μm filters. Store at 4°C. Before use, add EIPA to a final concentration of 30 μ*M*.

3. Methods

The method described below has been experienced with success in a variety of cultured cells including fibroblasts, smooth muscle cells, and vascular endothelial cells. These include HUVEC and two established cell lines derived respectively from mouse lung capillary endothelial cells (1G11) and HUVEC (Eahy 926).

3.1. Gene Transfer

The acid-load selection has been successfully applied following several gene transfer methods. Thus, for adherent cells such as vascular endothelial and smooth muscle cells, the transfection protocol yielding highest efficiency should be used. For all endothelial cells tested, DAC-30 lipofection gave positive transfectants whereas the classical $CaPO_4$ was totally inefficient.

1. On d 1: plate the cells in 100-mm Petri dishes at a cell density that allows them to reach 40–70% confluency at the time of transfection (usually 48 h after plating).
2. On d 3: 2 h prior to transfection, replace the medium of each plate with fresh culture medium.
3. Add DAC-30/DNA complex according to the protocol detailed in the technical bulletin (*see* **Note 2**).

3.2. Acid-Load Selection for Transient Expression

The time required is 2 h. All buffers should be prewarmed at 37°C before use.

3.2.1. Ammonium-Loading Step (see **Note 3**)

1. Remove the dishes from the CO_2 incubator.
2. Aspirate the culture medium and rinse once with 5 mL of ALB.
3. Add 10 mL of ALB per 100-mm dish.
4. Incubate at 37°C in a bacterial incubator (**no CO2**) for 1 h.

3.2.2. pH-Recovering Step

1. Aspirate the ALB.
2. Rinse twice with 10 mL of WB and quickly add 10 mL of RB (this operation should not exceed more than 15 s) (*see* **Note 4**).
3. Incubate for 1 h at 37°C in bacterial incubator (**no CO2**).
4. Aspirate the RB.
5. Rinse briefly with culture medium.
6. Add 10 mL of complete culture medium and place the dishes in the regular CO_2 incubator.

Within the next 2 h you could easily see by phase contrast microscopy nontransfected cells rounding up and either detaching from the dish or "dead-fixed" cells on the dish in response to the acute intracellular acidification. If one needs to perform biochemical analyses on the few transfected cells and thus eliminate the dead cells firmly fixed to the dish, trypsinize the surviving cells the next day and transfer them from a 100-mm dish to a 35- or 12-mm dish. After 4 h, aspirate the medium and rinse the attached cells gently. All cell debris and dead cells will be easily discarded.

3.3. Acid-Load Selection for Stable Expression

Proceed exactly as describe above for transient expression.

1. When cells have grown to near confluency in the initial 100-mm plate (or if there were only few transformants yielding clones visible by naked eye), apply a second acid-load selection (following exactly the same protocol as the first one), then apply a third selection 3–5 d later. Usually most of the clones that survive the third acid-load selection will survive a fourth selection. This usually takes about 2 wk.
2. Isolate the colonies for analysis and when interesting ones are expanded and passaged, apply the acid-load selection once or twice a month, in order to maintain the transgene in case of instability.

3.4. Controls

It is important to run parallel controls for each experiment to ensure that the saline solutions behave as expected and that the cells used do not express other NHE isoforms (*see* **Note 5**).

1. As controls, transfect two identical 100 mm dishes A and B without the selectable marker NHE1-R cDNA.
2. Treat dish A exactly as reported in **Subheading 3.2.**
3. Treat dish B exactly as reported in **Subheading 3.2.**, except omit EIPA from both WB and pHi-Recovery Buffer.

Expected results: All cells should die in dish A, whereas all cells should survive in dish B.

4. Notes

1. ALB and WB are Na-free isotonic saline solutions; therefore, they cannot be pH-adjusted with NaOH.
2. DNA consists of at least two expression vector plasmids in a ratio 2:1 or 3:1 (plasmid with the gene of interest : plasmid with selectable marker NHE1-R).
3. ALB does not acidify the cells per se. In fact this solution slightly alkalinizes the cells. However, when this saline solution is removed and rapidly washed out, NH_3 rapidly diffuses across the cell membrane out of the cell driving the

equilibrium ($NH_4^+ \leftrightarrow NH_3 + H^+$) rightward. Consequently, there is a rapid accumulation of H^+ proportional to the intracellular concentration of NH_4^+.

4. **VERY CRUCIAL:** If several dishes are transfected in parallel, which is often the case with controls, the washing step must be executed very quickly; therefore, handle one dish at a time. This step of washing aims to completely remove extracellular traces of NH_4^+. Since this step establishes the concentration of H^+ inside the cell[2] and the start of acidification, two rapid washes are required.

5. Some cells, particularly those from the gastrointestinal digestive tract and from the kidney proximal tubules, are known to express the amiloride- or EIPA- resistant NHE isoform, NHE3 (*see* **ref.** *1*). If a cell expresses such an isoform, the selection reported here is not possible. In that case, cells in the control dish A will survive the acid-load selection.

Acknowledgments

We thank Drs Josette Noël and Laurent Counillon for their valuable contribution in the preparation of the NHE1-R cDNA genetic marker, Dr. Ellen Van Obberghen-Schilling for carefully reading the manuscript, Dominique Grall for efficient assistance in cell culture, and all the members of the laboratory for fruitful discussions. This work was supported by research grants from CNRS (Centre National de la Recherche Scientifique), the University of Nice, INSERM (Institut National de la Santé et de la Recherche Médicale), ARC (Association pour la Recherche contre le Cancer), and the Ligue Nationale de la Recherche contre le Cancer.

References

1. Wakabayshi, S., Shigekawa, M., and Pouysségur, J. (1997) Molecular Physiology of vertebrate Na^+/H^+ exchangers. *Physiol. Rev.* **77**, 51–74.

2. Sardet, C., Franchi, A., and Pouysségur, J. (1989) Molecular cloning, primary structure, and expression of the human growth factor-activatable Na^+/H^+ antiporter. *Cell* **56**, 271–280.

3. Bussolino, F., Wang, J. M., Turrini, F., Alessi, D., Ghigo, D., Costamagna, C., Pescarmona, G., Mantovani, A., and Bosia, A. (1989) Stimulation of the Na^+/H^+ exchanger in human endothelial cells activated by granulocyte- and granulocyte-macrophage-colony-stimulating factor. Evidence for a role in proliferation and migration. *J. Biol. Chem.* **264**, 18,284–18,287.

4. Vigne, P., Ladoux, A., and Frelin, C. (1991) Endothelins activate Na^+/H^+ exchange in brain capillary endothelial cells via a high affinity endothelin-3 receptor that is not coupled to phospholipase. *J. Biol. Chem.* **266**, 5925–5928.

5. Faber, S., Lang, J. J., Hock, F. J., Scholkens, B. A., and Mutschler, E. (1998) Intracellular pH regulation in bovine aortic endothelial cells: evidence of both Na^+/H^+ exchange and Na^+-dependent $Cl^-/HCO3^-$ exchange. *Cell Physiol. Biochem.* **8**, 202–211.

6. Counillon, L., Franchi, A., and Pouysségur, J. (1993) A point mutation of the Na$^+$/H$^+$ exchanger gene (NHE1) and amplification of the mutated allele confer amiloride-resistance upon chronic acidosis. *Proc. Natl. Acad. Sci. USA* **90,** 4508–4512.
7. Van Obberghen, E., Vouret-Craviari, V., Haslam, R., Chambard, J. C., and Pouysségur, J. (1991) Cloning, functional expression and role in cell growth regulation of a hamster 5-HT2 receptor subtype. *Mol. Endocrinol.* **5,** 881–889.
8. Rivard, N., McKenzie, F., Brondello, J. M., and Pouysségur, J. (1995) The phosphotyrosine phosphatase PTP1D, but not PTP1C, is an essential mediator of fibroblast proliferation induced by tyrosine kinase and G protein-coupled receptors. *J. Biol. Chem.* **270,** 11,017–11,024.
9. Pagès, G., Brunet, A., L'Allemain, G., and Pouysségur, J. (1994) Constitutive mutant and putative regulatory serine phosphorylation site of mammalian MAP kinase kinase (MEK1). *EMBO J.* **13,** 3003–3010.
10. Pagès, G., Lenormand, P., L'Allemain, G., Chambard, J. C., Méloche, S., and Pouyssségur, J. (1993) The mitogen-activated protein kinases p42^{mapk} and p44^{mapk} are required for fibroblast proliferation. *Proc. Natl. Acad. Sci. USA* **90,** 8319–8323.
11. Chen, Y., Pouysségur, J., Courtneidge, S., and Von Obberghen-Schilling, E. (1996) Shc adaptor proteins are key transducers of mitogenic signaling mediated by the G protein-coupled thrombin receptor *EMBO J.* **15,** 1037–1044
12. Rivard, N., L'Allemain, G., Bartek, J., and Pouysségur, J. (1996) Abrogation of p27^{Kip1} by cDNA antisense suppresses quiescence (G$_0$ state) in fibroblasts. *J. Biol. Chem.* **271,** 18,337–18,341.
13. Ellis, L., Morgan, D. O., Clauser, E., Edery, M., Jong, S. M., Wang, L. H. Roth, R. A., and Rutter, W. J. (1996) Mechanisms of receptor-mediated transmembrane communication. *Cold Spring Harbor Symp.Quant. Biol.* **51,** 773–784.2

27

Use of Retroviruses to Express Exogenous Genes in Vascular Smooth Muscle Cells

Trevor D. Littlewood and Stella A. Pelengaris

1. Introduction

The ability to express cloned genes in mammalian cells has proved invaluable in the study of gene expression and function and in clinical applications for the correction of functional gene loss by gene therapy. Despite the wide use of DNA-mediated transfection of genes into eukaryotic cells, viruses possess several advantages for the transfer and expression of exogenous genes. Several types of relatively small viruses including the papovavirus SV40, papillomaviruses, adenoviruses, and retroviruses have been successfully employed. Vectors based on larger viruses such as Epstein-Barr, herpes simplex, and vaccinia are generally able to maintain infectivity in a wide range of cell types and have a greater capacity for foreign DNA. However, because most introduced cDNA sequences are relatively small these vectors have not been widely used.

Retroviruses exhibit several characteristics which render them excellent vehicles for the transfer and expression of exogenous genes (*see* **ref. *1*** for review). First, the relatively small genome of retroviruses is easily manipulated to allow the insertion of foreign genes and the ability to complement defects in viral replication *in trans* allows the use of replication-defective retroviruses. (This is an important consideration in limiting viral infection.) Second, the viruses can easily be produced at high titers in culture. Moreover, the efficiency of infection of susceptible cells is extremely high, approaching 100% in some cases. Third, retroviruses carry powerful transcriptional enhancer elements ensuring high levels of expression in a wide range of cell types.

The majority of retroviral vectors described to date are derived from either avian viruses or, more commonly, from the Moloney murine leukemia virus

From: *Methods in Molecular Medicine, Vascular Disease: Molecular Biology and Gene Therapy Protocols*
Edited by: A. H. Baker © Humana Press Inc., Totowa, NJ

(Mo-MuLV). Infection of target cells is mediated by the interaction of surface glycoproteins encoded by the viral *env* gene and poorly characterized cell surface receptors. The envelope proteins of MuLV-based viruses can be divided into different classes based on the particular cell-surface receptors with which they interact (*see* **ref. 2** for review). The host-range (tropism) of the virus is, therefore, restricted to those species that express the appropriate receptor. Thus, an ecotropic murine retrovirus can only infect mouse or rat cells, whereas an amphotropic virus has a broader host range, because its envelope proteins can interact with the host-cell receptors of a number of species. Although infection of a particular cell type may be restricted by the tissue-specific expression of cell receptors, this can be overcome by the prior expression of the appropriate receptor. Even if a target cell expresses the correct receptor, these receptors will be blocked if the host cell is already expressing the relevant envelope protein. Thus, a cell that is already infected with a replication-competent retrovirus expressing its *env* gene (NB many murine cells contain endogenous retroviruses) will be resistant to subsequent infection with a retrovirus of the same tropism. Although most retroviral vectors are based on MuLV, it is possible to extend their host range by packaging the genome of the retroviral vector in a virion particle bearing envelope proteins from an amphotropic virus (pseudotyping). "Packaging" cell lines harbor a defective provirus (e.g., one that lacks a packaging signal) that cannot itself be packaged into mature virions but, nonetheless, encodes viral proteins required for replication. Thus, DNA of a replication-defective provirus, when transfected into a packaging cell line, gives rise to retroviral RNA, which will be packaged by helper virus, proteins into mature "helper-free" virus and the source of the packaging *env* gene may be used to modify (pseudotype) the tropism of the recombinant virions (**Fig. 1**). Although the "helper-free" virus stock produced remains replication-defective, it is nonetheless, fully infectious. In the absence of helper viral gene products in the infected host cell, no further viral particles will be generated.

The packaging cell lines are susceptible to transfection by retroviral DNA using standard techniques (e.g., calcium phosphate or lipofection). Both transient and stable transfections have been employed typically giving viral titers of 10^3–10^6 infectious units per milliliter.

1.1. Retroviral Vectors for the Expression of Exogenous Genes in Mammalian Cells

The simplest retroviral vectors are those in which viral structural genes are deleted and replaced by sequences with one or more restriction enzyme sites to facilitate insertion of new sequences (**Fig. 2**). Although these vectors usually produce high titer virus stocks when transfected into a suitable packaging cell line, they are limited in use by the lack of a selectable marker. It is thus diffi-

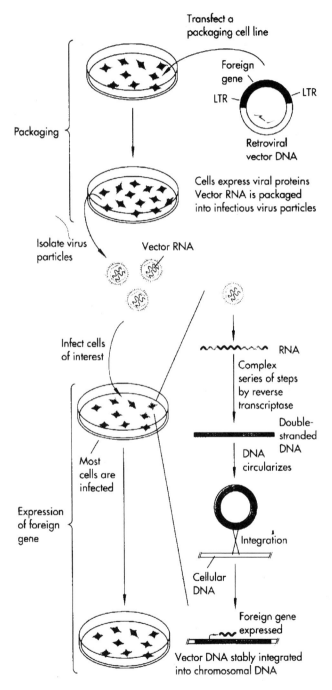

Fig. 1. Outline of the protocol for the production of infectious, replication-deficient retrovirus and the infection of host cells.

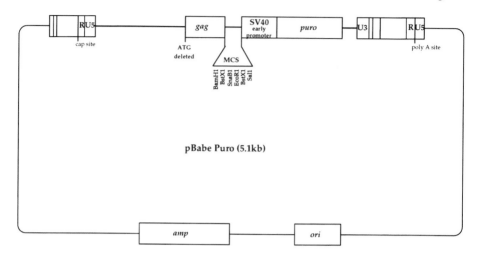

Fig. 2. Typical structure of a retroviral construct. Shown is the pBabe puro vector described by *(4)*. These vectors are also available with other markers for selection in mammalian cells such as hygromycin and neomycin. The retroviral *gag* gene does not generate a protein since the ATG is deleted. The viral LTR drives expression of the gene inserted into the multiple cloning site (MCS) and expression of the *puromycin* gene is from the SV40 early promoter. The vector also includes an origin of replication *(ori)* and the *ampicillin* gene *(amp)* for growth and selection in *E. coli*.

cult to identify transfected or infected cells harboring the recombinant virus if no selection exists for the expressed gene or there is no easily recognized phenotype. To overcome this problem, retroviral vectors that harbor genes encoding a selectable phenotype are commonly used. Genes encoding thymidine kinase *(tk)*, guanosine phosphoribosyl transferase *(gpt)* and dihydrofolate reductase *(dhfr)* have been used as selectable markers in retroviral vectors but require host cells that lack these activities. Vectors carrying *dhfr* have the advantage that the copy number of proviral sequences may be amplified by selection with methotrexate to give higher viral titers. However, the most widely used vectors are those which encode resistance to the drugs neomycin *(neo)*, hygromycin B *(hgr)*, puromycin *(puro)* and bleomycin/phleomycin *(bleo)*. These vectors may be used in a wide range of cell types, they do not require special media for selection and the drugs used for selection are readily available and fairly inexpensive. Alternatively, the retroviral vector can be engineered to express a cell surface marker such as CD20 or the green fluorescent protein from *Aequorea victoria* and the infected cells selected by FACS. This approach has proved to be particularly useful for selecting and tracking infected hematopoietic cells both in vitro and in vivo *(3–6)*. In general, of the vectors that carry two genes, the gene proximal to the 5' LTR is expressed from the genomic length viral RNA and the more distal gene is either expressed from a spliced subgenomic mRNA or from an internal promoter (e.g., herpes simplex *tk* promoter) inserted in the vector. All of the retroviral vectors also contain a gene encoding resistance to an antibiotic (most commonly ampicillin) for amplification in *Escherichia coli*. Because recombination is sometimes a problem during transformation of retroviral vectors into *E. coli*, those vectors that possess the *neo* or *hgr* genes may be co-selected with both ampicillin and either kanamycin (or neomycin) or hygromycin, respectively.

Most retroviral vectors of this type provide constitutive expression of the exogenous sequences. In some situations, however, this may not be desirable. For example, very high levels of some products may be toxic, or the product may restrict cell proliferation (e.g., when studying the effects of tumor suppressors) or induce apoptosis, making it difficult or impossible to establish cells that express the exogenous gene. To overcome these problems a number of inducible promoters have been developed. Some examples of such inducible promoters are the heat shock, metallothionien, growth hormone, and tetracycline *(7–11)* promoters, and the dexamethasone-dependent LTR of the mouse mammary tumor virus *(12)*. Others have rendered constitutively expressed proteins functionally hormone-dependent by fusion with the hormone-binding domain of certain steroid hormone receptors, notably the estrogen receptor *(13)*. Such fusion proteins are inactive in the absence of hormone because they are complexed with a variety of intracellular polypeptides, of which hsp90 is the prototype. Ligand binding releases the receptor from these inhibitory complexes.

1.2. Retroviral-Mediated Gene Delivery in the Vascular System

Cardiovascular disease and, in particular, arterial narrowing, is a major health problem of the developed world. Interventional techniques such as angioplasty have been used in an attempt to restore the diameter of the arterial lumen and hence blood flow. However, following angioplasty intimal hyperplasia and arterial remodeling often result in a renarrowing of the arterial lumen at the site of angioplasty—this is known as restenosis. Because intimal hyperplasia is largely the result of smooth muscle cell proliferation these cells are an inviting target for therapies aimed at limiting their proliferative capacity. Consequently, a considerable amount of effort has been directed at modifying the behavior of smooth muscle cells by the introduction of exogenous genes, and a variety of methods have been adopted for this purpose (*see* **refs.** *14–16* for review).

Although Semliki Forest, Sendai and adenovirus vectors and liposome-mediated methods have been widely used for the transfer of genes into vascular smooth muscle cells, retroviruses have also been successfully employed (*see* refs. *17–20* for review). For example, retroviral delivery and expression of antisense cyclin G_1 inhibits the proliferation of aortic smooth muscle cells in vitro and reduces neointima formation in vivo *(21)*. Similarly, retroviral transfer and expression have been used to investigate the role of oncoproteins and tumor suppressor proteins in the proliferation and apoptosis of vascular smooth muscle cells from normal and artherosclerotic plaques *(22–25)*. Retroviruses have also been used to express tissue plasminogen activator (tPA) *(26)*, interferon γ *(27)*, granulocyte colony-stimulating factor *(28)*, erythropoietin *(29)*, nitric oxide synthase *(30)*, and antisense molecules to the angiotensin II type 1 receptor *(31)* in vascular smooth muscle cells. Although replication-deficient retroviruses are relatively inefficient at gene transfer in vivo *(32)*, the genetically modified cells generated in vitro have, in some cases, been successfully reintroduced *(33)*. In addition, a modified retrovirus bearing a chimeric MoMuLV envelope protein incorporating a high-affinity collagen-binding domain has recently been used to target the retrovirus specifically to exposed collagen at sites of vascular injury in vivo *(34)*. Thus, retroviruses are useful vectors for the transfer and expression of exogenous genes into vascular cells both in vitro and in vivo.

1.3. Safety Considerations

If an amphotropic virus is involved, the need for effective containment is paramount. It is extremely important to ensure that no infectious virus is released. This may be achieved by verifying the absence of both reverse transcriptase activity and infectious virus in the culture medium of infected cells (*see* **Subheading 3.4.3.**). Some consideration should also be given to the nature of the inserted gene(s). For example, incorporation of the gene encoding a foreign glycoprotein into RSV virions yielded virus that could infect both avian and human cells with equal efficiency *(35)*. Particular attention should be paid to the insertion of oncogenes (including those whose protein products can interfere with the function of tumor suppressors) or genes encoding biologically active proteins (e.g., growth factors or cytokines) that may alter the proliferation, differentiation, or death of cells. Modifications to eukaryotic viral vectors not including genes whose products are potentially harmful may, nevertheless, give rise to harmful effects. For example, the inserted gene may lead to the alteration of tissue tropism or host range, increase in infectivity, recombination, or complementation of any disabling or attenuating feature of the vector or resistance to antiviral therapies. It is thus essential to seek the advice of the local safety representatives in the planning of experiments involving the use of retroviral vectors.

2. Materials

2.1. Insertion of Exogenous Genes into the Retroviral Vector

1. All of the reagents required for the isolation, cloning, amplification, and sequencing of DNA are available from suppliers of molecular biology reagents.
2. Antibiotics used for the selection of *E. coli* transformed with retroviral vectors are available from Sigma (St. Louis, MO).

2.2. Culture of the Retroviral Packaging Cell Line

2.2.1. Culture of the Retroviral Packaging Cell Line

Several retroviral packaging cell lines are available (*see* **Note 1**). The most commonly used in our laboratory for the production of ecotropic virus is the Bosc23 cell line and the materials and methods described below are adapted for the use of this cell line.

1. Bosc cell line: Available from the American Type Culture Collection (Rockville, MD) (www.atcc.org) or the European Collection of Cell Cultures (Salisburg, UK) (www.camr.org.uk/ecacc.htm).
2. DME growth medium: Dulbecco's modified Eagle's medium supplemented with 10% (v/v) heat-inactivated fetal bovine serum (FBS), 100 U/mL penicillin, 100 U/mL streptomycin, and 2 m*M* L-glutamine.
3. Hygromycin B (Calbiochem, Nottingham, UK, cat. no. 400051): supplied as a solution and can be used directly. Add to the growth medium and filter the complete medium (0.2-µm filter).
4. Mycophenolic acid (Sigma, cat. no. M3536): Prepare in 0.1 *M* NaOH, neutralize with HCl and store at 25 mg/mL in aliquots at –20°C. Add to the growth medium and filter the complete medium (0.2-µm filter).
5. Versene: 0.2 g/L EDTA prepared in PBS, autoclave, and store in aliquots at room temperature.
6. Trypsin (Difco, Detroit, MI): Prepare as a stock solution of 0.25% dissolved in versene, sterilize by filtration (0.2 µm), and store in aliquots at –20°C. Dilute 1/5 in versene prior to use.
7. Freezing solution: Complete growth medium supplemented with 10% (v/v) DMSO. This solution should be sterilized by filtration through a 0.2-µm filter before use. It can be stored at +4°C for several days.

2.2.2. Transfection of Retroviral Constructs into Suitable Packaging Cell Lines

1. 2X HBS: 50 m*M* HEPES, pH 7.05, 10 m*M* KCl, 12 m*M* dextrose, 280 m*M* NaCl, and 1.5 m*M* Na$_2$HPO$_4$. It is important that the final pH of the solution is pH 7.05 ± 0.05. Sterilize by filtering the solution through a 0.2-µm filter and store in aliquots at –20°C. To thaw, warm to room temperature and mix. Discard the aliquot after use.

2. 2 *M* CaCl$_2$. Prepare a 2 *M* solution, filter (0.2-μm filter), and store in aliquots at −20°C. To thaw, warm to room temperature and mix. Discard the aliquot after use.

3. Chloroquine. Prepare a 25 m*M* stock solution of chloroquine (Sigma, cat. no. C6628) in phosphate-buffered saline, filter through a 0.2-μm filter, and store in aliquots at −20°C. Discard each aliquot after use.

4. X-gal stock: 40 mg/mL prepared in DMSO. Store at −20°C.

5. β-gal buffer: For the determination of transfection efficiency, prepare as follows:

   PBS, pH 7.4   88 mL
   2 m*M* MgCl$_2$ 2 mL of 100 m*M* MgCl$_2$
   5 m*M* potassium ferricyanide   5 mL of 100 m*M* K$^+$ ferricyanide
   5 m*M* potassium ferrocyanide   5 mL of 100 m*M* K$^+$ ferrocyanide (pH 7.4)

6. NIH3T3 cells: Available from the American Type Culture Collection or the European Collection of Cell Cultures. Cultured in DME supplemented with 10% FBS.

2.3. Infection of Vascular Smooth Muscle Cells

1. Polybrene: Prepare a stock of 8 mg/mL polybrene (a registered trademark of Abbott Laboratories for hexadimethrine bromide, Sigma, cat. no. H9268) in phosphate-buffered saline, filter through a 0.2-μm filter, and store in aliquots at −20°C.

2. Puromycin (Sigma, cat. no. P 8833): Prepare as a 1 mg/mL stock solution in PBS, sterilised by filtration (0.2 μm) and stored at +4°C for 2–3 wk.

3. G418 (geneticin sulphate, Gibco-BRL, Grand Island, NY, cat. no. 11811–031): Add directly and filter sterilize the media.

4. Hygromycin B (Calbiochem, cat. no. 4000510): Add directly and filter-sterilize the media.

5. For the reverse transcriptase assay, prepare the 10X reaction buffer as follows:

   500 m*M* Tris.HCl, pH 8.3   (500 μL of 1 M stock)
   200 m*M* dithiothreitol (DTT)   (20 μL of 1 M stock)
   6 m*M* MnCl$_2$ (6 μL of 1 *M* stock)
   600 m*M* NaCl   (12 μL of 5 *M* stock)
   0.5% (v/v) NP-40   (50 μL of 10% v/v stock)

6. [α^{32}P]dTTP (Amersham, Buckinghamshire, UK AA0007) add distilled water to a final volume of 1 mL ("redivue," approx 3000Ci/mmol, 10 mCi/mL).

7. Poly(A) × (dT)$_{15}$ (polyadenylic acid × pentadecathymidylic acid) (Boehringer Mannheim, Lewes, UK, cat. no. 108677).

8. dTTP (Boehringer Mannheim, cat. no. 104286).

9. DE81 circles (Whatman).

10. Scintillant (e.g., aquasol, Dupont/NEN, Boston, MA).

3. Methods

3.1. Insertion of Exogenous Genes into the Retroviral Vector

1. Cleave the coding sequence (e.g., cDNA) with appropriate restriction nucleases, isolate by gel electrophoresis, and ligate into the multiple cloning site of the retroviral vector using standard molecular techniques *(36)*.

2. Transfect the recombinant DNA molecules are into a suitable *E. coli* bacterial strain and culture in the presence of antibiotics (e.g., ampicillin) to allow selection of bacteria containing the vector *(36)*. Many of the retroviral plasmids have the disadvantage of recombining when transformed into *E. coli.* Some vectors encode selective markers for mammalian cells that can also be used to select plasmid-transformed bacteria and selection with these reagents can be helpful in limiting recombination. For example, hygromycin B and kanamycin (added to the bacterial media at final concentrations of 25 and 50 μg/mL, respectively) can be used to select bacteria transformed with the appropriate retroviral constructs.

3.2. Culture and Transfection of the Retroviral Packaging Cell Line

3.2.1. Maintenance of the Packaging Cell Line

Several retroviral packaging cell lines are available. Although the procedures outlined below have been optimized for the use of the Bosc23 packaging line, they may also be used with other cell lines.

1. Maintain the Bosc23 cells in DME growth medium at 37°C and 5% CO_2. They should be passaged before reaching confluence and not diluted more than 1/5. Selection for expression of the *gag, pol,* and *env* genes is accomplished by addition to the growth medium of hygromycin B and mycophenolic acid at final concentrations of 200 and 25 μg/mL, respectively (*see* **Note 2**).
2. Remove the growth medium and gently wash the monolayer of cells with versene (*see* **Note 3**).
3. Remove the versene and add a small volume of diluted trypsin (1.5 mL is sufficient for a 10-cm dish).
4. Incubate at 37°C until the cells easily detach (approx 2 min).
5. Harvest the cells by gently pipeting with an equal volume of DME growth medium to form a single cell suspension and subculture into fresh dishes. Addition of fresh growth medium quenches the trypsin.

3.3.2. Freezing the Cells

1. Trypsinize the cells as described above (*see* **Subheading 3.2.1.**). It is essential that the cells are subconfluent prior to freezing.
2. Collect the cells and centrifuge at 500*g* for 4 min at room temperature.
3. Aspirate off the media, resuspend in freezing solution at approx 10^6 cells/mL and transfer 1 mL aliquots into cryogenic vials.
4. Place the vials in an insulated container (a small polystyrene box is ideal) and place at –70°C overnight (the cells can be left at –70°C for several days). Transfer to liquid nitrogen for long-term storage.
5. To thaw the cells, rapidly warm by placing in a water bath at 37°C, transfer the contents to a fresh tube, and slowly add with mixing 6 mL of growth medium. It is important to add the fresh medium slowly so as to avoid osmotic shock to the cells. Centrifuge at 500*g* for 4 min at room temperature, remove the medium, and gently resuspend in fresh growth medium before plating.

3.2.3. Transfection of Retroviral Constructs into Suitable Packaging Cell Lines

For the rapid production of high titre (10^5–10^7 infectious units/mL), helper-free retroviruses with ecotropic, amphotropic, and polytropic host ranges, a number of methods have been developed for the transient transfection of retroviral DNA into various packaging cell lines (*see* **Note 4**). In our experience the packaging cell line, Bosc23, is easy to transfect and routinely gives high retroviral titers.

1. On the day prior to transfection, plate 2.5×10^6 Bosc23 cells per 60-mm dish in 4 mL of DME growth medium (*see* **Note 5**).
2. Immediately prior to transfection, replace the medium with 4 mL of fresh DME growth medium containing 25 µM chloroquine. The addition of chloroquine can increase titers by twofold (*see* **Note 6**). The dish should be approx 80% confluent prior to transfection.
3. Prepare the transfection cocktail as follows: In a sterile 1.5-mL tube, add 6–10 µg DNA to sterile water to give a final volume of 438 µL and then add 62 µL of 2 M CaCl$_2$ to the DNA solution. Add 500 µL of 2X HBS (pH 7.05) and mix by gently bubbling air through the solution. Alternatively, the solution can be mixed by gently inverting the tube 4–5 times.
4. As soon as possible after mixing add the DNA solution to the cells and gently rock the dish to ensure uniform mixing. It is important to add the solution immediately after mixing, as any delay may reduce the transfection efficiency and subsequent retroviral titers.
5. Approximately 10 h after adding the transfection cocktail, remove the medium and gently replace (by slowly adding the medium to the side of the dish) with 3 mL of fresh DME growth medium.
6. Approximately 24 h later harvest the retroviral supernatant (*see* **Subheading 3.3.**).

3.2.4. Determination of Transfection Efficiency

When performed correctly, transfection efficiencies for Bosc23 cells should be about 60% (*see* **Note 7**). In order to monitor transfection efficiencies, a retroviral vector expressing an easily assayable marker, such as *lacZ*, should be used, and transfected cells should be subsequently stained for β-gal activity.

1. Wash transfected cells once in PBS at room temperature.
2. Fix cells for 5 min at room temperature in 0.5% glutaraldehyde prepared in PBS (2 mL per 60-mm dish).
3. Wash cells twice with PBS.
4. Incubate cells at 37°C in β-gal buffer containing 1 mg/mL of X-gal until intracellular staining is easily detectable (usually between 4 h and overnight). Count the number of blue cells to determine the proportion of transfected cells.

3.3. Harvesting and Titration of Recombinant Retrovirus

3.3.1. Harvesting and Storage of Recombinant Retrovirus

Recombinant retrovirus is secreted from the packaging cell line into the culture medium (*see* **Note 8**). When the packaging cells reach confluence (usually 48 h posttransfection), the culture supernatant containing the recombinant retrovirus should be harvested (*see* **Note 9**).

1. Harvest the culture media containing the recombinant virus from the packaging cell line, filter through a 0.45-µm filter and either use immediately or store as described below (*see* **Note 10**).
2. For short-term storage (up to 1 wk) store the viral supernatant be at +4°C. The culture media containing the viral stock should contain FBS (10% FBS is usual)—if not FBS, an alternative carrier protein such as bovine serum albumin (BSA) should be added.
3. For long-term storage snap-freeze the viral stock (containing FBS or BSA) in a dry ice/ethanol bath and store at -70°C. In order to avoid repeated freeze/thawing, store the viral stock in appropriately-sized aliquots (in our experience 1-mL aliquots are optimal).

3.3.2. Determination of Viral Titer (see **Note 11**)

1. For determination and comparison of viral titer, infect 5×10^5 NIH3T3 cells with the harvested virus as described in **Subheading 3.4.**
2. At 24 h postinfection, split the NIH3T3 cells 1/5, 1/10, and 1/50 into the appropriate selective media and refeed every 3 d.
3. Count the surviving colonies after 10 d and estimate the viral titer from the average number of surviving colonies corrected for the number of cells infected (assuming one population doubling in the absence of selective drug) and dilution of the infectious virus stock.

3.4. Infection of Vascular Smooth Muscle Cells

3.4.1. Infection of Vascular Smooth Muscle Cells (VSMC)

1. Approximately 12–18 h prior to infection, plate 5×10^5 VSMC in DME growth medium (or another appropriate growth medium) on a 100-mm dish.
2. For each infection prepare 3 mL of an infection cocktail containing the retroviral supernatant and polybrene (final concentration of 4–8 µg/mL) in growth medium (*see* **Note 12**). If the titer of the virus stock is unknown, it should be used undiluted, otherwise the viral stock may be diluted with fresh growth medium. To thaw frozen retroviral stock, warm for a minimal period of time at 37°C. Filter the infection cocktail through a 0.45-µm filter before use.
3. Remove the medium from the VSMC and add the infection cocktail to the cells.
4. Incubate at 37°C for at least 3 h.

5. Add 7 mL of growth medium to the cells and culture overnight. Alternatively, the retroviral infection cocktail may be left on the target cells overnight and then replaced with 10 mL of fresh growth medium.

6. At this stage the cells may be processed directly for various analyses including determination of exogenous gene expression or, alternatively, selected to generate stable clones (*see* **Subheading 3.4.2.**).

3.4.2. Selection of Infected Cells

In order to generate stably expressing clones the cells are selected with the appropriate reagent (*see* **Note 13**).

1. Split the cells 24 h after the infection 1/5, 1/10, and 1/50 into the appropriate selective media and refeed every 3 d.

2. Depending on the mode of selection, the surviving colonies can be isolated and harvested 3–10 d later.

3. If clones are required, isolate 10–20 surviving colonies with cloning rings (*see* **Note 14**) and transfer to fresh tissue culture dishes.

4. Rinse the dish containing the colonies to be picked with versene.

5. Dip cloning rings in sterile Vaseline and place over individual colonies.

6. Add trypsin/versene.

7. Harvest the detached cells with fresh growth medium and transfer to fresh dishes containing medium supplemented with the selective reagents. Alternatively, a pool of infected cells is obtained by replating all of the colonies into selective media.

3.4.3. Assays for the Secretion of Infectious Virus

3.4.3.1. Assay for Reverse Transcriptase

The ability of the retrovirally encoded reverse transcriptase enzyme (RNA-dependent DNA polymerase) to incorporate radioactive dNTPs into DNA using an RNA template is a unique attribute of retroviruses. Determination of reverse transcriptase activity is a simple method for detecting the presence of retrovirus in media from cells in culture (*see* **Note 15**). This assay may be adapted, with appropriate standardization, to assess viral titer. It is also very useful as a preliminary screen to exclude the possibility of the release of retrovirus from infected host cells. However, other assays to exclude amphotropic viral release must be conducted before the infected cells are used in the general laboratory (*see* **Subheading 3.4.3.2.** and **Note 8**).

1. Prepare fresh 10X reaction buffer.

2. Prepare the reaction mix by combining the following components in order. The quantities shown are sufficient for one sample only.

10X reaction buffer	5 µL
poly(A) × (dT)$_{15}$ (5 A$_{260}$ U/mL)	5 µL
100 µM dTTP	5 µL

Water   20 µL
      Finally add 1 µCi [α^{32}P]dTTP.
3. Aliquot 35 µL of the reaction mix into a 96-well plate and add 15 µL of the medium to be assayed.
4. Mix gently and incubate the plate at 37°C for 60–90 min. The test medium should be assayed in triplicate in conjunction with both a negative (noninfected cells) and a positive control (e.g., medium harvested from the transfected packaging cells).
5. Meanwhile prepare sufficient DE81 filter circles as follows: spot 25 µL of 100 m*M* EDTA (pH 8.0) onto each filter and allow to dry and number with a pencil.
6. At the end of the reaction spot 10 µL of each sample onto a prepared DE81 circle and allow to dry.
7. Wash the circles three times in 2X SSC (**ref. *36***; 200 mL per wash, approx 5 min each) and then rinse twice with absolute ethanol.
8. Allow to air-dry, put into scintillation vials, add an appropriate volume of scintillant and determine the level of radioactive incorporation with a suitable scintillation counter.

3.4.3.2. Assay for Infectious Viral Particles

Although determination of reverse transcriptase activity is a fairly sensitive indicator of the presence of retrovirus, it is essential when working with amphotropic retroviruses to employ an additional assay. The most convenient method is to harvest culture media from the infected host cells and test this for retrovirus by using it to infect either the same cell line or another cell line known to be sensitive to retroviral infection.

3.5 Analysis of Infected Cells

Lysates of transiently infected (24–48 h postinfection) or stable, selected cells can be analyzed for expression of the exogenous sequences by a variety of standard protocols including Western blotting, immunoprecipitation, and immunocytochemistry *(37)*.

4. Notes

1. Several retroviral packaging cell lines have been developed (*see* **ref. *38*** for review). Recombination between the transfected retroviral vector (which lacks these genes) and the helper-virus (which lacks a packaging signal) generates infectious but replication defective virus. The helper-virus genes are transfected into the packaging cell and their presence maintained by selection. In order to reduce the possibility of recombination with endogenous viral elements that could generate replication-competent virus, packaging cell lines have been generated with separate *gag*, *pol*, and ecotropic *env* genes with minimal sequence overlap and decreased sequence homology due to "codon wobbling" (the use of rarely-used codons to introduce silent mutations in the sequence without altering the amino acid sequence) *(39–41)*. Those regularly used in our laboratory are listed below:

GP+E-86 ecotropic packaging cell line derived from NIH3T3 murine fibroblasts *(32,42)*.

GP+envAM12 amphotropic packaging cell line derived from NIH3T3 murine fibroblasts *(43)*.

Bosc23: ecotropic packaging cell line derived from the 293/T cell line (a variant of the 293 adenoviral transformed human kidney cell line into which a temperature-sensitive SV40 large T antigen had been introduced) *(44)*.

2. Bosc23 cells were generated by sequential cotransfection of a *gag* and *pol* encoding plasmid with one encoding resistance to hygromycin B and a plasmid encoding an ecotropic *env* gene with one encoding guanine phosphoribo-syltransferase (gpt). Thus, retention of the transfected helper-virus genes in Bosc23 cells is achieved by selection with hygromycin B and mycophenolic acid (gpt resistance). The most convenient strategy is to select the cells, ascertain their efficacy of viral production, and freeze a large number of aliquots. The frozen selected cells may be thawed and used for several passages without further selection, thus providing a supply of packaging cells that should generate uniform viral titers.

3. Bosc23 cells are derived from 293 cells and are much less adherent than other fibroblast cell lines. They are easily detached by trypsin and care must be taken to avoid detaching the cells by over-vigorous pipeting when changing the medium, etc.

4. Transient retroviral production has several advantages over stable production, such as higher infectious titers and minimal potential toxic effects of the introduced gene products. In order to maximize the viral titer, the packaging cell line may be infected with recombinant virus. This may be achieved by the sequential use of two different packaging cell lines such that virus produced by transfection of the first is used to infect the second *(45,46)*. However, this requires the use of an amphotropic packaging cell line that, because of need for stricter biological containment, may not be desirable. Alternatively, the resistance of the packaging cells to infection with virus of the same tropism (viral interference) may be overcome by treatment with tunicamycin (which inhibits the glycosylation of many membrane proteins including retroviral receptors; *47*). In cases where the efficiency of infection of the target cells remains low, the target cells can be cocultivated with the packaging cells. Although, the latter still produce virus for several days, they can be killed by prior treatment with mitomycin C.

5. The initial plating of the cells is one of the most important steps in successfully obtaining high retroviral titers. Therefore, it is extremely important that the cells are at the correct density—the dish should be approx 80% confluent prior to transfection and, ideally, 95–100% confluent 24 h after transfection. In order to prevent clumping, it is essential that the cells are not allowed to become overconfluent. Otherwise, it will be necessary to split them 1:2 or 1:3 for several passages prior to plating for transfection.

6. It is important not to leave the chloroquine longer than 12 h as this will cause a large decrease in titer.

7. Other transfection methods may also be used. For example, we have successfully used lipofectamine (Gibco-BRL) and Superfect (Qiagen, Chatsworth, CA) to transfect the GP+E-86 packaging cell line.

8. The viral supernatants produced by these methods might contain potentially hazardous recombinant constructs. For example, replication-competent viruses have been detected in some instances *(48,49)*. Therefore, caution must be exercised in the production, use, and storage of retroviral virions, especially those with amphotropic and polytropic host ranges. Appropriate guidelines should be followed in the use of recombinant retrovirus production systems.

9. The optimum time after transfection of the retroviral vector DNA to harvest the infectious virus depends on several parameters. For example, the efficiency of the transfection may affect the kinetics of maximal viral production. In addition, the proliferation rate and optimum density may differ between different packaging cell lines. However, most experiments do not require extremely high viral titers and, in most cases, the titer is optimal at 36–72 h posttransfection when the packaging cells should be confluent. If the cells are not confluent by 72 h, then it may be necessary to decrease the amount of DNA transfected and/or increase the number of initially plated cells in order to obtain a confluent dish by 48 h posttransfection. The retroviral titer begins to drop after 72 h.

10. Although the highest infectious viral titers are obtained with viral supernatants freshly harvested from the packaging cell line this is not always convenient and it is possible to store the viral stock for later repeated use. The storage condition depends largely on how long the virus will be stored. At +4°C the viral titer drops by 50% every 5–6 d (at 37°C the titer drops by 50% in approx 5 h). If the viral stock is stored frozen, freeze/thawing reduces the viral titer by about 30–50% and repeated freeze/thawing should be avoided.

11. The titer of retrovirus generated by transient transfection of Bosc23 cells is generally sufficiently high and may even be diluted in fresh growth medium. Nonetheless, where a high titer is required (e.g., for in vivo applications) the titer can be increased by up to 10-fold by centrifugation *(50)* or ultrafiltration *(51–53)* and increases in titer of 20-fold have been achieved.

12. Polybrene is often used to increase retroviral infection and a concentration of 8 μg/mL appears to be optimum. Others have used DEAE-Dextran at 10 μg/mL instead of polybrene to good effect *(51)*.

13. The speed and efficacy of selection of resistant cells depends on the host cell type and the selective reagent. In general, puromycin will eliminate sensitive cells within three to five population doublings (about 2–3 d for most cell types), whereas hygromycin B and G418 (for neomycin selection) take approx 4–5 and 10 d, respectively. For VSMC the following concentrations are suitable: 1–2 μg/mL puromycin, 100–150 μg/mL hygromycin B, and 0.5–1 mg/mL G418. For other selective reagents, a titration should be performed on uninfected cells and the lowest concentration which gives 100% killing used.

14. Cloning rings can be easily made by cutting off the lid and bottom of a 0.5-mL centrifuge tube. The resulting cylinders are sterilized by autoclaving.

15. For the reverse transcriptase assay the medium should be used fresh, because retroviruses are susceptible to freeze/thaw conditions. The culture medium is harvested from near confluent populations of cells and clarified at 500g for 5 min before use. Typical results of quadruplicate assays from one experiment are as follows:

Sample	CPM (±sd)
Negative control (reaction mix alone)	71 (9.5)
Negative control (mock infected host cells)	85 (15.6)
Positive control (transfected GP+envAM12 packaging cells)	836 (89.8)
Test sample (infected host cells)	92 (8.2)

References

1. Vile, R. G., and Russell, S. J. (1995) Retroviruses as vectors. *Br. Med. Bull.* **51,** 12–30.
2. Miller, A. D. (1996) Cell-surface receptors for retroviruses and implications for gene transfer. *Proc. Natl. Acad. Sci. USA* **93,** 11,407–11,413.
3. Limon, A., Briones, J., Puig, T., Carmona, M., Fornas, O., Cancelas, J. A., et al. (1997) High-titer retroviral vectors containing the enhanced green fluorescent protein gene for efficient expression in hematopoietic cells. *Blood* **90,** 3316–3321.
4. Bierhuizen, M. F., Westerman, Y., Visser, T. P., Dimjati, W., Wognum, A. W., and Wagemaker, G. (1997) Enhanced green fluorescent protein as selectable marker of retroviral- mediated gene transfer in immature hematopoietic bone marrow cells. *Blood* **90,** 3304–3315.
5. Bierhuizen, M. F., Westerman, Y., Visser, T. P., Wognum, A. W., and Wagemaker, G. (1997) Green fluorescent protein variants as markers of retroviral-mediated gene transfer in primary hematopoietic cells and cell lines. *Biochem. Biophys. Res. Commun.* **234,** 371–375.
6. Lybarger, L., Dempsey, D., Franek, K. J., and Chervenak, R. (1996) Rapid generation and flow cytometric analysis of stable GFP-expressing cells. *Cytometry* **25,** 211–220.
7. Lindemann, D., Patriquin, E., Feng, S., and Mulligan, R. C. (1997) Versatile retrovirus vector systems for regulated gene expression in vitro and in vivo. *Mol. Med.* **3,** 466–476.
8. Vlach, J., Hennecke, S., Alevizopoulos, K., Conti, D., and Amati, B. (1996) Growth arrest by the cyclin-dependent kinase inhibitor p27Kip1 is abrogated by c-Myc. *EMBO J.* **15,** 6595–6604.
9. Paulus, W., Baur, I., Boyce, F. M., Breakefield, X. O., and Reeves, S. A. (1996) Self-contained, tetracycline-regulated retroviral vector system for gene delivery to mammalian cells. *J. Virol.* **70,** 62–67.
10. Bohl, D. and Heard, J. M. (1997) Modulation of erythropoietin delivery from engineered muscles in mice. *Human Gene Ther.* **8,** 195–204.
11. Yu, J. S., Sena-Esteves, M., Paulus, W., Breakefield, X. O., and Reeves, S. A. (1996) Retroviral delivery and tetracycline-dependent expression of IL-1beta-

converting enzyme (ICE) in a rat glioma model provides controlled induction of apoptotic death in tumor cells. *Cancer Res.* **56,** 5423–5427.

12. Mee, P. J. and Brown, R. (1990) Construction and hormone regulation of a novel retroviral vector. *Gene* **88,** 289–292.

13. Mattioni, T., Louvion, J. F.,and Picard, D. (1994) Regulation of protein activities by fusion to steroid binding domains. *Meth. Cell. Biol.* **43 Pt A,** 335–352.

14. Chang, M. W. and Leiden, J. M. (1996) Gene therapy for vascular proliferative disorders. *Semin. Interv. Cardiol.* **1,** 185–193.

15. Nabel, E. G. (1995) Gene therapy for vascular diseases. *Atherosclerosis* **118 Suppl,** S51–56.

16. Finkel, T. and Epstein, S. E. (1995) Gene therapy for vascular disease. *FASEB J.* **9,** 843–851.

17. Feldman, L. J., Tahlil, O., and Steg, P. G. (1996) Adenovirus-mediated arterial gene therapy for restenosis, problems and perspectives. *Semin. Interv. Cardiol.* **1,** 203–208.

18. Yang, Z., Simari, R. D., Tanner, F., Stephan, D., Nabel, G. J., and Nabel, E. G. (1996) Gene transfer approaches to the regulation of vascular cell proliferation. *Semin. Interv. Cardiol.* **1,** 181–184.

19. Pickering, J. G., Takeshita, S., Feldman, L., Losordo, D. W., and Isner, J. M. (1996) Vascular applications of human gene therapy. *Semin. Interv. Cardiol.* **1,** 84–88.

20. Smith, R. C. and Walsh, K. (1997) Prospects for intravascular gene therapy. *J. Clin. Apheresis.* **12,** 140–145.

21. Zhu, N. L., Wu, L., Liu, P. X., Gordon, E. M., Anderson, W. F., Starnes, V. A., and Hall, F. L. (1997) Downregulation of cyclin G1 expression by retrovirus-mediated antisense gene transfer inhibits vascular smooth muscle cell proliferation and neointima formation. *Circulation* **96,** 628–635.

22. Bennett, M. R., Evan, G. I., and Newby, A. C. (1994) Deregulated expression of the c-myc oncogene abolishes inhibition of proliferation of rat vascular smooth muscle cells by serum reduction, interferon-gamma, heparin, and cyclic nucleotide analogues and induces apoptosis. *Circ. Res.* **74,** 525–536.

23. Bennett, M. R., Evan, G. I., and Schwartz, S. M. (1995) Apoptosis of rat vascular smooth muscle cells is regulated by p53- dependent and -independent pathways. *Circ. Res.* **77,** 266–273.

24. Bennett, M. R., Littlewood, T. D., Schwartz, S. M., and Weissberg, P. L. (1997) Increased sensitivity of human vascular smooth muscle cells from atherosclerotic plaques to p53-mediated apoptosis. *Circ. Res.* **81,** 591–599.

25. Bennett, M. R., Macdonald, K., Chan, S. W., Boyle, J. J., and Weissberg, P. L. (1998) Cooperative interactions between RB and p53 regulate cell proliferation, cell senescence, and apoptosis in human vascular smooth muscle cells from atherosclerotic plaques. *Circ. Res.* **82,** 704–712.

26. Ekhterae, D. and Stanley, J. C. (1995) Retroviral vector-mediated transfer and expression of human tissue plasminogen activator gene in human endothelial and vascular smooth muscle cells. *J. Vasc. Surg.* **21,** 953–962.

27. Stopeck, A. T., Vahedian, M., and Williams, S. K. (1997) Transfer and expression of the interferon gamma gene in human endothelial cells inhibits vascular smooth muscle cell growth in vitro. *Cell Transplant.* **6**, 1–8.

28. Lejnieks, D. V., Han, S. W., Ramesh, N., Lau, S., and Osborne, W. R. (1996) Granulocyte colony-stimulating factor expression from transduced vascular smooth muscle cells provides sustained neutrophil increases in rats. *Human Gene Ther.* **7**, 1431–1436.

29. Osborne, W. R., Ramesh, N., Lau, S., Clowes, M. M., Dale, D. C., and Clowes, A. W. (1995) Gene therapy for long-term expression of erythropoietin in rats. *Proc. Natl. Acad. Sci. USA* **92**, 8055–8058.

30. Tzeng, E., Shears, L. L. N., Robbins, P. D., Pitt, B. R.,. Geller, D. A, Watkins, S. C., et al. (1996) Vascular gene transfer of the human inducible nitric oxide synthase: characterization of activity and effects on myointimal hyperplasia. *Mol. Med.* **2**, 211–225.

31. Martens, J. R., Reaves, P. Y., Lu, D., Katovich, M. J., Berecek, K. H., Bishop, S. P., et al. (1998) Prevention of renovascular and cardiac pathophysiological changes in hypertension by angiotensin II type 1 receptor antisense gene therapy. *Proc. Natl. Acad. Sci. USA* **95**, 2664–2669.

32. Laitinen, M., Pakkanen, T., Donetti, E., Baetta, R., Luoma, J., Lehtolainen, P., et al. (1997) Gene transfer into the carotid artery using an adventitial collar: comparison of the effectiveness of the plasmid-liposome complexes, retroviruses, pseudotyped retroviruses, and adenoviruses. *Human Gene Ther.* **8**, 1645–1650.

33. Plautz, G., Nabel, E. G., and Nabel, G. J. (1991) Introduction of vascular smooth muscle cells expressing recombinant genes in vivo. *Circulation* **83**, 578–783.

34. Hall, F. L., Gordon, E. M., Wu, L., Zhu, N. L., Skotzko, M. J., Starnes, V. A., and Anderson, W. F. (1997) Targeting retroviral vectors to vascular lesions by genetic engineering of the MoMLV gp70 envelope protein. *Human Gene Ther.* **8**, 2183–2192.

35. Dong, J., Roth, M. G., and Hunter, E. (1992) A chimeric avian retrovirus containing the influenza virus hemagglutinin gene has an expanded host range. *J. Virol.* **66**, 7374–7382.

36. Sambrook, J., Fritsch, E. F., and Maniatis, T. (1989) *Molecular Cloning, A Laboratory Manual.* Cold Spring Harbor Laboratory Press.

37. Harlow, E. and Lane, D. (1988) *Antibodies, A Laboratory Manual.* Cold Spring Harbor Laboratory Press.

38. Miller, A. D. (1990) Retrovirus packaging cells. *Human Gene Ther.* **1**, 5–14.

39. Soneoka, Y., Cannon, P. M., Ramsdale, E. E., Griffiths, J. C., Romano, G., Kingsman, S. M., and Kingsman, A. J. (1995) A transient three-plasmid expression system for the production of high titer retroviral vectors. *Nucleic Acids Res.* **23**, 628–633.

40. Markowitz, D., Hesdorffer, C., Ward, M., Goff, S., and Bank, A. (1990) Retroviral gene transfer using safe and efficient packaging cell lines. *Ann. NY Acad. Sci.* **612**, 407–414.

41. Morgenstern, J. P. and Land, H. (1990) Advanced mammalian gene transfer: high titre retroviral vectors with multiple drug selection markers and a complementary helper-free packaging cell line. *Nucleic Acids Res.* **18**, 3587–3596.

42. Markowitz, D., Goff, S., and Bank, A. (1988) A safe packaging line for gene transfer: separating viral genes on two different plasmids. *J. Virol.* **62**, 1120–1124.

43. Markowitz, D., Goff, S., and Bank, A. (1988) Construction and use of a safe and efficient amphotropic packaging cell line. *Virology* **167**, 400–406.

44. Pear, W. S., Nolan G. P., Scott, M. L., and Baltimore, D. (1993) Production of high-titer helper-free retroviruses by transient transfection. *Proc. Natl. Acad. Sci. USA* **90**, 8392–8396.

45. Kim, Y. S., Lim, H. K., and Kim, K. J. (1998) Production of high-titer retroviral vectors and detection of replication-competent retroviruses. *Mol. Cells.* **8**, 36–42.

46. Cosset, F. L., Girod, A., Flamant, F., Drynda, A., Ronfort, C., Valsesia, S., et al. (1993) Use of helper cells with two host ranges to generate high-titer retroviral vectors. *Virology* **193**, 385–395.

47. Miller, D. G. and Miller, A. D. (1992) Tunicamycin treatment of CHO cells abrogates multiple blocks to retrovirus infection, one of which is due to a secreted inhibitor. *J. Virol.* **66**, 78–84.

48. Chong, H., Starkey, W., and Vile, R. G. (1998) A replication-competent retrovirus arising from a split-function packaging cell line was generated by recombination events between the vector, one of the packaging constructs, and endogenous retroviral sequences. *J. Virol.* **72**, 2663–2670.

49. Martinez, I. and Dornburg, R. (1996) Partial reconstitution of a replication-competent retrovirus in helper cells with partial overlaps between vector and helper cell genomes. *Human Gene Ther.* **7**, 705–712.

50. Zelenock, J. A., Welling, T. H., Sarkar, R., Gordon, D. G., and Messina, L. M. (1997) Improved retroviral transduction efficiency of vascular cells in vitro and in vivo during clinically relevant incubation periods using centrifugation to increase viral titers. *J. Vasc. Surg.* **26**, 119–127.

51. Lee, S.-G., Kim, S., and Kim, B.-G. (1996) Optimization of environmental factors for the production of retrovirus, in *Cell Culture Engineering* (Robinson, V. D., ed.), Kluwer Academic Publishers, San Diego, CA.

52. Parente, M. K. and Wolfe, J. H. (1996) Production of increased titer retrovirus vectors from stable producer cell lines by superinfection and concentration. *Gene Ther.* **3**, 756–760.

53. Paul, R. W., Morris, D., Hess, B. W., Dunn, J., and Overell, R. W. (1993) Increased viral titer through concentration of viral harvests from retroviral packaging lines. *Human Gene Ther.* **4**, 609–615.

28

Embryonal Stem (ES) Cell–Derived Macrophages

A Cellular System that Facilitates the Genetic Dissection of Macrophage Function

Kathryn J. Moore and Mason W. Freeman

1. Introduction

The monocyte/macrophage (Mø) contributes to atherosclerotic lesion initiation and progression through a variety of interactions with cells of the artery wall that depend on the elucidation of a host of cytokines and growth factors by cells residing in the intima. The number and complexity of these interactions make it difficult to determine which cellular functions are contributing to the progression of atherosclerosis and which might be exploited to interrupt that progression. Studies of macrophage functions in atherosclerosis have been hindered by the limitations of available macrophage cell lines and primary cultures, including poor transfectability and the transformed state of immortal cell lines. Recent studies have demonstrated that pluripotential mouse embryonic stem cells can be differentiated down specific hematopoietic lineages in vitro, including lines that give rise to macrophages *(1)*. This technique provides a genetically tractable cellular system for studying myeloid cell function. Macrophages arising from this differentiation system demonstrate cell surface presentation of classic macrophage markers and macrophage functions including phagocytosis and responses to inflammatory stimuli. There are several important advantages inherent in using embryonic stem (ES) cell derived macrophages as a cell culture system for studying Mø function. As the cells are not transformed, and the progenitor cells arising from ES cells are capable of reconstituting the entire hematopoietic compartment of a mouse, they represent a cell culture system that appears to retain the physiologic regulation on growth and differentiation that is absent from transformed myelomonocytic

From: *Methods in Molecular Medicine, Vascular Disease: Molecular Biology and Gene Therapy Protocols*
Edited by: A. H. Baker © Humana Press Inc., Totowa, NJ

cell lines. In addition, the ease of transfection of ES cells may overcome some of the obstacles to gene expression studies that are now impeded by the notoriously inefficient transfections of monocytic cell culture lines. While these attributes are valuable, it is the ability to inactivate genes in a single allele in an ES cell line, and then examine phenotypic alterations in ES differentiated macrophage function in vitro, that is the greatest strength of this system.

ES cells can be readily targeted by homologous recombination to eliminate expression of a gene product *(2)*. Using increasing concentrations of the selection drug G418, the single allele targeted event can be converted to a homozygous deletion, thus creating an ES cell that lacks the gene of interest *(3)*. Subsequent in vitro differentiation of the targeted ES cell line produces a "knock-out" macrophage that can be used for studies without the time and expense associated with the generation of a mouse. This technique is of particular value in cases where homozygous deletions of key genes results in embryonic lethality in the mouse, and cannot be studied by generating a whole animal. Thus, the differentiated ES cell system makes it possible to study many of the targeted deletions that are otherwise not accessible to investigation, a problem that is particularly acute when deletions of key molecules in signal transduction pathways are generated. The differentiated ES cell system is also applicable to investigations of gene regulation in the macrophage. Permanent ES cell lines harboring transfected transcriptional units or endogenous genes mutated by the "knock-in" strategy could be employed to characterize gene regulatory systems without the many drawbacks of the use of transformed monocyte/macrophage cell lines. Thus, differentiation of ES cells into macrophages opens the door to genetic manipulation of the macrophage in vitro, providing a powerful research tool for studies of gene expression or targeted gene deletion in the macrophage that will be useful in dissecting many complex disease pathways, including atherosclerosis.

We have recently characterized in vitro differentiated ES macrophages as a model system for studying atherosclerosis-associated macrophage functions *(4)*. ES macrophages express all of the currently identified modified LDL receptors, form foam cells in vitro, and secrete matrix metalloproteinases that are thought to play a role in plaque remodeling or rupture. Our results suggest the possibility that several genes expressed in atherosclerotic macrophages might be targeted for elimination in ES cells. Using multiple selection strategies in order to inactivate multiple genes, investigators should be able to characterize the dependence of critical macrophage functions on several genes whose redundant functions would render a single gene knockout uninformative. For example, the systematic elimination of all known scavenger receptor family members from macrophages could provide insights into the importance of foam cell formation on altering macrophage function in vitro. If multitargeted ES cell lines can also retain their ability to reconstitute a mouse when reimplanted into blastocysts, then in vivo studies of such genetically deficient mice could dramatically facilitate the elucidation of the macrophage's contributions to atherosclerosis. This chapter will outline the methods for gene targeting of ES cells by homologous recombination and their subsequent differentiation into macrophages.

2. Materials

ES cells are very sensitive to impurities in culture, which can affect differentiation. To optimize culture conditions and consistency, all media, water, and buffers should be of the highest quality. To eliminate contamination from detergents, LPS, etc., all bottles and instruments used should be prepackaged, sterile plastic for cell culture use.

2.1. Culture of Embryonic Stem Cells

1. Embryonic stem (ES) cell line (e.g., CCE or J1) *(5,6)*.
2. STO fibroblasts *(7,8)*.
3. 0.2% gelatin (Type A: porcine skin), autoclaved.
4. Leukemia inhibitory factor-D (LIF-D) (*see* **Note 1**).
5. EF culture media: Dulbecco's modified Eagle's medium (DMEM) containing 4500 mg/L glucose supplemented with 10% fetal bovine serum (FBS) (heat inactivated), 2 mM L-glutamine, 50 U/mL penicillin, and 50 mg/mL streptomycin.
6. ES culture media: DMEM containing 4500 mg/L glucose supplemented with 15% FBS (heat inactivated), 2 mM L-glutamine, 50 U/mL penicillin, 50 mg/mL streptomycin, 1.5×10^{-4} M monothioglycerol (MTG), and 0.7% LIF-D.
7. Phosphate-buffered saline (PBS), pH 7.4, calcium and magnesium free.
8. 0.05% trypsin, 0.53 mM EDTA.

2.2. Gene Targeting and ES Cell Transfection

1. Gene targeting vector, approx 50 µg (*see* **Fig. 1** and **Note 2**).
2. Neutral-buffered phenol.
3. Phenol:chloroform: isoamyl alcohol (25:24:1).
4. Ethyl ether.
5. 3 M NaOAC, pH 5.2.
6. 100% EtOH, ice-cold.
7. TE: 10 mM Tris-HCl pH 8.0, 1 mM EDTA, sterile.
8. 4 mm gap electroporation cuvets.
9. Electroporation buffer: 20 mM HEPES, 137 mM NaCl, 5 mM KCl, 0.7 mM Na$_2$HPO$_4$, 6 mM glucose, and 0.1 mM β-mercaptoethanol.
10. Electroporator (e.g., Gene Pulser from Bio-Rad, Hercules, CA).
11. G418.
12. Gancyclovir.

Positive selection of homologous recombinants:

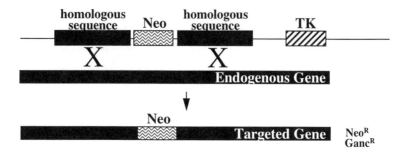

Negative selection of non-homologous recombinants:

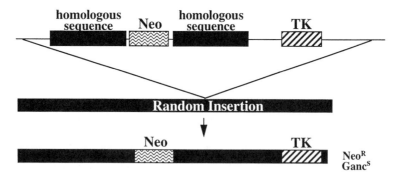

Fig. 1. Gene targeting by homologous recombination. A typical gene targeting vector contains >2 kb stretches of DNA of the gene of interest interrupted by a drug resistance gene (e.g., Neomycin) as a positive selectable marker, and a negative selectable marker (e.g., thymidine kinase) outside of the region of homology to eliminate nonhomologous recombinants. ES cells transfected with the targeting vector are doubly selected with G418 and gancyclovir. Homologous recombination of the gene targeting construct will generate ES cells that are resistant to G418 (Neo^R) and gancyclovir (TK^R). Random insertion of the targeting vector into the genome will render the ES cells sensitive to gancyclovir (TK^s), thus eliminating any nonhomologous recombinants.

2.3. Isolation and Expansion of Selected ES Cell Clones

1. 24-well tissue culture plates.
2. Dimethylsulfoxide (DMSO).
3. DNA extraction buffer: 10 mM EDTA pH 8.0, 20 mM Tris-HCl, 10 mM NaCl, 50 µg/mL proteinase K, and 1% SDS.
4. Saturated NaCl.
5. Isopropanol.
6. 1–5 µL glass pipets (Fisher Scientific, Pittsburgh, PA).

2.4. ES Cell Differentiation into Embryoid Bodies

1. Interleukin-3 (IL-3) (*see* **Note 3**).
2. L929 conditioned medium (LCM) (*see* **Note 4**).
3. Interleukin-1 (IL-1) (R & D Systems, Minneapolis, MN).
4. Insulin: 10 mg/mL in PBS (Sigma, St. Louis, MO).
5. Powdered Iscove's modified Dulbecco's medium (IMDM) for making 2X IMDM.
6. Methyl cellulose (Fluka BioChemika, Switzerland).
7. Sterile 2-L Erlenmeyer flask and magnetic stir bar.
8. Ultrapure, sterile H_2O.
9. Bacterial grade 35-mm Petri plates (Greiner Labortechnik, Germany, also distributed by Intermountain, UT).

2.5. Embryoid Body Differentiation into Macrophages

1. Macrophage differentiation media: IMDM supplemented with 10% FBS (heat inactivated), 2 mM L-glutamine, 50 U/mL penicillin, 50 mg/mL streptomycin, 10% LCM, 5 % IL-3, and 100 U/mL IL-1.

3. Methods

3.1. Culture of Embryonic Stem Cells

3.1.1. Fibroblast Feeder Layers

1. Coat 10-cm tissue culture plates with 4 ml of 0.2% gelatin for 10–30 min (*see* **Note 5**).
2. Aspirate residual gelatin immediately prior to plating of STO fibroblasts.
3. Culture STO fibroblasts on gelatin coated plates in 8–10 mL of EF culture medium.
4. Harvest cells when they reach approx 85% confluence.
5. Aspirate medium from STO fibroblasts and wash the cell layer with PBS.
6. Add 2 mL of trypsin and incubate at 37°C for 4 min. While cells are incubating, prepare new gelatin coated plates.
7. Collect the cells by vigorously rinsing the plate with EF culture medium.
8. Centrifuge cells at 200g for 5 min to pellet and resuspend in EF culture medium.
9. Mitotically inactivate cells by gamma-irradiation (3000 rad).
10. Replate irradiated STO fibroblasts on fresh gelatin coated plates (*see* **Note 6**).
11. Incubate for 2 h to overnight before using for ES cell culture.

3.1.2. ES Cell Culture

1. Seed ES cells at $2 \times 10^4/cm^2$ onto the irradiated feeder layer in 10 mL of ES media.
2. Change media daily to replenish LIF-D and to prevent acidification. ES cell colonies will be visible as raised cell clusters on the fibroblast layer.
3. Subculture ES cells on d 2 or 3 when colonies appear to be 50–75% confluent (*see* **Note 7**).
4. Prior to passaging ES cells, prepare irradiated fibroblast feeder plates (*see* **Subheading 3.1.1.**).

5. Passage the cells by rinsing the ES cell layer with PBS, adding 2.5 mL of prewarmed (37°C) 0.05% trypsin-EDTA, and incubating at 37°C for 5 min.
6. Using a sterile Pasteur pipet, vigorously pipette trypsin solution to create a single cell suspension, and add to 10 mL of ES media.
7. Centrifuge at 200*g* for 5 min to pellet cells and resuspend in PBS.
8. Repeat centrifugation in **step 7**, and resuspend cell pellet in ES media.
9. Split ES cells 1:2 onto irradiated fibroblast feeder layers. ES cells will be ready for electroporation in 48 h.
10. On d 1, prepare 10 10-cm plates of irradiated STO fibroblasts (*see* **Subheading 3.1.1.**).
11. On d 2, transfer irradiated STO fibroblasts into ES media.

3.2. Gene Targeting and ES Cell Transfection

3.2.1. Preparation of Targeting Vector DNA

1. Linearize 50 μg of targeting vector DNA (200 μL reaction volume) using a unique restriction enzyme located outside of the homologous regions. Allow DNA to digest for 2–4 h.
2. To purify DNA, add 200 μL of neutral-buffered phenol to the DNA digest.
3. Mix well by repeated inversion and centrifuge at 14,000*g* for 10 min.
4. Transfer upper phase to a new Eppendorf tube and add 200 μL of phenol:chloroform:isoamyl alcohol.
5. Mix well by repeated inversion and centrifuge at 14,000*g* for 10 min.
6. Transfer upper phase to a new Eppendorf tube and add 200 μL ethyl ether. This step should be done in a fume hood.
7. Mix well by repeated inversion and allow the upper ether layer to evaporate. To ensure complete evaporation of ether, place the tube with the cap open at 37°C for 5 min.
8. Add 20 μL of 3 *M* NaOAC, pH 5.2. Mix well.
9. Add 500 μL of ice-cold 100% EtOH. Mix well and incubate at –70°C for 1 h.
10. Centrifuge at 14,000*g* for 20 min to pellet precipitated DNA.
11. Wash pellet once with 70% EtOH and allow to air-dry to remove residual EtOH.
12. Resuspend DNA in 30 μL of sterile TE and determine DNA concentration by measuring absorbance at 260 nm.

3.2.2. ES Cell Transfection

1. Add fresh media to ES cells 4 h prior to electroporation.
2. Prepare a single cell suspension by trypsinization as described in **Subheading 3.1.2.**
3. Wash ES cells twice in ES Media.
4. Resuspend 1 × 10^7 ES cells in 5 mL of electroporation buffer. Centrifuge at 200*g* for 5 min.
5. Resuspend in 0.8 mL of electroporation buffer.
6. Add 30 μg of linearized targeting vector DNA, and mix well.
7. Transfer ES cells to a 4 mm gap electroporation cuvet and incubate for 10 min at room temperature.

8. Electroporate ES cells at 250 V, 250 µF. Incubate for 10 min at room temperature.
9. Add 4.2 mL of ES media to electroporated ES cells and plate 0.5 mL per 10-cm dish of irradiated STO fibroblasts. Incubate for 24 h.
10. Change media to ES Media containing G418 (200 µg/mL) and gancyclovir (2 µM). Continue to change media daily for 8 d.

3.2.3. Isolation and Expansion of Selected ES Cell Clones

1. Prepare 8–12 24-well plates of irradiated STO fibroblasts on d 7 of G418/gancyclovir selection. Change media in 24-well plates prior to use to ES media containing G418 and gancyclovir.
2. Pick 200–300 ES colonies from the G418 and gancyclovir selected plates. Using an autoclaved pipet tip gently lift off the ES colony and transfer it into 20 µL of trypsin (37°C) for 5 min.
3. Pipet vigorously to disrupt the ES cell colony and transfer into the 24-well plate.
4. Incubate for 3–4 d until well formed colonies are visible. Monitor cultures closely to ensure that colonies do not become too large, as it is critical at this point that colonies do not differentiate.
5. Split ES cells 1:2 into 24-well plates containing fibroblast feeder layers. One set of ES cells will be used for DNA extraction and the other set of ES cells will be frozen.
6. On d 2–3, freeze ES cell cultures by removing ES media and replacing with ES media:FCS (50:50) containing 10% DMSO. Wrap plates well in Saran Wrap and store in zip-lock bags at –70°C.
7. Extract DNA from remaining 24-well plates. Add 300 µL of extraction buffer per well and place plates in a sealed container containing moistened paper towel.
8. Incubate at 55°C on a rocking platform shaker overnight.
9. Add 150 µL of saturated NaCl per well and mix on shaker for 3 min.
10. Add 500 µL of isopropanol and mix on shaker for 10 minutes.
11. Pick up precipitated DNA with a 1–5 µL glass pipette.
12. Dip the glass pipet briefly in 70% EtOH and allow the DNA to air-dry for 10 min.
13. Carefully break off the tip of the glass pipet containing the DNA into a Eppendorf tube and add 50 µL of TE. Incubate overnight at 55°C.
14. Determine DNA concentration by measuring absorbance at 260 nm.
15. Screen ES cell clones by Southern blot analysis to identify homologous recombinants.

3.2.4. Creation of a Homozygous Mutant ES Cell Line

1. Thaw identified heterozygously targeted ES cell line from frozen 24-well plates.
2. Add 1 mL of prewarmed ES media to each well and incubate at 37°C for 5 min.
3. Transfer ES cells to a 15-mL tube containing 5 mL of ES Media. Centrifuge at 200g for 5 min.
4. Resuspend ES cells in 4 mL of ES media containing 200 µg/mL G418 and culture in 6-cm dishes on irradiated STO fibroblast layers until confluent (2–3 d).
5. Split ES cells into three 10-cm plates and culture in 2, 4, or 6 mg/mL G418.

6. Incubate ES cells for 8–10 d, changing media daily.
7. Isolate and expand selected colonies as described in **Subheading 3.2.3.**
8. Screen ES cell clones by Southern blot to detect doubly targeted ES cells (*see* **Note 8**).

3.3. ES Cell Differentiation into Embryoid Bodies

3.3.1. Preparation of Methyl Cellulose Medium (MCM)

1. Prepare 2X IMDM by reconstituting the amount of powdered IMDM intended for a 500 mL volume in 250 mL of ultrapure sterile water.
2. Add the recommended amount of sodium bicarbonate for a 500 mL solution, as this 2X solution will later be diluted to 1X.
3. Filter sterilize the 2X IMDM and store at 4°C until use.
4. Place 230 mL of ultrapure sterile water and a magnetic stirrer in a sterile 2-L Erlenmeyer, and record the total weight.
5. Gently boil water on a magnetic hot plate for 5–10 min.
6. While stirring, slowly add 10 g of methyl cellulose to form a slurry, avoiding the formation of lumps. The slow addition of the methyl cellulose is critical to achieve the proper consistency of the methyl cellulose media.
7. Cover and boil for 10–12 min to sterilize. Watch the methyl cellulose mixture carefully to ensure that it does not boil over.
7. Allow the methyl cellulose mixture to cool to less than 40°C.
8. While stirring rapidly, add 250 mL of sterile 2X IMDM media.
9. Weigh the Erlenmeyer containing the methyl cellulose/2X IMDM mixture, and adjust the final net weight to 506 g with sterile H_2O.
10. Aliquot the methyl cellulose medium (MCM) in 50-mL conical tubes and store at –20°C until use. Once thawed, the MCM can be stored at 4°C for up to 1 wk.

3.3.2. Primary Differentiation: Embryoid Body (EB) Formation

1. Prior to differentiation, passage ES cells once or twice in the absence of EF feeder layers on gelatinized tissue culture plates to create feeder-free ES cultures (*see* **Note 9**).
2. To prime ES cells for differentiation, 2–4 h prior to harvesting replenish feeder-free ES cultures with ES media <u>minus</u> LIF-D.
3. Prepare the EB differentiation medium by combining in a 50-mL conical tube: 10 mL MCM, 2 mL FBS (heat inactivated), 6 mL 1X IMDM containing 50 U/mL penicillin, 50 mg/mL streptomycin, and 2 mM L-glutamine, 2 mL LCM, 1 mL IL-3 (X63 IL-3 supernatant), 20 µL of 10 mg/mL insulin, 100 U/mL rIL-1β, and 60 µL of 600 µM monothioglycerol (MTG) (25 µL in 2 mL media, filter) (*see* **Note 10**).
4. Mix EB differentiation media well by inverting 10 times.
5. Trypsinize the LIF-free ES cultures and prepare a single cell suspension as described in **Subheading 3.1.2.**
6. Wash ES cells twice in PBS and resuspend in a minimal volume of ES media <u>minus</u> LIF-D.

7. Add 10^3 to 5×10^3 ES cells/mL to EB differentiation media and mix well by repeatedly inverting the tube.
8. Using a syringe fitted with an 16–18-gage needle, seed 4 mL of EB differentiation media containing ES cells into 6-cm bacteriologic Petri plates.
9. Place two 6-cm Petri plates inside a 150×25 mm tissue culture dish with a third 6-cm dish containing water to reduce evaporation during incubation.
10. Culture 10–12 d at 37°C with a minimum amount of disturbance.

3.3.3. Progression of Embryoid Body Differentiation

The following changes should be apparent. On d 2–3, the EB formation should be visible as clusters consisting of 5–10 cells (*see* **Note 11**). On d 4 EB should reach a diameter of 100–500 µm (*see* **Fig. 2A**). By d 8, EB should be visible to the naked eye, and should have become globinized giving them the appearance of having dark centers (*see* **Note 12** and **Fig. 2B**). By d 11–12, the expansion of erythroid cells will fade, and there will be a rapid expansion of macrophages from the EB (*see* **Fig. 2C**).

3.4. Embryoid Body Differentiation into Macrophages

3.4.1. Secondary Differentiation: Macrophages

1. Harvest EB on d 11–12 during the rapid expansion of hematopoietic cells.
2. Add 4 mL of PBS per 6-cm dish, gently swirl to dilute the MCM, and transfer to a 50-mL conical tube using a wide bore pipet.
3. Dilute the methyl cellulose further by adding an equal volume of PBS, and centrifuge at 200*g* for 5 min.
4. Aspirate off the medium and gently resuspend EB in PBS for a second wash, being careful not to disrupt EB structure.
5. Resuspend EB in IMDM containing myeloid growth factors.
6. Split EB from a single 6-cm plate to 1–4 6-cm bacteriologic Petri plates.
7. Macrophages will be "shed" from EB and preferentially attach to bacteriologic plastic. By d 10, a nearly confluent layer of macrophages can be obtained (*see* **Note 13**).

3.4.2. Harvesting of Macrophages from Bacteriologic Petri Dishes

1. Aspirate off culture media and rinse in PBS without calcium or magnesium.
2. Add 2.5 mL of ice-cold PBS without Ca or Mg to cover the surface of the dish and incubate at 4°C for 20 min *(9)*.
3. Using a flat-edged cell scraper, gently and thoroughly scrape the surface of the Petri plate.
4. Centrifuge supernatants and resuspend macrophages in DMEM containing 15% FCS and 10% LCM (*see* **Note 14**).

4. Notes

1. To maintain their pluripotent, undifferentiated state, ES cells must be cultured in the presence of LIF-D *(10)*. LIF-D is commercially available, or can be prepared

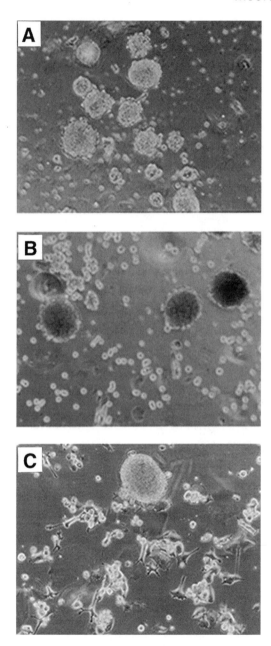

Fig. 2. Myeloid differentiation of ES cells. (**A**) After 4 d of culture semi-solid methyl cellulose medium embryoid bodies should reach a diameter of 100–500 µm. (**B**) By d 8, EB are visible to the naked eye, and have become globinized. (**C**) EB harvested at d 11 and transferred to medium containing myeloid growth factors are producing macrophages which adhere to the bacteriologic plastic. Magnification: 400×.

by collecting cell culture supernatants from CHO 8/24 720LIF-D cells (Genetics Institute Inc., Cambridge, MA). Culture CHO 8/24 720 LIF-D cells in 75 cm² tissue culture flasks in α-MEM medium supplemented with 10% dialyzed, heat-inactivated FCS, 2 mM L-glutamine, 50 U/mL penicillin, 50 mg/mL streptomycin, and 0.1 μM methotrexate. Cell culture supernatants are collected after 4–5 d, filtered through a 0.22-μm membrane and stored at –20·C until use.

2. Detailed protocols for the design of targeting vectors and screening of homologous knock-outs should be consulted prior to beginning *(11)*. Special attention should be paid to the design of the screening strategy, as this will often cause the most problems.

3. IL -3 containing cell culture supernatants can be prepared from X63–Ag8 653 myeloma cells carrying the IL-3 expression plasmid (Genetics Institute, Cambridge, MA). Culture X63–AG8 cells in 75 cm² tissue culture flasks in DMEM supplemented with 5% heat-inactivated fetal calf serum (CS,) 50 U/mL penicillin, 50 mg/mL streptomycin, 25 mM HEPES, 2 mM L-glutamine, and 1 mg/mL G418. Once cells reach confluence (2×10^6 cells/mL), centrifuge cell suspension at 400 x g for 4 minutes. Wash pelleted cells three times in PBS and resuspend 2×10^8 cells in 500 mL of DMEM supplemented with 2% heat-inactivated FCS, 50 U/mL penicillin, 50 mg/mL streptomycin, 25 mM HEPES, and 2 mM L-glutamine. Culture cells in 175 cm² tissue culture flasks for several days until the media turns yellow. To collect the supernatants, centrifuge the cell suspension at 200g for 4 min, filter through a 0.22-μm membrane, and store at –20°C until use.

4. LCM is used as a source of Macrophage Colony Stimulating Factor (M-CSF). Culture L929 fibroblasts (ATCC, Rockville, MD) in 75 cm² flasks until 90% confluent in DMEM supplemented with 5% heat-inactivated FCS, 50 U/mL penicillin, 50 mg/mL streptomycin, 2 mM L-glutamine, and 25 mM HEPES. The cell monolayer is rinsed gently with PBS and replenished with IMDM (0.1 mL/cm²) supplemented with 2% heat-inactivated FCS, 50 U/mL penicillin, 50 mg/mL streptomycin, and 2 mM L-glutamine. Supernatants are collected after 3 d, centrifuged at 400g for 4 min, and filtered through a 0.22-μm membrane. The cell layer can be replenished with fresh media and reused twice. To promote consistency, pool all three batches of LCM and store aliquots at –20°C until use. Once thawed, store LCM at 4°C for up to 1 wk.

5. As an alternative to gelatin coating, Primaria tissue culture plastic (Falcon Labs, Los Angeles, CA) can be used. Primaria tissue cultureware is slightly more expensive, however, this method is simpler and more time efficient if dealing with large numbers of ES cell cultures.

6. For convenience, irradiated STO fibroblasts can be frozen in 10% DMSO and thawed 2–3 h prior to use. Primary cultures of embryonic fibroblasts can be used in place of STO cells *(7,12)*. The primary embryonic fibroblasts have a limited culture lifespan, which ensures that feeder cells do not later contaminate ES cell cultures and inhibit embryoid body formation. However, because of their limited lifespan in culture, this method is also labor intensive.

7. A critical component of successful ES cell culture is maintaining the undifferentiated state of ES cell. If ES cell colonies reach a high density in monolayers, or ES cultures do not contain sufficient LIF-D in the medium, they can spontaneously differentiate to various cell types. Spontaneous differentiation will lead to contamination of cultures by cells that can later inhibit embryoid body formation and macrophage differentiation.

8. If homozygous knock-out ES cells are not detected, increase concentration of G418 and repeat selection and screening.

9. ES cells do not grow as vigorously in the absence of EF feeder layers, and should not be split too thin at this stage. The percentage of LIF-D in ES cell media can be increased up to 10–30% to ensure that ES cells do not differentiate. Contaminating feeder cells will inhibit differentiation of ES cells into embryoid bodies. If ES cells have spontaneously differentiated and cultures are contaminated with mature cells, these can be eliminated by preplating single cell ES cultures (*see* **Subheading 3.1.2.**) onto nongelatin-treated tissue culture plates for 1 h. Differentiated cells will preferentially adhere, and the supernatant containing the ES cells can be transferred to gelatinized or Primaria brand tissue culture plates.

10. The methyl cellulose medium is extremely viscous and is most easily and accurately dispensed using a syringe fitted with an 16–18-gauge needle. The ES cell differentiation medium can be prepared several days in advance, however, the MTG must be prepared fresh and added just prior to use.

11. The optimal EB plating density is 25–50 EB/mL of methyl cellulose differentiation media. If the EB are cultured too densely, the media will not be able to provide sufficient nutrients for 10–12 d. If the media appears yellow after several days, EB bodies can be removed using a wide-bore 25-mL pipet and added to fresh ES differentiation media.

12. To optimize for macrophage differentiation, different batches of FCS should be tested for EB formation and blood island development. Batches of FCS can be scored for EB globinization using dark-field illumination microscopy using a white light source (halogen light) combined with a pale blue filter. Globinized EB will glow red and can then easily be counted *(13)*. Small amounts of several batches of serum can be requested from a commercial supplier and tested simultaneously. Once a "good" batch of serum has been identified, larger quantities of this batch can be ordered. Bottles of serum can be stored for up to 2 yr at –20°C.

13. Macrophages should selectively adhere to bacterial Petri plates to the exclusion of other cell types, making macrophages easy to isolate. If macrophage cultures become contaminated with other cell types, various sorting methods can be used to obtain a pure culture including FACS analysis and magnetic cell sorting. These two methods are covered in detail in a review by Faust *(14)*.

14. Macrophages can be identified by immunochemical staining of macrophage-specific antigens such as F4/80, CD68, macrophage scavenger receptor, and CD11b. Detection of F4/80 Ag is perhaps the most commonly used because of the availability of the F4/80 hybridoma cell line (ATCC) and the high level of F4/80 on the surface of macrophages *(15)*. Other methods of macrophage identification

include May–Grunwald–Giemsa staining by which macrophages can be identified by their highly vacuolated appearance, and phagocytosis assays in which macrophages are fed stained latex beads *(9)*.

References

1. Wiles, M. V. and Keller, G. (1991) Multiple hematopoietic lineages develop from embryonic stem (ES) cells in culture. *Development* **111**, 259–267.
2. Bradley, A., Evans, M., Kaufman, M. H., and Robertson, E. (1984) Formation of germ-line chimeras from embryo-derived teratocarcinoma cell line. *Nature* **309**, 255–256.
3. Mortensen, R. M., Conner, D. A., Chao, S., Geisterfer-Lowrance, A. A., and Seidman, J. G. (1992) Production of homozygous mutant ES cells with a single targeting construct. *Mol. Cell. Biol.* 122, 2391–2395.
4. Moore, K. J., Fabunmi, R. P., Andersson, L. P., and Freeman, M. W. (1998) *In vitro* differentiated embryonic stem (ES) cell macrophages: a model system for studying atherosclerosis-associated macrophage functions. *Aterioscl. Thromb. Vasc. Biol.* **18**, 1647–1654.
5. Martin, G. R. (1981) Isolation of a pluripotent cell line from early mouse embryos cultured in medium conditioned by tertocarcinoma stem cells. *Proc. Natl. Acad. Sci. USA* **78**, 7634–7638.
6. Robertson, E. J. (1991) Using embryonic stem cells to introduce mutations into the mouse germ line. *Biol. Reprod.* **44**, 238–245.
7. Robertson, E. J. (1987) in *Teratocarcinomas and Embryonic Stem Cells: A Practical Approach*, (Robertson, E. J., ed.), IRL Press, Oxford, pp. 71–112.
8. Ware, L. M. and Axelrad, A. A. (1972) Inherited resistance to N- and B-tropic murine leukemia viruses *in vitro*: evidence that congenic mouse strains SIM and SIM.R differ at the Fv-1 locus. *Virology* **50**, 339–348.
9. Moore, K. J., Turco, S. J., and Matlashewski, G. (1994) Leishmania donovani infection enhances macrophage viability in the absence of exogenous growth factor. *J Leukoc Biol.* **55**, 91-98.
10. Williams, R. L., Hilton, D. J., Pease, S., Willson, T. A., Stewart, C. L., Gearing, D. P., Wagner, E. F., Metcalf, D., Nicola, N. A., and Gough, N. M. (1988) Myeloid leukaemia inhibitory factor maintains the developmental potential of embryonic stem cells. *Nature* **336**, 684-687.
11. Ausubel, F. M., Brent, R., Kingston, R. E., Moore, D. D., Seidman, J. G., Smith, J. A., and Struhl, K. (1994) (Janssen, K., ed.), Wiley, New York, NY.
12. Evans, M. (1994) in *Cell Biology: A Laboratory Handbook,* Academic Press, pp. 54–67.
13. Wiles, M. V. (1993) *Methods in Enzymology*, Vol. 225, (Wasserman, P. M. and DePamphilis, M. L., eds.), Academic Press, San Diego, CA, pp. 900–918.
14. Faust, N., Konig, S., Bonifer, C., and Sippel, A. E. (1997) in *Human Genome Methods*, CRC Press, Boca Raton, FL, pp. 185–205.
15. Austyn, J. M. and Gordon, S. (1981) F4/80, a monoclonal antibody directed specifically against the mouse macrophage. *Eur. J. Immunol.* **11**, 805–815.

29

Delivery of Recombinant Adenoviruses to Human Saphenous Vein

Sarah J. George and Andrew H. Baker

1. Introduction

The human saphenous vein is the most commonly used conduit for coronary artery bypass grafting owing to its ready availability, ease of harvesting, and favorable surgical handling *(1)*. However, it suffers from a progressive decline in patency, resulting in a graft failure rate of 50% after 10 yr *(2,3)*. This high failure rate is caused by either early thrombosis occlusion, which occurs in the first year after graft implantation, or the later development of intimal thickening and superimposed atherosclerosis *(1–3)*.

Genetic manipulation of cells in human saphenous vein grafts aimed at preventing graft failure is a promising application of gene therapy in cardiovascular disease. The surgical technique provides a unique opportunity for gene transfer, because the vein is removed from the patient's leg and is subjected to surgical preparation. Surgical preparation involves adventitial stripping, side-branch ligation and distension with heparinized blood. The vein is then placed in heparinized blood for up to 45 min while the chest is prepared. It is therefore clinically feasible to use this time period to carry out gene transfer.

The human saphenous vein organ culture model provides a reproducible, well-characterized model of intimal thickening *(4,5)*. A neointima of vascular smooth muscle cells (VSMC) forms during 14 d of culture due to migration and proliferation of VSMC *(4)*. Therefore, using this model, the effect of gene transfer on the processes of VSMC migration and proliferation that lead to intimal thickening can be studied in human tissue in the absence of a deleterious immune response to the delivery vehicle.

Molecular techniques such as those described in previous chapters have identified candidate genes that may be useful for prevention of vein graft failure.

From: *Methods in Molecular Medicine, Vascular Disease: Molecular Biology and Gene Therapy Protocols*
Edited by: A. H. Baker © Humana Press Inc., Totowa, NJ

These include antiproliferative genes, antithromobolytic genes, antimigratory genes, and suicide genes. We have used recombinant adenoviruses to deliver antimigratory genes to the vein wall since adenoviruses are highly efficient and infect both dividing and nondividing cells. Additionally, the viral DNA is not integrated, resulting in transient recombinant gene expression. The production of recombinant adenoviruses and other gene transfer vehicles is described in detail in other chapters (*see* Chapters 22 and 25).

2. Materials

All solutions and equipment used should be sterile.

2.1. Vein Collection and Preparation for Adenoviral Infection

Collection medium: RPMI 1640 tissue culture medium containing 20 mM HEPES-buffered, 5 µg/mL amphotericin B, and 20 IU/mL sodium heparin. Store in 20 mL aliquots at –20°C. Prewarm to 37°C, immediately before use add 0.225 mg/mL papaverine hydrochloride (McCarthy Medical, Wrexham, UK).

2.2. Infection with Recombinant Adenovirus

1. Wash medium: RPMI 1640 tissue culture medium containing 20 mM HEPES, 2 mM L-glutamine, 8 µg/mL gentamicin, 100 IU/mL penicillin, and 100 µg/mL streptomycin. Store at 4°C. Prewarm to 37°C before use.
2. 18-gauge × 32 mm catheter needle (Abbocath®-T, Venisystems™, Abbott Ireland, Sligo, Republic of Ireland).
3. Vessel cannula with 3 mm beveled tip and one-way valve (DLP Inc, Grand Rapids, MI).
4. 4/0 Mersilk™ braided silk suture (Ethicon Ltd, Edinburgh, UK).
5. Lockable three-way stopcock (Vygon, Ecouen, France).

2.3. Organ Culture

1. Serum-free incubation medium: RPMI 1640 tissue culture medium containing 2 g/L bicarbonate, 2 mM L-glutamine, 8 µg/mL gentamicin, 100 IU/mL penicillin, and 100 µg/mL streptomycin.
2. Incubation medium: To a 50-mL Falcon tube containing 35 mL of serum-free incubation medium add 15 mL of filtered foetal calf serum (FCS). Store at –20°C. Prewarm to 37°C before use.
3. Phosphate-buffered saline (PBS): 0.15 M NaCl, 7.5 mM Na$_2$HPO$_4$, and 1.9 mM NaH$_2$PO$_4$, pH 7.4.
4. 10% buffered formal saline: Add 100 mL of 30% fomaldehyde solution to 900 mL of PBS.
5. Organ culture dishes: To a 45-mm glass Petri dish (BDH, Poole, UK) add 5 mL of Sylgard resin (BDH) mixed 1:10, place at 37°C overnight to set. Sterilize in autoclave.

6. Polyester mesh (size P500, G. Bopp & Co. Ltd, Derbyshire, UK) cut into 15×15 mm squares and sterilize in an autoclave.
7. Minuten pins (size A1, Natkins and Doncaster, Kent, UK): Sterilize by autoclaving.

3. Methods

3.1. Vein Collection and Preparation for Adenoviral Infection

1. Obtain "surgically prepared" human saphenous vein segments (approx 8–10 cm long), from coronary artery bypass patients after adventitial stripping, side branch ligation, gentle manual distension, and storage in heparinized blood for 60–120 min, at the completion of the bypass procedure (*see* **Notes 1** and **2**).
2. Collect veins in 20 mL of prewarmed collection medium.
3. In a laminar flow hood, place vein segments in a 16-cm glass Petri dish containing 75 mL of wash medium. Using microscissors and forceps dissect the remaining adventitia and then bisect the vein transversely (*see* **Note 3**).
4. Place one piece into a small Petri dish containing 5 mL of wash medium to serve as the uninfected control.

3.2. Infection with Recombinant Adenovirus

1. Remove the sheath of an 18-gauge $\times$ 32 mm catheter needle from the catheter needle and trimmed to 2 cm in length with scissors (*see* arrow in **Fig. 1B**).
2. Insert the catheter sheath into the lumen of the piece of vein to be infected (*see* **Notes 4** and **5**).
3. Hold the catheter sheath in place with forceps and check for the presence of obstructing valves by injecting 0.5 mL of wash medium into the vein lumen via the catheter sheath using a 1 mL sterile syringe. If the wash medium does not flow through the vein segment, this process should be repeated at the other end of the vein (*see* **Note 6**).
4. When unobstructed flow of wash medium is observed, insert a vessel cannula with 3 mm beveled tip and one-way valve into the lumen of the other end of the vein.
5. Cut a 10 cm length of sterile 4/0 Mersilk™ braided silk suture with microscissors.
6. Place the suture around the end of the vein with the vessel cannula inserted.
7. Using two pairs of sterile forceps tie two knots in the silk suture to secure the vessel cannula (**Fig. 1A**) (*see* **Note 7**).
8. Insert the catheter cannula into the other end of the vein segment.
9. Cut another 10 cm length of sterile 4/0 Mersilk™ braided silk suture with microscissors.
10. Secure the catheter sheath in place with the silk suture in a similar fashion as described above for the vessel cannula (**Fig. 1C**).
11. While still in their sterile wrapping, twist the taps of two three-way stopcocks to close the stopcocks.
12. Remove both stopcocks from the wrapping and place into the Petri dish containing the vein and wash medium.
13. Attach one stopcock to the vessel cannula (**Fig. 2A**).

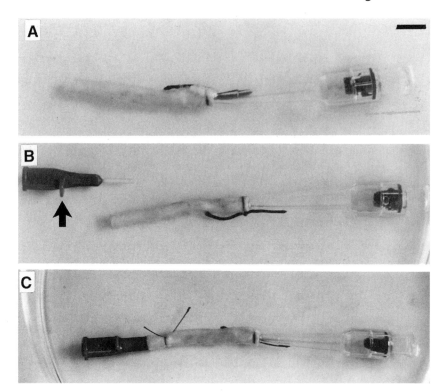

Fig. 1. Stages of adenoviral infection protocol I. (**A**) Vein segment with vessel cannula inserted and secured in one end. (**B**) Vein segment with vessel cannula secured, trimmed catheter sheath is placed in medium (see arrow). (**C**) Vein segment with vessel cannula and catheter sheath inserted into both ends. Scale bar in panel (A) applies to all panels and represents 1 cm.

14. Using a 1 mL sterile syringe medium inject wash medium through the catheter sheath until it just enters the distal cannula.
15. Briefly microfuge the cryovial containing the adenovirus to ensure that the 100 μL is at the bottom of the tube.
16. Take up 100 μL of recombinant adenovirus solution at 1.2×10^{10} pfu/mL into another 1 mL sterile syringe (*see* **Note 8**).
17. Hold the catheter sheath vertically at the place of the Nylon suture knot with sterile forceps.
18. Insert the syringe containing the adenovirus into the catheter sheath and inject the contents into the lumen of the vein proximal cannula without increased pressure (**Fig. 2B**) (*see* **Note 9**).
19. Carefully remove the 1 mL syringe from the catheter sheath, and using forceps attach the other stopcock to the catheter sheath (**Fig. 2C**) (*see* **Note 10**).
20. Remove the wash medium and replace with fresh medium.

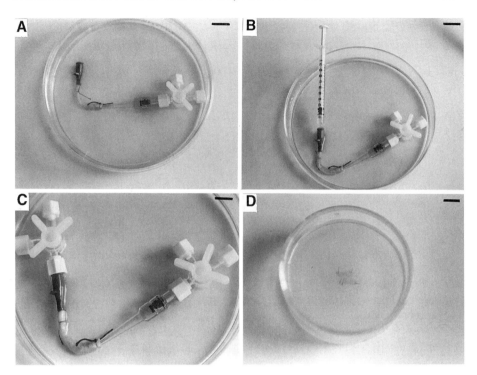

Fig. 2. Stages of adenoviral infection protocol II. **(A)** Vein segment with vessel cannula and catheter sheath inserted and one closed stop cock attached to the vessel cannulae. **(B)** Vein segment with a 1 mL syringe inserted into the catheter sheath. **(C)** Vein segment with stop cocks inserted into both ends. **(D)** Vein set up as an organ culture. Scale bars in panels (A) and (B) represent 1.25 cm, scale bar in (C) represents 2 cm, and scale bar in panel (D) represents 0.5 cm.

21. Incubate the infected and uninfected vein segments for 1 h at room temperature in the laminar flow hood (*see* **Notes 11** and **12**).

3.3. Organ Culture

1. After incubation, remove the cannulae by cutting the vein segment at the end of the cannula with microscissors.
2. Place the infected region of the vein into a small glass Petri dish containing set Sylgard resin and 10 mL of wash medium.
3. Using microscissors cut the vein longitudinally to open it out and then transversely into three 5–10 mm segments (*see* **Note 13**).
4. Divide the control vein similarly.
5. Pin each vein segment down, endothelial surface uppermost on a 15 × 15 mm square of polyester mesh resting on set Sylgard resin in glass Petri dishes with minuten pins (**Fig. 2D**).

6. Wash the segment twice with 5 mL of wash media.
7. Add 5 mL of incubation medium and then culture for up to 14 d at 37°C under 95% air/5% CO_2.
8. Every 2 d remove incubation medium, wash vein segment twice with 5 mL aliquots of wash medium, and add 5 mL of fresh incubation medium.
9. At the required time point, remove vein segments (*see* **Notes 14** and **15**).

4. Notes

1. Ensure that vein used is of good quality by collecting as soon as possible after the completion of the bypass surgery. Vein that is not fresh will have poor intimal formation.
2. Check that the vein has some remaining endothelial cells by immunocytochemistry as the presence of endothelial cells is essential for intimal thickening in this model.
3. When removing the adventitia be careful to avoid cutting small holes in the vessel wall.
4. When choosing the segment of vein for gene transfer, avoid areas of vein with side branches because these may be a source of leakage and because valves are commonly situated around the side branches.
5. Although this method describes the use of human saphenous vein, it could also be used to infect animal veins or arteries or human arteries. However, if other vessels are used, it may be necessary to change the size of vessel cannulae and catheter sheath.
6. Take care to avoid vein segments with valves, because these can obstruct the entry of adenovirus into the lumen of the entire length of the vein segment.
7. When tying the knots in the silk suture to secure the vessel cannula and catheter sheath, check that these are secure and that they are not too close to the end of the vein or the cannulae, as the injection of the adenovirus may dislodge them.
8. When taking the adenovirus up into the 1 mL syringe avoid bubbles.
9. Always ensure that a little air is taken into the 1 mL syringe before the adenovirus (approx 200 μL of volume). This will propel the virus through the catheter sheath and into the lumen of the vein.
10. After insertion of the second stopcock and during the 1 h incubation period, the vein can be gently massaged with sterile forceps to mix the contents of the vein lumen.
11. During the 1 h incubation it must be ensured that the vein segment is completely immersed in wash medium so that the surface of the vein does not dry out.
12. If the vein appears deflated and the lumen contents have leaked out, the vein segment should be discarded because infection of nonlumenal cells may have occurred.
13. When cutting the infected vein segment into three 5–10 mm segments, the position from which the vein segment was taken should be noted. This will allow the identification of problematic regional infections.
14. After required culture period, wash the vein segments twice with PBS. To detect luminal reporter gene, expression, fix the vein segment *in situ* and stain. Typical

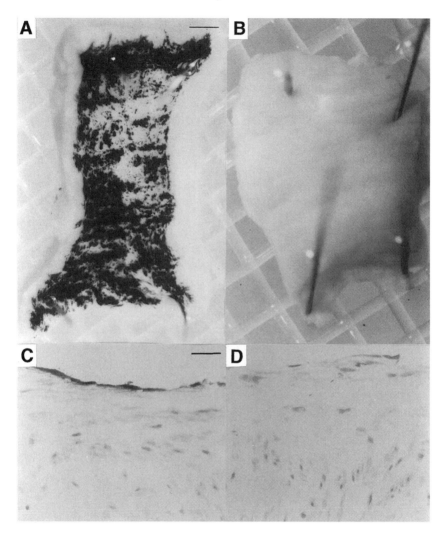

Fig. 3. Detection of the reporter gene β-galactosidase in vein segments after 7 d of culture. (**A**) Typical *en face* staining of infected vein segment, dark color indicates cells expressing β-galactosidase. (**B**) Control vein segment with no (β-galactosidase expression. (**C**) Transverse section of infected vein segment, dark color on luminal surface cells indicates cells expressing β-galactosidase. (**D**) Transverse section of control vein segment with no β-galactosidase expression. Scale bar in panel (A) applies to panels (A and B), and represents 0.1 cm and scale bar in panel (C) applies to panels (C and D) and represents 25 μm.

luminal detection of β-galactosidase expression is shown in **Fig. 3A**. Then paraffin wax embed the vein segment and cut transverse sections. Typical

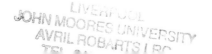

β-galactosidase expression in a transverse section is shown in **Fig. 3B**. To detect specific protein expression and examine the effect of the gene transfer on neointimal thickening, fix the vein segment in 10% formal buffered saline and paraffin wax embed or freeze in isopentane, and store at –70°C. Cut paraffin or frozen sections and carry out histological staining and immunocytochemistry *(5,6)*.

15. We have used this organ culture model to maintain vein segments for a maximum of 14 d without loss of cell viability. Prolonged incubation after 14 d or use of large vein segments in culture will lead to loss of cell viability and distortion of data.

References

1. Bryan, A. J. and Angelini, G. D. (1994) The biology of saphenous vein graft occlusion: etiology and strategies for prevention. *Curr. Opin. Cardiol.* **9,** 641–649.
2. Campeau, L., Enjalbert, M., Lesperance, J., Bourassa, M. G., Kwiterovich, P., Jr., Wacholder, S., and Snideman, A. (1984) The relation of risk factors to the development of atherosclerosis in saphenous-vein bypass grafts and the progression of disease in the native circulation. *N. Eng. J. Med.* **311(21),** 1329–1332.
3. Lytle, B. W., Loop, F. D., Cosgrove, D. M., Ratliff, N.B., Easly, K., and Taylor, P. C. (1985) Long term (5 to 12 years) serial studies of internal mammary artery and saphenous vein coronary bypass grafts. *J. Thorac. Cardiovasc. Surg.* **89,** 248–258.
4. Soyombo, A. A., Angelini, G. D., Bryan, A. J., Jasani, B., and Newby, A. C. (1990) Intimal proliferation in an organ culture of human saphenous vein. *Am. J. Pathol.* **137(6),** 1401–1410.
5. George, S. J., Williams, A., and Newby, A. C. (1996) An essential role for platelet derived growth factor in neointima formation in human saphenous vein *in vitro*. *Atherosclerosis* **120,** 227–240.
6. George, S. J., Johnson, J. L., Angelini, G. D., Newby, A. C., and Baker, A. H. (1998) Adenovirus-mediated gene transfer of the human TIMP-1 gene inhibits SMC migration and neointima formation in human saphenous vein. *Human Gene Ther.* **9,** 867–877.

VII

IN VIVO VASCULAR GENE TRANSFER PROTOCOLS

30

An In Vivo Angiogenesis Assay to Study Positive and Negative Regulators of Neovascularization

Maurizio C. Capogrossi and Antonino Passaniti

1. Introduction

The formation of new blood vessels from existing blood vessels has been referred to as angiogenesis to distinguish the process from *de novo* embryonic vessel formation or vasculogenesis *(1)*. This chapter will describe an in vivo assay to measure angiogenesis. There are several important reasons to study and measure angiogenesis in vascular disease. First, it is necessary to try to understand proliferative angiogenesis as it occurs in tumors and in diabetic complications and devise strategies to inhibit it. Second, there is intense interest in improving angiogenesis after ischemia or in chronic wounds *(2)*. Third, many potential modulators of angiogenesis need to be evaluated to determine their effects on blood vessel development.

To determine which angiogenic factors or inhibitors to use and which responses to analyze in a given assay, a consideration of the major temporal events in a tumor angiogenic response is instructive (**Fig. 1**). In response to secreted tumor cytokines such as fibroblast growth factor (FGF), vascular endothelial growth factor (VEGF), and others, degradation of basement membrane components by collagenases, metalloproteinases, and plasminogen activators can occur *(3)*. Endothelial cells (EC) may provide some of these enzymes in response to growth factor stimulation o·r they may be secreted by the tumor cells or host stromal cells. Several defined methods which are not the topic of this chapter, have been devised to study the expression of these enzymes or their effects on cells in culture including protein zymograms *(4)* and cellular invasion chambers *(5)*.

Endothelial cell migration can occur on tissue matrix because of specific cell surface receptors (integrins) that are activated in response to angiogenic

From: *Methods in Molecular Medicine, Vascular Disease: Molecular Biology and Gene Therapy Protocols*
Edited by: A. H. Baker © Humana Press Inc., Totowa, NJ

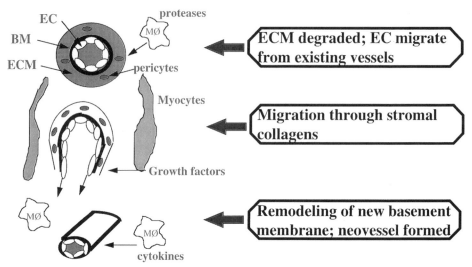

Fig. 1. Steps in angiogenesis illustrating the role of various cells, cytokines, and proteases. ECM = extracellular matrix; EC = endothelial cells, MF = macrophages; BM = basement membrane. For details, refer to text.

stimuli (6). Chemoattractants released from mast cells also appear to be important in the activation of cell surface cytokine receptors. Some cytokines released by stromal and tumor cells can also directly increase endothelial cell proliferation. Increased cell number allows the formation of new blood vessels to proceed. Because heparin is a cofactor for many of these cytokines (including FGF and VEGF), mast cells are also believed to play an important role in this process (7). Proliferative indices using proliferating cell nuclear antigen (PCNA) expression in vivo or DNA synthesis and growth assays in vitro have been used to verify endothelial cell proliferation. In general, growth factors such as FGF are very mitogenic for endothelial cells. However, VEGF mitogenic activity is relatively low, whereas the ability of VEGF to increase vascular permeability and blood flow is very potent (8). Associated with increased numbers of endothelial cells is the capacity for branching, which appears to be highly regulated by the balance of proliferative and antiproliferative signals in combination with recently described angiopoietins (9).

Maturation of blood vessels involves the process of endothelial cell differentiation characterized by growth arrest and secretion of basement membrane components. The recruitment of pericytes leads to their association with the immature vessel and subsequent resolution of the response (10). This latter phase involves extensive cell contact (between endothelial cells) and subsequent vessel maturation in response to many cytokines, but, in particular, transforming growth factor-β (TGFβ), which regulates matrix expression. Some of these processes can be mimicked in vitro using a variety of collagenous (collagen I gels, Matrigel) and stromal (fibrin clots) substrates. In some cases, artificial lumen formation can be observed even without the presence of associated pericytes *(11)*.

It is clear from extensive studies on pathogenic angiogenesis that the presence of natural inhibitors of angiogenesis play an important role in attenuating the process. When angiogenesis is associated with inflammatory phenomena, the expression of interleukin-8 can lead to the down-regulation of adhesion receptors, which prevents further vessel instability *(12)*. The recruitment of pericytes to inhibit the angiogenic response appears to involve the expression of the Tie-2 receptor and interaction with angiopoietin-1 and angiopoietin-2 *(13)*. The migration of smooth muscle cells and pericytes to the neovascular environment coincides with basement membrane synthesis and the assembly of fibronectin and thrombospondin crosslinks, which also stabilize the formation of a vessel lumen. More recently, the demonstration that naturally occurring inhibitors of endothelial cells such as angiostatin, derived from plasminogen *(14)*, and endostatin, derived from collagen 18 *(15)*, inhibit tumor angiogenesis suggests that these molecules may also be involved in normal vessel maturation.

Assays to study angiogenesis consist of several in vitro and in vivo methods (*see* **Table 1** for summary) *(16–29)*. Although migration, chemotaxis, and invasion assays have been used to assess the response of EC to various agents *(5)*, the growth arrest, morphological changes, and expression of markers typical of neovascular EC undergoing differentiation are features of several in vitro assays that more closely mimic the in vivo situation. Of these, the culture of EC on collagenous substrates leads to spontaneous morphological differentiation *(19,26)*. Differentiation is not limited to collagen substrates, as fibrin clots will also support EC differentiation *(20)*. More complex mixtures of basement membranes have been used as support matrix for EC differentiation including amniotic membrane *(24)*. Other developments led to the use of basement membrane extracts of the EHS mouse tumor (Matrigel) to enhance cellular differentiation *(21)*. It was found that certain components of Matrigel, especially laminin and several laminin peptides, were responsible for some of the biological activity associated with differentiation *(23)*.

In vivo assays to study angiogenesis have been of interest because of the advantage of studying the complete process in a physiological setting and for the testing of therapeutic compounds. Advances and pitfalls in the analysis of results from in vivo angiogenesis assays have recently been reviewed *(29)*. Some of the earliest studies relied on the implantation of angiogenic vehicles in slow release carriers placed in the limbic area of rabbit or rodent corneas

Table 1
Chronology of Angiogenesis Assays[a]

Year	Assay	In vitro	In vivo	Citation	Ref
1974	rabbit cornea		+	Gimbrone, *JNCI* **52,** 413	*(16)*
1975	CAM[b]		+	Ausprunk, *Am. J. Pathol.* **79,** 597	*(17)*
1979	mouse cornea		+	Muthudaruppan, *Science* **205,** 1416	*(18)*
1980	monolayer[c]	+		Folkman, *Nature* **288,** 551	*(19)*
1987	rat aorta[d]	+		Nicosia, *Am. J. Pathol.* **128,** 78	*(20)*
1988	Matrigel[e]	+		Kubota, *J. Cell Biol.* **107,** 1589	*(21)*
1988	Gelfoam		+	Thompson, *Science* **241,** 1349	*(22)*
1989	laminin	+		Grant, *Cell* **58,** 933	*(23)*
1989	amnion[f]	+		Mignatti, *J. Cell. Biol.* **108,** 671	*(24)*
1990	alginate gels		+	Plunkett, *Lab. Invest.* **62,** 510	*(25)*
1991	collagen gels	+		Iruela-Arispe, *Lab. Invest.* **64,** 174	*(26)*
1992	Matrigel[g]		+	Passaniti, *Lab. Invest.* **67,** 519	*(27)*
1996	human placenta[h]	+		Brown, *Lab. Invest.* **75,** 539	*(28)*

[a]For recent review of other methods, *see (29)*.
[b]Chick allantoic membrane.
[c]Spontaneous differentiation of bovine aortic endothelial cells.
[d]Fibrin clot or collagen gel.
[e]Basement membrane extracellular matrix from the EHS tumor.
[f]Human amniotic membrane.
[g]Matrigel sc implants in rodents.
[h]Fibrin clot.

(16,18). The chick allantoic membrane has also been used as an ex vivo method *(17)*. Alginate gels impregnated with EC growth factors or tumor cells have resulted in potent angiogenic responses *(25)* as have Gelfoam implants *(22)*.

In our studies we have taken advantage of the ability of EC to attach to basement membrane matrix and of the affinity of angiogenic cytokines for basement membrane components, such as heparin sulfate proteoglycans, to develop an assay using Matrigel impregnated with EC growth factors *(27)*. Basal lamina consists predominantly of the proteins laminin and collagen IV crosslinked in a dense matrix with heparin sulfate proteoglycan. Linker molecules such as nidogen/entactin are also present. Vascular endothelium is often seen in direct contact with basal lamina, which is believed to provide rigid support for thin capillaries lacking pericytes. The assay described in this chapter, utilizing the basement membrane proteins found in EHS matrix (Matrigel), has allowed the testing of a variety of angiogenic and antiangiogenic factors and is being used to investigate basic mechanisms of angiogenesis.

2. Materials

1. 10% formalin: Prepare by diluting formaldehyde (37.7% stock, Mallinkrodt Baker Inc., Paris, KY) with phosphate-buffered saline (PBS) to a final concentration of 3.77. Add glutaraldehyde fresh to the formalin from a 25% stock (Sigma, St. Louis, MO) for a final 1% concentration.

2. Cytokines: Typically, fibroblast growth factors (bovine basic FGF, FGF-2, or acidic FGF, FGF-1, R&D, Minneapolis, MN) contain buffer salts and carrier protein. Store at –20°C if dry. Reconstitute 25 µg protein with 0.5 mL H_2O or media salts (Dulbecco's modified Eagle's medium, [DMEM]) to make 50 µg/mL stocks. Store 0.1-mL aliquots at -20°C in a noncycling freezer. Thaw a maximum of two times for dilution in the assay described below. Frozen FGF is stable for up to 6 mo.

3. Heparin (Gibco-BRL, Gaithersburg, MD): prepare as a stock of 10,000 U/mL. Store at –20°C.

4. Adenovirus vectors: The preparation of adenovirus vectors as well as their purification and the determination of viral titers have been described in other chapters (*see* Chapters 22 and 25). For the in vivo studies described below, the AdCMV.NLSβGal (expresses a nuclear localized β-galactosidase) and AdCMV.null (expresses no transgene) vectors were used as controls. The AdCMV.FGF-1 (expresses FGF-1), AdCMV.sp+FGF-1 (expresses FGF-1 with a signal peptide for secretion), and the AdCMV.VEGF (expresses VEGF) vectors were used to promote an angiogenesis response. The AdCMV.p53 (express p53) and AdCMV.TIMP2 (expresses tissue inhibitor of metalloproteinase-2, TIMP2) vectors are used to inhibit an angiogenesis response.

5. Cell lines: 3T3 fibroblasts (obtained from the American Type Culture Collection, Rockville, MD) for adenoviral infection studies and cultured in DMEM containing 10% FBS and antibiotics.

6. Animals: Female C57BL/6 mice (Jackson Laboratories, Bar Harbor, ME) are used at 6–8 wk of age. In some studies, male mice from the Gerontology Research Center (National Institute on Aging) between 3 and 24 mo of age were used. These animals were maintained on standard chow throughout the lifespan.

7. Buffers: Prepare in 2 L portions (*31*). Buffer A contains 397 g NaCl (3.4 *M*), 12.1 g Tris base (0.05 *M*), 3.0 g EDTA (0.004 *M*), and 0.05 g NEM (0.002 *M*), pH 7.4 with HCl. Buffer B contains 240 g urea (2.0 *M*), 12.1 g Tris Base (0.05 *M*), 18.0 g NaCl (0.15 *M*), pH 7.4 with HCl. Buffer C contains 12.1 g Tris Base (0.05 *M*), 18.0 g NaCl (0.15 *M*), pH 7.4 with HCl.

8. Phosphate-buffered saline (PBS): 0.02 *M* phosphate, 0.15 *M* NaCl, pH 7.4.

9. Penicillin (Gibco-BRL).

10. Streptomycin (Gibco-BRL).

11. 10 m*M* EDTA.

12. Dialysis tubing (12,000 MW cut-off). Pretreat with EDTA, boil and rinse in dH_2O.

13. Chloroform.

14. DMEM with or without phenol red.

15. Xylene.

16. Masson's Trichrome stain.
17. X-gal (5-bromo-4-chloro-3-indolyl β-D-galactopyranoside): 50 mg/mL in DMSO:diethylpyrocarbonate water (50:50).
18. X-gal stain: 35 mM potassium ferricyanide, 1 mM MgCl$_2$, 0.02% NP-40, and 0.01% deoxycholate stock solution, 1 mg/mL X-Gal.

3. Methods

There are several discrete steps in performing an in vivo angiogenesis assay: preparation of the Matrigel/cytokine mixtures, injection and processing of gel plugs containing neovessels, and analysis/quantitation of the results. This section will describe the specific protocols and expected results with particular emphasis on the variety of applications of the assay to study angiogenic and antiangiogenic factors.

3.1. Matrigel Preparation and Extraction of Matrix Proteins

An abundant source of basement membrane proteins is a mouse tumor (Englebreth/Holm/Swarm, EHS) which was described in 1963, that secretes laminin, collagen IV, and proteoglycans *(30,31)*. The tumor was originally isolated from Balb/c mice, but has been adapted to grow in C57BL mice. EHS tumor cells do not grow in culture and, therefore, passage of the tumor necessitates transplantation of tumor pieces between mice.

3.1.1. EHS Tumor Maintenance

1. Excise tumor tissue from young mice (9–11 wk of age) with 2–4-g tumors.
2. Wash three times to remove serum with PBS containing penicillin (50 µg/µL) and streptomycin (50 U/mL).
3. Extrude the tumor tissue through a 16-gage needle to remove dense, fibrous pieces that clog the syringe.
4. Normally, inject 100 mg (0.5 mL) of tumor suspension im in the soleus muscle of the hind limb of each mouse.
5. The tumor will be visible after two weeks and can be harvested between the third and fourth week after transplantation. Occasionally, tumors are propagated sc to increase the proportion of extracellular matrix to cells, but growth rates are about 1/3 reduced from the im implantation site. For the methods described in this chapter only tumors harvested from the im implantation sites were used.

3.1.2. Extraction of Matrix Proteins

Perform all procedures at 4°C, unless stated. Total time for preparation of EHS matrix is 3 d. All volumes assume 100-g tumor tissue for each preparation. On d 1, tumor tissue is washed with a high-salt buffer to remove blood and matrix proteins are extracted with urea:

1. Homogenize tumor with a polytron in 200 mL of Buffer A.
2. Centrifuge at 16,000g Sorvall GSA rotor, for 15 min and discard the supernatant.
3. Repeat twice more, discard the final supernatant.
4. Homogenize the tumor pellet in 100 mL of Buffer B.
5. Stir in the cold overnight.

On d 2, urea-extracted proteins are dialyzed to remove urea.

6. Aliquot the tumor extract (in 2 *M* urea) into centrifuge tubes and centrifuge at 23,000g in a Sorvall SS34 rotor, for 20 min.
7. Save the supernatants and reextract the tumor pellets with 50 mL of Buffer B, stirring for 30 min.
8. Centrifuge at 23,000g as in **step 6** and combine the supernatants with the previous urea supernatants.
9. Filter the extracted proteins in the supernatants over a 4 × 4 gauze and place in dialysis tubing.
10. Dialyze versus Buffer C (900 mL) containing 5 mL chloroform (to sterilize). Stir overnight in the cold.

On d 3, dialysis to remove urea continues and the final EHS matrix is isolated.

11. Invert the dialysis bags to mix insoluble material.
12. Change dialysate to Buffer C without chloroform for 2 h.
13. Dialyze the samples once more with Buffer C for 2 h and then with media salts (DMEM or DMEM without phenol red or Buffer C again) for 2 h.
14. Remove the dialysis bags, place on ice, and spray with 70% ethanol to sterilize the outside of the bags.
15. Cut the bags with scissors rinsed in ethanol and remove the matrix proteins with a sterile 10 mL pipet.
16. Combine the matrix material from all dialysis bags, aliquot, and freeze at –20°C (noncycling freezer) in 15-mL conical tubes (*see* **Note 1**).
17. Determine protein concentrations using the Bradford method. Routinely, preparations of 5–10 mg/mL are obtained (*see* **Note 2**).

3.2. Preparation of Gel Mixtures

3.2.1. Gels Containing Cytokines

1. Thaw frozen EHS matrix (Matrigel) and maintain as a liquid at 4°C on ice (*see* **Note 3**). This is the vehicle for delivery of angiogenic cytokines.
2. Typically, prepare an angiogenic cytokine (25 µg) such as FGF-2 (bovine basic FGF) before the experiment by resuspending the lyophilized factor and carrier protein (provided by the manufacturer) in 0.5 mL of DMEM buffer to a final concentration of 50 µg/mL. If heparin is needed for subsequent hemoglobin analysis (*see* **Notes 4** and **5**), prepare as a 1000X stock, typically 10,000 U/mL in DMEM.
3. Usually, for a group of five mice, place 3.0 mL of Matrigel in a 15-mL sterile conical tube.

4. In some cases, angiogenic antagonists can be included within the gel at the time of injection. In a separate sterile Eppendorf centrifuge tube, combine 9 µL of FGF-2 and 150 µL of DMEM just before use. If needed, include 3 µL of heparin with various amounts of inhibitors and adjust the volume to 150 µL with DMEM. Add aliquots (50 µL) of the FGF mixture in the Eppendorf tube separately to the 3 mL of Matrigel and mixed rapidly by inverting the 15-mL conical tube between each addition. This allows even distribution of the proteins within the Matrigel. The final concentrations of FGF and heparin are 150 ng/mL and 10 U/mL, respectively.
5. Store the mixtures on ice until mice are injected.

3.2.2. Gels Modified with Recombinant Adenoviruses

1. Prepare 5–10-µL aliquots of recombinant adenovirus containing 1×10^7 to 1×10^9 plaque forming U/mL (pfu/mL) in PBS.
2. Combine with FGF-2 (150 ng/mL) and heparin (10 U/mL) in DMEM as described above (**Subheading 3.2.1.**).
3. Mix 50-µL aliquots with Matrigel as described above (**Subheading 3.2.1.**).

3.3. Injection of Mice and Processing of Gels

At least five mice (*see* **Note 6**) per data point are normally used. The animals are injected sc with 0.5 mL liquid Matrigel containing FGF and other components (heparin, inhibitors as needed). Because of the high viscosity of the Matrigel, mixtures of 3 mL are sufficient for one treatment group of five mice.

3.3.1. Gels Containing Cytokines

1. Place the Matrigel/FGF solutions in 3-mL syringes to inject each group of five mice.
2. Insert a 25-gage needle and inject 0.5 mL sc on the abdominal midline of each mouse (*see* **Note 7**). Injections at other sites can lead to poor recovery of the gels (*see* **Note 8**). The injection site should form a distinct "bump" that persists as the gel hardens in response to the higher body temperature (40°C) of the mouse. The injection site is easily identified during the course of the response and solid gels persist for up to 3 wk.
3. Sacrifice animals usually at 1–2 wk after injection (*see* **Note 9**).
4. At this time, treat the area of the implant with 70% ethanol. This allows clear identification of the gel plug.
5. Excise the perimeter of the plug including skin and peritoneal muscle with sterile scissors. Make no attempt to cut the gel, because, this would result in loss of structure.
6. Place the intact skin, gel, and muscle in tubes containing PBS-buffered 10% formalin.

3.3.2. Injection with Recombinant Adenoviruses

To analyze adenovirus-mediated gene expression on angiogenesis, an alternative to mixing recombinant adenovirus with the Matrigel is to inject the virus sc prior to Matrigel injection.

1. Prepare 0.5 mL of recombinant adenovirus (total 5×10^7 pfu) in PBS.
2. Inject into mice sc at the same site to be used for Matrigel injection.
3. Allow transgene expression to proceed for at least 3 d.
4. Inject 0.5 mL of Matrigel as described above (*see* **Subheading 3.3.1.**).

3.4. Analysis of Data: Vessel Staining and Quantitation

3.4.1. Histological Analysis of Endothelial Cells

1. After overnight incubation in formalin, the gel plugs are prepared for histological stains or antibodies by progressive dehydration in increasing ethanol concentrations.
2. Embed in paraffin under vacuum *(27)*.
3. Deparaffinize sections (5 µm) with xylene, rehydrate with decreasing ethanol concentrations, and stain with Masson's Trichrome stain or specific antibodies (*see* **Note 10** and **ref. *32***).
4. Quantify the histological sections with an image analysis system with a CCTV or digital camera and appropriate software (*see* **Note 11**).
5. Set threshold values to subtract background stain (light blue with Masson's Trichrome) and detect specific cellular areas (dark blue or black).
6. Quantitate as a percent of total image area (*see* **Note 12**).

3.4.2. Analysis of Intact Vessels

1. To visualize intact vessels in the gel plug, resect the overlying skin and place the gel in a Petri plate.
2. Visualize under a dissection scope at low power (6×–10×).
3. To improve visibility, squashes of the tissue can be prepared by placing a glass slide over the gel plug and photographing the surface vessels. With direct illumination the small, tortuous vessels within the gel plug can be observed.

3.4.3. Hemoglobin Analysis

Lysis of RBC releases hemoglobin, which can be separated from the gel and tissue by brief centrifugation.

1. For hemoglobin analysis, separate the gel plugs containing low amounts of heparin from surrounding skin while retaining the peritoneal muscle.
2. Transfer the tissue to Eppendorf tubes containing 0.5 mL dH_2O.
3. Incubate overnight at 37°C.
4. Crush the tissue with a syringe barrel.
5. Centrifuge at 200*g* for 10 min to remove tissue debris.

6. Measure the hemoglobin in the soluble supernatant using the Drabkin method (Sigma) and express relative to total protein in the supernatant or the weight of the original gel plug (*see* **Note 13**).

3.4.4. Analysis of Adenoviral Infection

In some applications using adenovirus vectors containing the *lacZ* gene, β-galactosidase staining was used to visualize infected cells surrounding the gel plugs.

1. Cut the tissue into several pieces.
2. Fix for 2–3 h in fresh 10% formalin buffered with PBS.
3. Wash samples three times for 30 min each in PBS.
4. Stain at 30°C in X-gal solution:
5. After 3 d, wash tissue in PBS until the rinse solution is colorless.
6. Process for paraffin embedding and sectioning.

3.5. Applications of the Assay: Analysis of Data and Expected Results

Time course and histological studies with FGF have shown that after an initial (2–6 h) neutrophil response, cells begin to invade the gel within 24 h *(27)*. By 72 h, capillary-sized vessels are readily apparent inside the gel. Persistent vessels with clear lumens surrounded by fenestrated endothelial cells are readily apparent up to 3 wk following injection of the mice. vWF staining of tissue sections also revealed increases in factor staining within 24 h of implantation. Hemoglobin content increases from 2 –6 d after injection.

Initial studies with the in vivo Matrigel angiogenesis assay utilized both angiogenic and antiangiogenic factors. Cytokines (FGF, TNF, TGFβ, HGF), adenoviral vectors (FGF, VEGF), tumor cells (LNCaP, 3T3 infected with Ad.FGF-1), and other molecules (IL-15, NO, thrombin) have all been used to stimulate blood vessel formation (**Table 2**) *(27,33–51)*. Notably absent from this list is VEGF protein, which has been shown to be important in sustaining, but not initiating, tumor angiogenesis *(52)*. Numerous attempts utilizing recombinant VEGF165 (both human and mouse) have failed to elicit an angiogenic response (personal communications; unpublished observations) (*see* **Note 14**). Interestingly, VEGF gene delivery with recombinant adenoviral vectors has resulted in potent angiogenic responses, perhaps because of activation of existing vascular cells after viral coat adhesion to angiogenic receptors. Nude mice, rats, SCID mice, and Balb/c mice have all been used and routinely respond to a variety of angiogenic stimuli.

Inhibitors of angiogenesis used in this assay (*see* **Note 15**) have included antiproliferative cytokines (TGFβ, IL-1, IP-10), protease inhibitors (Batimastat), glycosidase inhibitors (CST, castanospermine), and adenoviral vectors coding for tumor suppressor genes (Ad.p53). Expression of p53 *(51)* was induced by

Table 2
Angiogenic Modulators in the Matrigel Angiogenesis Assay[a]

Factor[b]	Activity[c]	Year	Citation	Ref
FGF, TNFα	+	1992	Passaniti, *Lab. Invest.* **67,** 519	(27)
TGFβ, PDGF-BB,				
IL-1β, IL-6, TIMP	–	1992	Passaniti, *Lab. Invest.* **67,** 519	(27)
SIKVAV	+	1992	Kibbey, *JNCI* **84,** 1633	(33)
Linomide	–	1992	Vukanovic, *Cancer Res.* **53,** 1833	(34)
HGF	+	1993	Grant, *PNAS* **90,** 1937	(35)
Age	–	1994	Pili, *JNCI* **86,** 1303	(36)
CST	–	1995	Pili, *Cancer Res.* **55,** 2920	(37)
Ad.VEGF	+	1995	Muhlhauser, *Circulation Res.* **77,** 1077	(38)
Ad.FGF-1[d]	+	1995	Muhlhauser, *Human Gene Ther.* **6,** 1457	(39)
Batimastat	–	1995	Taraboletti, *JNCI* **87,** 293	(40)
IP-10	–	1995	Angiolillo, *J. Exp. Med.* **182,** 155	(41)
PAF	+	1995	Bussolino, *J. Clin. Invest.* **96,** 940	(42)
	+	1995	Camussi, *J. Immunol.* **154,** 6492	(43)
Tat	+	1996	Corallini, *AIDS* **10,** 701	(44)
Anti-Fas Ab	+	1997	Biancone, *J. Exp. Med.* **186,** 147	(45)
Thrombin	+	1997	Haralabopoulos, *Am. J. Physiol.* **273,** 239	(46)
IL-15	+	1997	Angiolillo, *BBRC* **233,** 231	(47)
NO, PAF, TNFα	+	1997	Montrucchio, *Am. J. Pathol.* **151,** 557	(48)
LNCaP	+	1997	Wilson, *Anatomical Rec.* **249,** 63	(49)
3T3 (Ad.FGF-1)	+	1997	Pili, *Int. J. Cancer* **73,** 258	(50)
Ad.p53	–	1998	Riccioni, *Gene Ther.* **5,** 747	(51)

[a]Angiogenic or anti-angiogenic factors tested in the Matrigel in vivo assay.
[b]Acidic (FGF-1) or basic (FGF-2) bovine fibroblast growth factor; tumor necrosis factor (TNFα); transforming growth factor (TGFβ); platelet-derived growth factor (PDGF-BB); interleukin-1 (IL-1β); interleukin-6 (IL-6); Tissue inhibitor of metalloproteinases-1 (TIMP); Laminin peptide (SIKVAV); Quinoline-3-carboxamide (Linomide); Hepatocyte growth factor (HGF); Castanospermine (CST, glycosidase inhibitor); Adenovirus coding for vascular endothelial growth factor (Ad.VEGF) or acidic fibroblast growth factor (Ad.FGF-1); Proteinase inhibitor (Batimastat); Interferon-inducible protein 10 (IP-10); Platelet activating factor (PAF); AIDS viral transactivating protein (tat); Interleukin-15 (IL-15); Nitric oxide (NO); Human prostate tumor cells (LNCaP); 3T3 fibroblasts infected with Ad.FGF-1 (3T3Ad.FGF-1); Adenovirus coding for p53 tumor suppressor gene (Ad.p53).
[c]Proangiogenic, +; Antiangiogenic, –.
[d]Includes wild-type and signal peptide, secreted, recombinant FGF.

prior inoculation of the angiogenic implant site, resulting in inhibition of FGF-mediated angiogenesis (**Fig. 2**). In cell culture studies, overexpression of p53 in adenovirus-infected endothelial cells was found to inhibit cell differentiation without affecting cell proliferation. Although most studies have employed mice between 2 –3 mo of age, the angiogenic responses of older

FGF Induction   **Ad.p53 Inhibition**

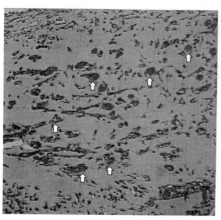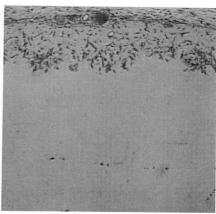

Fig. 2. Inhibition of angiogenesis in vivo by targeted delivery of a tumor suppressor gene with a recombinant adenoviral vector. Athymic nude mice were injected sc at a dorsal site with 5×10^7 pfu of Ad.p53 in 0.5 mL of PBS to infect local tissue and elicit p53 expression. Three days after infection, FGF-2 (150 ng/mL) within Matrigel was injected at the site of viral infection and 7 d later the gel plug was dissected. FGF induction of blood vessels was evident in mice pretreated with saline, while inhibition of angiogenesis occurred in mice preinfected with Ad.p53. Staining was Masson's Thrichrome. Arrows indicate functional neovessels in cross-section containing RBC. (From **ref. 51**)

mice (24–30 mo of age) are often compromised (**Fig. 3**; **36**). This "inhibitor" effect of age appears to involve a slower and less intense response to FGF since the angiogenic response does improve in a 2-wk assay, although not to the extent as in young mice.

4. Notes

1. Before freezing, matrix material may be centrifuged briefly to remove insoluble fragments.
2. Preparation of growth factor-reduced (GFR) Matrigel is often an advantage, especially for use in in vitro assays. This involves treatment of the final Matrigel with 20% ammonium sulfate (from a saturated solution) for 1 h at 4°C. Collect the insoluble material by centrifugation at 23,000g for 20 min in an SS-34 rotor. Resuspend the pellet in Tris-saline and dialyze as described for Matrigel preparations.
3. Matrigel is thawed carefully at room temperature (not in a 37°C water bath) to prevent gelling prior to preparation of cytokine solutions. The frozen Matrigel is rotated in the palms of the hands until ice crystals melt. It is then immediately placed on ice for the addition of cytokines.

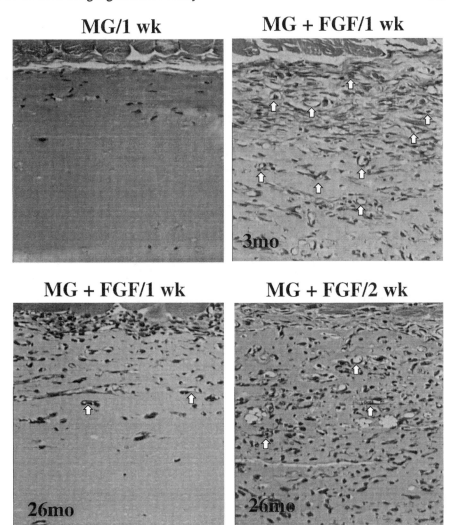

Fig. 3. Effect of age on angiogenesis. Mice of different ages were injected sc with FGF (150 ng/mL) within a Matrigel vehicle and dissected 1 wk or 2 wk after implantation. More extensive vessel formation was evident in 3-mo old mice than in 26-mo old mice at 1 wk. A slower and less intense response was evident in 26-mo old mice. Matrigel vehicle alone (MG) failed to elicit an angiogenic response. Arrows indicate neovessels within the Matrigel

4. It is important to maintain a constant source and preparation lot of heparin from a single manufacturer because quality varies from lot to lot. Frozen aliquots of concentrated heparin can be stored at −70°C almost indefinitely. Heparin in these

assays is more than a cofactor for FGF. It serves as an anticoagulant that allows vessel permeability and increases the deposition of RBC from the neovessels inside the gel. Neovessels are more sensitive to the anticoagulant effects of heparin than existing vessels.

5. Heparin is not necessary if histology is used to determine the neovascular response.
6. C57BL/6 mice were used to illustrate this protocol. However, athymic nude mice, SCID, and rats can also be used with the assay. In rat studies *(34)* up to 2 mL of Matrigel can be injected per rat and it is often advantageous to pregel the Matrigel/ FGF mixtures within the syringe prior to injection.
7. The abdominal mid-line, just below the sternum, has been described *(53)* to be a preferred site for rapid and reproducible growth of transplantable tumors, which might be related to the improved neovascular response. Because of variable responses at other sites, only one injection per mouse is used. Failure to see a distinct "bump" during injection usually results in an intraperitoneal implant which cannot be recovered. Injection at an intradermal site occurs rarely, but is indicated by high back pressure on the syringe which leads to injection of only 50 μL of solution.
8. Injections near the inguinal area tend to diffuse into the subcutaneous fat pad and do not form a distinct, recoverable "bump" on the animal.
9. This depends on the specific angiogenic factor used. For FGF, potent responses are observed after 7 d, whereas for HGF, implants are maintained for 14 d.
10. Factor VIII-related antigen (vWF) is routinely used for detection of endothelial cells (Dako, Carpinteria, CA) although this often requires signal amplification. Briefly, treat peroxide and pronase-treated slides with vWF antibody (1:1000 dilution) at 4°C (16 h) in PBS containing a blocking agent such as nonfat dry milk or bovine serum albumin. Use the Vector ABC kit (biotin/avidin/HRP) to visualize the reaction product (Vector, Burlingame, CA). Alternatively, use antibodies to PECAM (CD-31) *(32)*. Certain lectins, such as Ulex europas and Griffonia simplificans, although not specific for endothelial cells, can also be used to visualize blood vessels.
11. Use of image analysis allows enhancement of neovessels within the gel.
12. Usually, the angiogenic response proceeds from the dermal interstitial collagens or the peritoneal muscle. Scan these interfaces with the Matrigel for the appearance of linear or cross-sectional structures with RBC within the lumen, indicative of functional vessels.
13. The hemoglobin determination requires sufficient extraction of hemoglobin from the gel plugs. Low levels of heparin allow some neovessel leakage into the gel in vivo, which can then be extracted from the gel plug in vitro. It is important to use gels lacking FGF as controls.
14. However, use of the short form of VEGF (VEGF121) in combination with FGF can stimulate in vivo angiogenesis. In fact, synergistic effects can be investigated by mixing cytokines within the Matrigel prior to injection. Although bovine basic FGF-2 is a potent angiogenic factor, recombinant human FGF- 2 has been a poor angiogenic factor in these assays.

15. Strategies for delivery of inhibitors are dependent on the experimental design, the pharmacokinetics and molecular weight of the drug, and the endpoints of the study. For example, for systemic delivery of low-molecular-weight, water soluble inhibitors such as castanospermine *(37)*, frequent injections ip were necessary. Alternatively, these types of drugs are amenable to delivery by Alzet mini-pump. However, it is difficult to achieve high daily dosages of large proteins in mini pumps and, therefore, ip injections are preferred. If systemic delivery is not required, mixing of inhibitors and angiogenic factors with the Matrigel prior to implantation is often the best way to achieve inhibition of angiogenesis. An added advantage is that relatively low concentrations of inhibitors (equivalent to culture conditions) are usually sufficient to inhibit angiogenesis.

References

1. Folkman, J. (1995) Angiogenesis in cancer, vascular rheumatoid and other diseases. *Nat. Med.* **1**, 27–30.
2. Melillo, G., Scoccianti, M., Kovesdi, I., Safi, J. Jr., Riccioni, T., and Capogrossi, M. C. (1997) Gene therapy for collateral vessel development. *Cardiovasc. Res.* **35**, 480-489.
3. Knighton, D. R. and Fiegel, V. D. (1991) Regulation of cutaneous wound healing by growth factors and the micro-environment. *Invest. Radiol.* **26**, 604–611.
4. Quesada, A. R., Barbacid, M. M., Mira, E., Fernandez-Resa, P., Marquez, G., and Aracil, M. (1997) Evaluation of fluorometric and zymographic methods as activity assays for stromelysins and gelatinases. *Clin. Exp. Metastasis* **15**, 339,340.
5. Albini, A., Iwamoto, Y., Kleinman, H. K., Martin, G. R., Aaronson, S. A., Kozlowski, J. M., and McEwan, R. N. (1987) A rapid in vitro assay for quantitating the invasive potential of tumor cells. *Cancer Res.* **47**, 3239–3245.
6. Varner, J. A., Brooks, P. C., and Cheresh, D. A. (1995) REVIEW: the integrin alpha V beta 3: angiogenesis and apoptosis. *Cell. Adhes. Commun.* **3**, 367–374.
7. Norrby, K. (1997) Mast cells and de novo angiogenesis: angiogenic capability of individual mast-cell mediators such as histamine, TNF, IL-8 and bFGF. *Inflamm. Res.* **46**, S7,8.
8. Brown, L. F., Detmar, M., Claffey, K., Nagy, J. A., Feng, D., Dvorak, A. M., and Dvorak, H. F. (1997) Vascular permeability factor/vascular endothelial growth factor: a multifunctional angiogenic cytokine. *EXS* **79**, 233–269.
9. Maisonpierre, P. C., Suri, C., Jones, P. F., Bartunkova, S., Wiegand, S. J., Radziejewski, C., et al. (1997) Angiopoietin-2, a natural antagonist for Tie2 that disrupts in vivo angiogenesis. *Science* **277**, 55–60.
10. Klagsbrun, M. and D'Amore, P. A. (1991) Regulators of angiogenesis. *Annu. Rev. Physiol.* **53**, 217–239.
11. Grant, D. S., Tashiro, K., Segui-Real, B., Yamada, Y., Martin, G. R., and Kleinman, H. K. (1989) Two different laminin domains mediate the differentiation of human endothelial cells into capillary-like structures in vitro. *Cell* **58**, 933–943.
12. Yoshida, S., Ono, M., Shono, T., Izumi, H., Ishibashi, T., Suzuki, H., and Kuwano, M. (1997) Involvement of interleukin-8, vascular endothelial growth factor, and basic fibroblast growth factor in tumor necrosis factor alpha-dependent angiogenesis. *Mol. Cell. Biol.* **17**, 4015–4023.

13. Hanahan, D. (1997) Signaling vascular morphogenesis and maintenance. *Science* **277,** 48–50.

14. O'Reilly, M. S., Holmgren, L., Shing, Y., Chen, C., Rosenthal, R. A., Moses, M., et al. (1994) Angiostatin: a novel angiogenesis inhibitor that mediates the suppression of metastases by a Lewis lung carcinoma. *Cell* **79,** 315–328.

15. O'Reilly, M. S., Boehm, T., Shing, Y., Fukai, N., Vasios, G., Lane, W. S., et al. (1997) Endostatin: an endogenous inhibitor of angiogenesis and tumor growth. *Cell* **88,** 277–285.

16. Gimbrone, M. A., Cotran, R. S., Leapman, S. B., and Folkman, J. (1974) Tumor growth and neovascularization: an experimental model using the rabbit cornea. *J. Natl. Cancer Inst.* **52,** 413.

17. Ausprunk, D. H., Knighton, D. R., and Folkman, J. (1975) Vascularization of normal and neoplastic tissues grafted to the chick chorioallantois: role of host and pre-existing graft blood vessels. *Am. J. Pathol.* **79,** 597.

18. Muthukaruppan, V. R. and Auerbach R. (1979) Angiogenesis in the mouse cornea. *Science* **205,** 1416.

19. Folkman, J. and Haudenschild, C. (1980) Angiogenesis in vitro. *Nature* **288,** 551–556.

20. Nicosia, R. F. and Madri, J. A. (1987) The microvascular extracellular matrix: developmental changes during angiogenesis in the aortic ring-plasma clot model. *Am. J. Pathol.* **128,** 78–90.

21. Kubota, Y., Kleinman, H. K., Martin, G. R., and Lawley, T. J. (1988) Role of laminin and basement membrane in the differentiation of human endothelial cells into capillary-like structures. *J. Cell. Biol.* **107,** 1589–1597.

22. Thompson, J. A., Anderson, K. D., DiPietro, J. M., Zwiebel, J. A., Zametta, M., Anderson, W. F., and Maciag, T. (1988) Site-directed neovessel formation in vivo. *Science* **241,** 1349–1352.

23. Gran,t D. S., Tashiro, K., Segui-Real, B., Yamada, Y., Martin, G. R., and Kleinman, H. K. (1989) Two different laminin domains mediate the differentiation of human endothelial cells into capillary-like structures in vitro. *Cell* **58,** 933–943.

24. Mignatti, P., Tsuboi, R., Robbins, E., and Rifkin D. B. (1989) In vitro angiogenesis on the human amniotic membrane: requirement for basic fibroblast growth factor-induced proteinases. *J. Cell Biol.* **108,** 671–682.

25. Plunkett, M. L. and Hailey, J. A. (1990) An in vivo quantitative angiogenesis model using tumor cells entrapped in alginate. *Lab. Invest.* **62,** 510–517.

26. Iruela-Arispe, M. L., Hasselaar, P., and Sage, H. (1991) Differential expression of extracellular proteins is correlated with angiogenesis in vitro. *Lab. Invest.* **64,** 174–186.

27. Passaniti, A., Taylor, R. M., Pili, R., Guo Y., Long, P. V., Haney, J.A., Pauly, R. R., Grant, D. S., and Martin, G. R. (1992) A simple, quantitative method for assessing angiogenesis and anti-angiogenic agents using reconstituted basement membrane, heparin, and FGF. *Lab. Invest.* **67,** 519–528.

28. Brown, K. J., Maynes, S. F., Bezos, A., Maguire, D. J., Ford, M. D., and Parish, C. R. (1996) A novel in vitro assay for human angiogenesis. *Lab. Invest.* **75,** 539–555.

29. Jain, R. K., Schlenger, K., Hockel, M., and Yuan, F. (1997) Quantitative angiogenesis assays: progress and problems. *Nature Med.* **3,** 1203–1208.

30. Swarm, R. L. (1963) Transplantation of a murine chondrosarcoma in mice of different inbred strains. *J. Natl. Cancer Inst.* **31**, 953–974.
31. Kleinman, H. K., McGarvey, M. L., Hassell, J. R., Star, V. L., Cannon, F. B., Laurie, G. W., and Martin, G. R. (1986) Basement membrane complexes with biological activity. *Biochemistry* **25**, 312–318.
32. DeLisser, H.. M, Christofidou-Solomidou, M., Strieter, R. M., Burdick, M. D., Robinson, C. S., Wexler, R. S., et al. (1997) Involvement of endothelial PECAM-1/CD31 in angiogenesis. *Am. J. Pathol.* **151**, 671–677.
33. Kibbey, M. C., Grant, D. S., and Kleinman, H. K. (1992) Role of the SIKVAV site of laminin in promotion of angiogenesis and tumor growth: an in vivo Matrigel model. *J. Natl. Cancer Inst.* **84**, 1633–1638.
34. Vukanovic, J., Passaniti, A., Hirato, T., Traysman, R. J., and Isaacs, J. T. (1992) Antiangiogenic effects of the Quinoline-3-carboxamide, linomide. *Cancer Res.* **53**, 1833–1837.
35. Grant, D. S., Kleinman, H. K., Goldberg, I. D., Bhargava, M. M., Nickoloff, B. J., Kinsella, J. L., et al. (1993) Scatter factor induces blood vessel formation in vivo. *Proc. Natl. Acad. Sci. USA* **90**, 1937–1941.
36. Pili, R., Guo, Y., Chang, J., T., Nakanishi, H., Martin, G. R., and Passaniti, A. (1994) Altered angiogenesis underlying age-dependent changes in tumor growth. **86**, 1303–1314.
37. Pili, R., Chang, J., Partis, R. A., Mueller, R. A., Novick, T., Chrest, F. J., and Passaniti, A. (1995) The α-glucosidase inhibitor castanospermine alters endothelial cell glycosylation, prevents angiogenesis, and inhibits tumor growth. *Cancer Res.* **55**, 2920–2926.
38. Muhlhauser, J., Merrill, M. J., Pili, R., Maeda, H., Bacic, M., Bewig, B., Passaniti, A., et al. (1995) VEGF165 expressed by replication deficient recombinant adenovirus vector induces angiogenesis in vivo. *Cir. Res.* **77**, 1077–1086.
39. Muhlhauser, J., Pili, R., Merrill, M.J., Maeda, H., Passaniti, A., Crystal, R. G., and Capogrossi, M. C. (1995) In vivo angiogenesis induced by recombinant adenovirus vectors coding either for secreted or non-secreted forms of acidic fibroblast growth factor. *Human Gene Ther.* **6**, 1457–1465.
40. Taraboletti, G., Garofalo, A., Belotti, D., Drudis, T., Borsotti, P., Scanziani, E., Brown, P, D., and Giavazzi R. (1995) Inhibition of angiogenesis and murine hemangioma growth by batimastat, a synthetic inhibitor of matrix metalloproteinases. *J. Natl. Cancer Inst.* **87**, 293–298.
41. Angiolillo, A. L., Sgadari, C., Taub, D. D., Liao, F., Farber, J. M., Maheshwari, S., et al. (1995) Human interferon-inducible protein 10 is a potent inhibitor of angiogenesis in vivo. *J. Exp. Med.* **182**, 155–162.
42. Bussolino, F., Arese, M., Montrucchio, G., Barra, L., Primo, L., Benelli, R., et al. (1995) Platelet activating factor produced in vitro by Kaposi's sarcoma cells induces and sustains in vivo angiogenesis. *J. Clin. Invest.* **96**, 940–952.
43. Camussi, G., Montrucchio, G., Lupia, E., De Martino, A., Perona, L., Arese, M., et al. (1995) Platelet-activating factor directly stimulates in vitro migration of endothelial cells and promotes in vivo angiogenesis by a heparin-dependent mechanism. *J. Immunol.* **154**, 6492–6501.

44. Corallini, A., Campioni, D., Rossi, C., Albini, A., Possati, L., Rusnati, M., et al. (1996) Promotion of tumour metastases and induction of angiogenesis by native HIV-1 Tat protein from BK virus/tat transgenic mice. *AIDS* **10**, 701–710.
45. Biancone, L., Martino, A. D., Orlandi, V., Conaldi, P. G., Toniolo, A., and Camussi, G. (1997) Development of inflammatory angiogenesis by local stimulation of Fas in vivo. *J. Exp. Med.* **186**, 147–152.
46. Haralabopoulos, G. C., Grant, D. S., Kleinman, H. K., and Maragoudakis, M. E. (1997) Thrombin promotes endothelial cell alignment in Matrigel in vitro and angiogenesis in vivo. *Am. J. Physiol.* **273**, 239–245.
47. Angiolillo, A. L., Kanegane, H., Sgadari, C., Reaman, G. H., and Tosato, G. (1997) Interleukin-15 promotes angiogenesis in vivo. *Biochem. Biophys. Res. Commun.* **233**, 231–237.
48. Montrucchio, G., Lupia, E., de Martino, A., Battaglia, E., Arese, M., Tizzani, A., Bussolino, F., ad Camussi, G. (1997) Nitric oxide mediates angiogenesis induced in vivo by platelet-activating factor and tumor necrosis factor-alpha. *Am. J. Pathol.* **151**, 557–563.
49. Wilson, M. J. and Sinha, A. A. (1997) Human prostate tumor angiogenesis in nude mice: metalloprotease and plasminogen activator activities during tumor growth and neovascularization of subcutaneously injected matrigel impregnated with human prostate tumor cells. *Anat. Rec.* **249**, 63–73.
50. Pili, R., Chang, J., Muhlhauser, J., Crystal, R. G., Capogrossi, M. C., and Passaniti, A. (1997) Adenovirus-mediated gene transfer of fibroblast growth factor-1: angiogenesis and tumorigenicity in nude mice. *Int. J. Cancer* **73**, 258–263.
51. Riccioni, T., Cirielli, C., Wang, X., Passaniti, A., and Capogrossi, M. (1998) Adenovirus-mediated wild-type p53 overexpression inhibits endothelial cell differentiation in vitro and angiogenesis in vivo. *Gene Ther.* **5**, 747–754.
52. Skobe, M., Rockwell, P., Goldstein, N., Vosseler, S., and Fusenig, N. E. (1997) Halting angiogenesis suppresses carcinoma cell invasion. *Nat. Med.* **3**, 1222–1227.
53. Auerbach, R., Morrissey, L. W., and Sidly, Y. A. (1978) Regional differences in the incidence and growth of mouse tumors following intradermal or subcutaneous inoculation. *Cancer Res.* **38**, 1739–1744.

31

Efficient Liposome-Mediated Gene Transfer to Rabbit Carotid Arteries In Vivo

Michael-Christopher Keogh and Daxin Chen

1. Introduction

Methods for gene delivery in vivo vary dramatically in their relative efficiencies. The most efficient to date involve the use of recombinant viruses, most notably adenoviruses, adeno-associated viruses (AAVs), or retroviruses (*see* Chapters 32 and 34). The creation of these recombinant constructs is laborious and requires specialized techniques, however. A technique that can efficiently deliver simple plasmids containing the gene of interest in vivo allows the screening of gene constructs to determine their effects prior to embarking on the creation of recombinant viruses.

This protocol utilizes the cationic liposome Tfx™-50, commercially available from Promega (Madison, WI) (*1*), for in vivo delivery of the luciferase reporter gene to rabbit carotid arteries. The luciferase gene was chosen as a marker protein for its ease of detection enzymatically and immunohistochemically, while the rabbit carotid was chosen for its relative accessibility and absence of side branches. The protocol describes the procedures used in our laboratory for the introduction of liposome-plasmid conjugates and immunohistochemical detection of the resulting cytoplasmic protein (*2,3*). It should be noted that liposome-mediated gene transfection generally requires extensive optimization to achieve efficient gene delivery—this cannot be overstressed (*see* **Note 1**). The transfection conditions described here have been optimized for gene delivery to rabbit vascular smooth muscle cells (VSMCs) (*see* **Fig. 1**). If delivery to rabbit endothelial cells is desired, for example, optimization for this lineage will be required.

From: *Methods in Molecular Medicine, Vascular Disease: Molecular Biology and Gene Therapy Protocols*
Edited by: A. H. Baker © Humana Press Inc., Totowa, NJ

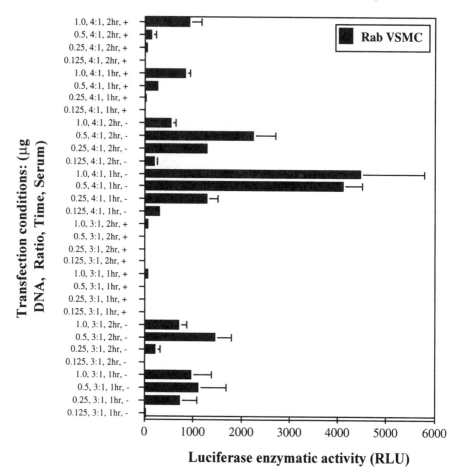

Fig. 1. Optimization of Tfx™-50 transfection conditions in rabbit vascular smooth muscle cells (VSMCs) in vitro. Cells were transfected in triplicate in 24 well plates utilising the conditions shown. Rabbit VSMCs for transfection were plated in at 5×10^4 cells/well in 24-well plates 2 d prior to transfectiion to allow them to adhere. On the day of transfection the media was aspirated and the cells were washed twice in serum-free M199. Triplicate cultures were then incubated with 200 µL of transfection complexes according to the conditions shown (Promega, 1995). Conditions are expressed as follows: µg DNA (per 200 µL), ratio of Tfx™-50 to DNA, transfection time (in hours), presence (+) or absence (–) of serum. After the appropriate length of time, 1.0 mL of 10% M199 was added per well and cells cultured for 48 h before assaying for luciferase activity enzymatically *(2)*. Data points are expressed as the mean of triplicates of luciferase enzymatic activity with the standard error of the mean (*see* **Note 1**).

Cationic liposomes possess a number of properties that make them attractive candidates for facilitating gene delivery over viral systems. Their main advantage is the ability to facilitate the delivery of a range of nucleic acids including oligonucleotides *(4–6)*, RNA *(7,8)*, and DNA in forms as diverse as simple plasmids or chromosomal fragments *(9–12)*. Other advantages include the possibility of cell-specific targeting (based on the narrow efficiency windows for different cell lineages *[2]*); reduced safety concerns relative to those associated with viral genomes, and less propensity to induce an immune response in vivo *(13–19)*. However, many of these advantages are outweighed by the low transfection efficiency of the majority of cationic liposome protocols.

Cationic liposomes mediate their activity by neutralizing the negative charge of the DNA intended for transfection. This results in a condensation reaction and the formation of stable complexes with a net positive charge, which can then associates with the negatively charged surface of the cell *(20,21)*. This complex then either fuses with, or causes a transient destabilization of, the cell membrane. The net result is macromolecule delivery to the cytoplasm while avoiding fusion with lysosomes and subsequent degradation *(22)*.

The Tfx™-50 reagent (Promega UK) is a mixture of the synthetic; cationic lipid molecule (*N,N,N',N'*-tetramethyl-*N,N'*-bis(2-hydroxyethyl)-2,2,-dioleoyloxy-1,4-butane-diammonium–iodide) and L-dioleoylphosphatidylethanolamine (DOPE) *(1)*. The use of DOPE is common to many cationic liposome formulations and its role is to facilitate the membrane fusion or destabilization step in macromolecule delivery *(22,23)*. Tfx™-50 mediated gene transfection is not mediated by acidic endocytotic vesicles *(24)*. Hence, it is classed as a "cytofectin," which describes the ability of a compound to facilitate macromolecule entry into living cells while avoiding the lysosomal pathway *(6,22)*.

2. Materials

All buffers and reagents for transfections are sterile at time of use. All manipulations for the preparation of reagents are performed in a laminar flow hood under aseptic conditions unless stated otherwise. The in vivo experiments described require the worker to have an animal licence, appropriate training, and access to an animal facility.

2.1. Materials for Transfection

1. Tfx™-50 (E1811; Promega UK, Southampton, UK): Store at –20°C. Reconstitute the day before required with 200 µL of sterile endotoxin-free ddH$_2$O per vial. Leave to stand for 4 h at room temperature (RT) with vortexing every hour. Store at 4°C after reconstitution where it is stable for up to 1 mo.

2. Cesium chloride (CsCl) banded plasmid vectors (e.g., pGL3) (*see* **Note 2**).
3. Microvascular vessel dilator.
4. Atraumatic microvascular clamps.
5. Microscissors (Aescular Ltd., Sheffield, UK). Sterlize by autoclaving.
6. Microforceps (Aescular Ltd.). Sterlize by autoclaving.
7. Rabbits (Harlan Sera-Labs Ltd., Crawley Down, UK, or Charles River UK Ltd., Kent, UK).
8. Phenol red-free M199 media (Gibco Life Technologies, Renfrewshire, UK).

2.2. Materials for Transgene Detection

1. Directly conjugated polyclonal rabbit antiLuciferase FITC (Europa Research Products, Cambridge, UK).
2. Goat antirabbit IgG FITC (Sigma Chemicals, Dorset, UK).
3. Polyclonal antivon Willebrand factor (vWf) (Dako Ltd., High Wycombe, UK).
4. Heat-inactivated foetal calf serum (FCS, Harlan Sera-Labs Ltd.).
5. Frosted slides and coverslips.
6. Bovine serum albumin (BSA).
7. Tween-20 (Polyoxyethylene sorbitan monolaurate).
8. Triton X-100.
9. 0.2% Triton X-100 in PBS.
10. Normal horse serum.
11. Blocking solution: 0.1% BSA and 0.1% Tween-20 in PBS.
12. Vectashield mounting medium with DAPI (Vector Labs., Peterborough , UK).
13. Optimal cutting temperature (OCT) embedding medium.

3. Methods
3.1. Transfection of Rabbit Carotid Arteries In Vivo

1. To 1 mL of serum-free medium M199 without phenol red add 2.5 µg plasmid vector (pGL3 Control) and 7.5 µL Tfx™-50 (final charge ratio 4:1 - *see* **Note 1**) and incubate for 30 min at RT. Although the volume of the isolated segment (*see below*) is generally no larger than 300 µL, 1 mL of transfection solution is made up per rabbit to allow for leakage (*see* **step 8**).
2. While the transfection solution is incubating, induce a 16–18 wk old male rabbit (brown half-lop or New Zealand White—mean weight approx 3 kg, *see* **Note 3**) with 10 mg of Brietal sodium (methohexitone sodium) intravenously (iv) via the ear vein and anesthetize with Halothane (2%) (fluranisone 10 mg/mL and fentanyl citrate 0.315 mg/mL) in nitrous oxide/oxygen via nosecone or endotracheal tube.
3. Systemically anticoagulate the rabbit with heparin (300 U/kg) by iv 5 min prior to isolation of the carotid segment for infusion.
4. Surgically expose the **right** common carotid artery and dissect free of the vagus nerve (**Fig. 2A**). Either side can be used but be sure to note which vessel was transfected.

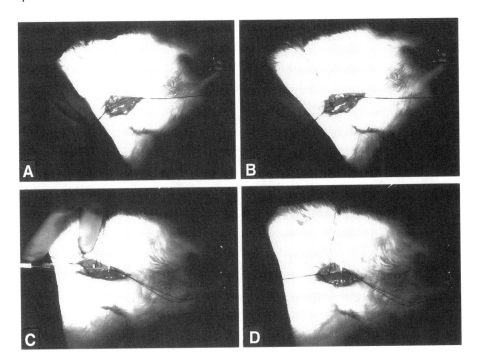

Fig. 2. Dissection protocol for the dwell technique to rabbit carotid arteries. The different steps are described in **Subheading 3.1.** (**A**) Surgical exposure of the common carotid artery. (**B**) Isolation of the vessel segment for gene delivery with nontraumatic vessel clamps. (**C**) Injection of the plasmid:liposome transfection solution. (**D**) Presence of transfection complexes indicated by inflation of the artery.

5. Isolate the experimental segment (approx 2 cm in length) by means of soft, nontraumatic microvascular clamps (**Fig. 2B**).
6. Flush with serum-free phenol red-free M199 (ensure all of the smaller branches attached to the segment have been ligated [*see* **Notes 3** and **4**]).
7. Placing suture ties around the vessel flanking the treated segment will aid in its identification when the segment is removed for analysis (note their presence in the figures). Ensure the sutures are not tight enough to restrict blood flow.
8. Directly instill the transfectant solution into the isolated vessel segment with a 30-gauge needle.
9. Leave for 30 min (the "dwell" technique, **Fig. 2C**). Inject as much as possible to replace the serum free medium injected in **step 4**.
10. Ensure there is no leakage from the isolated segment and a sufficient amount of transfection solution remains in the vessel during the gene transfer (**Fig. 2D**) (*see* **Note 5**).

11. After the incubation period remove the microvessel clamps and restore free flow of blood to the vessel (*see* **Note 6**). This will wash the remaining transfection complexes into the circulation.
12. Close the wound with 4.0 subcutaneous Vicryl sutures and dust the area with Aureomycin (2% chlortetracycline hydrochloride) antibiotic powder (*see* **Note 7**).
13. Allow the rabbit to recover from anesthesia and return to the cage.
14. After surgery, water is allowed immediately, but food is withheld for 10 h. Analgesia is given as required.

3.2. Removal, Fixation, and Sectioning of Vessel Segments

1. After the desired incubation period (2 d for these experiments), premedicate the rabbits with 0.25 mg of intramuscular (im) Hypnorm (fluanisone 10 mg/mL) and 0.3 mL of iv heparin (5000 IU/mL).
2. Kill by standard iv barbiturate overdose (8 mL pentabarbitone sodium, 60 mg/mL).
3. Remove the experimental vessel segment as defined by the loose suture ties.
4. Clean with PBS for examination by histochemical analysis. The negative control for each rabbit is the untreated left common carotid vessel.
5. Cut the arteries into three or four serial segments each approx 3 mm in length.
6. Embed in OCT embedding medium.
7. Freeze immediately in isopentane cooled with liquid N_2.
8. For immunocytochemical staining, cut 8–10 µm cryosections on to glass slides and air-dry for 1 h at RT.
9. Rinse three times for 5 min each with PBS, fix for 30 min in methanol (at –20°C), and store desicated at –20°C until use.

3.3. Immunohistochemical Analyses

1. Equilibrate frozen sections to room temperature for 30 min before staining.
2. Briefly wash three times in PBS.
3. Dry the area of slide immediately around the sections with a lint-free tissue, being careful not to disturb the sections.
4. Using a Dako-pen, draw an aqueous-repellent circle around the sections—this will hold the antibody solution in place during staining.
5. Permeabilize the tissues for 30 min by addition of 0.2% Triton X-100 in PBS.
6. Rinse slides in PBS, and remove as much liquid as possible by tapping gently edgeways on tissue paper.
7. Block tissue sections for 1 h with 5% horse serum in blocking solution and drain thoroughly.
8. Add 50 µL of directly conjugated antiluciferase FITC antibody diluted in blocking solution with 5% horse serum and incubate in darkness overnight at 4°C (*see* **Note 8**).
9. Wash slides five times by 5 min in blocking solution.
10. Mount in Vectashield with DAPI.
11. Cover with a coverslip (sealing the edges with nail varnish).
12. Visualize by confocal microscopy (*see* **Note 9**).

4. Notes

1. As with all physical methods of gene transfer, extensive optimization is essential if efficient gene delivery is to be achieved. **Figure 1** shows the experimental transfection conditions tested in vitro to determine those which are optimal for rabbit VSMCs, protocols for these have been previously published *(2,3)*. The conditions tested vary: the amount of plasmid DNA, the ratio of plasmid to Tfx™-50, the time of complex exposure to the cells, and the presence or absence of serum. The variability in transfection efficiency is striking—conditions outside those optimal can result in a dramatic reduction of luciferase activity.
   Optimal conditions chosen from this profile are: 0.5 µg DNA (per 200 µL), ratio 4:1, 1 h, serum-free medium. The addition of 1 µg plasmid DNA gives slightly higher luciferease activity in the profile shown, but this would require a concomitant increase in the amount of Tfx™-50 used, increasing expense. Although 1 h is the optimal transfection time observed in vitro, a 30-min incubation was performed on the rabbits to reduce the length of time under anesthesia. Time course experiments under otherwise optimal conditions show approx 30% efficiency at this time *(2)*.

2. This protocol utilises the luciferase plasmid *pGL3 Control* (Promega UK), although the delivery of any plasmid is possible. *pGL3 Control* contains the luciferase gene under the regulation of the SV40 promoter and enhancer and directs high levels of expression in mammalian cells. Plasmid DNA intended for transfection must be of CsCl grade or equivalent—we typically transform plasmids into *Escherichia coli* (JM109) using standard techniques *(25)* and purify on Qiagen-500™ columns (Qiagen, Surrey, UK) as per manufacturers instructions. Precipitated plasmid is dissolved in endotoxin free ddH$_2$O, concentration and purity calculated by absorbance at OD 260 nm/280 nm and made to 0.5 mg/mL, and stored at 4°C.

3. The rabbit is chosen for an animal model because of its relatively large size (relative to the rat), which makes the operations technically more simple. In the rabbit, the common carotid artery is chosen for its relative accessibility and absence of side branches. Ligation of any visible side branches is essential, however, to prevent drain off of the instilled transfection solution.

4. Complete flushing of blood from the vessel is essential for optimal transfection efficiency. This can be visualized by the fact that the run-off from the flushing will run clear and the vessel will appear white in color.

5. Leakage will be visualized by deflation of the vessel as run-off escapes through the injection site or collateral vessels.

6. It is important that blood flow is reestablished to the main branch of the common carotid following gene-delivery. The most common cause of failure is clotting. However it is also important to ensure that the suture ties used to define the transfected segment are not tightened.

7. This is sufficient prophylaxis if a 2 or 3 d incubation period is to be used prior to further analyses. If longer periods are intended additional prophylaxis with 0.5 mL Tribrissen 24% (trimethoprim 40 mg/mL, sulphadiazine 200 mg/mL), subcutaneous antibiotic is recommended.

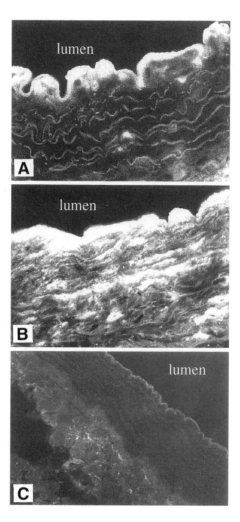

Fig. 3. Immunocytochemical analyses of rabbit carotid arteries following Tfx™-50 mediated transfection in vivo. (A) Luciferase expression localized to the immediate endothelial and intimal smooth muscle cell layers. (B) Deep penetrance of luciferase expression as occasionally seen. (C) Nontransfected vessels (negative controls) show no detectable luciferase expression. Magnification: (A,B), X130; (C), X80.

8. Optimal dilution determined as 1:50, but will need to be verified for each antibody and/or batch.
9. The majority of transfected vessels exhibit luciferase expression localized to the intimal layer (**Fig. 3A**). Luciferase expression that penetrates the internal elastic lamina into the media is seen in some vessels, however (**Fig. 3B**). The degree of penetrance appears to be due to the integrity of the endothelial layer such that

when the layer is removed, deep penetrance is observed: colocalization of von Willebrand factor (vWf) (a marker of endothelial cells) and luciferase expression is observed in vessels which exhibit luciferase expression localized to the intima (data not shown) *(2)*. Nontransfected vessels show no detectable staining (**Fig. 3C**). The presence of an intact endothelium appears to restrict the penetrance of the transfection complexes in this protocol. Thus, damaging the endothelium prior to incubation with the transfection complexes can increase efficiency. Methods to achieve this can include the insertion and inflation of a foley catheter or crush trauma. Either could be performed prior to the protocol.

Acknowledgments

These studies were supported by funding from the Garfield Weston Foundation.

References

1. Promega Corporation. *Tfx™-10, Tfx™-20 and Tfx™-50 reagents for the transfection of eukaryotic cells, Technical Bulletin TB216*.
2. Keogh, M.-C., Chen, D., Lupu, F., Shaper, N., Schmitt, J. F., Kakkar, V. V., and Lemoine, N. R. (1997) High efficiency reporter gene transfection of vascular tissue *in vitro* and *in vivo* using a cationic lipid-DNA complex. *Gene Ther.* **4,** 162–171.
3. Chen, D., Lupu, F., Shaper, N., Schmitt, J. F., Lemoine, N. R., and Keogh, M.-C. (1998) Tfx-50 reagent and high efficiency transfection of vascular tissue *in vitro* and *in vivo*. *Promega Notes* **65,** 19–26.
4. Wagner, R. (1994) Gene inhibition using antisense oligodeoxynucleotides. *Nature* **372,** 333–335.
5. Bennett, M. R., Anglin, S., McEwan, J. R., Jagoe, R., Newby, A. C., and Evan, G. I. (1994) Inhibition of vascular smooth muscle cell proliferation *in vitro* and *in vivo* by c-*myc* antisense oligodeoxynucleotides. *J. Clin. Invest.* **93,** 820–828.
6. Lewis, J. G., Lin, K.-Y., Kothavale, A., Flanagan, W. M., Matteuchi, M. D., DePrince, R. B., et al. (1996) A serum-resistant cytofectin for cellular delivery of antisense oligodeoxynucleotides and plasmid DNA. *Proc. Natl. Acad. Sci. USA* **93,** 3176–3181.
7. Malone, R. W., Felgner, P. L., and Verma, I. M. (1989) Cationic-liposome mediated RNA transfection. *Proc. Natl. Acad. Sci. USA* **86,** 6077–6081.
8. Lu, D., Benjamin, R., Kim, M., Conry, R., and Curiel, D. (1994) Optimization of methods to achieve mRNA-mediated transfection of tumour cells *in vitro* and *in vivo* employing cationic liposome vectors. *Cancer Gene Ther.* **1,** 245–252.
9. Felgner, P. L., Gadek, T. R., Holm, L., Roman, R., Chan, H. W., Wenz, M., Northrop, J. P., Ringold, G. M., and Danielsen, M. (1987) Lipofection: a highly efficient lipid-mediated DNA-transfection procedure. *Proc. Natl. Acad. Sci. USA* **84,** 7413–7417.
10. Nabel, E. G., Facc, G. P., and Nabel, G. J. (1991) Gene transfer into vascular cells. *JACC* **17,** 189B–194B.
11. Stewart, M. J., Plautz, G. E., Del Buono, L., Yang, Z. Y., Lu, L., Gao, X., Huang, X., Nabel, E. G., and Nabel, G. J. (1992) Gene transfer *in vivo* with DNA-liposome complexes: safety and acute toxicity in mice. *Hum Gene Ther.* **3,** 267–275.

12. Ghoumari, A. M., Rixe, O., Yarouvi, S. V., Zerrouki, A., Mouawad, R., Poynard, T., Opolon, P., Khayat, D., and Soubrane, C. (1996) Gene transfer in hepatocarcinoma cell lines: *in vitro* optimization of a virus-free system. *Gene Ther.* **3,** 483–490.
13. Yang, Y., Nunes, F. A., Berencsi, K., Furth, E. E., Gönczöl, E., and Wilson, J. M. (1994) Cellular immunity to viral antigens limits E1-deleted adenoviruses for gene therapy. *Proc. Natl. Acad. Sci. USA* **91,** 4407–4411.
14. Zabner, J., Petersen, D. M., Puga, A. P., Graham, S. M., Couture, L. A., and Keyes, L. D. (1994) Safety and efficacy of repetitive adenovirus-mediated transfer of CFTR cDNA to airway epithelia of primates and cotton rats. *Nature Genetics* **6,** 75–83.
15. Simon, R. H., Engelhardt, J. F., Yang, Y., Zepeda, M., Weber-Pendleton, S., Grossman, M., and Wilson, J. M. (1993) Adenovirus-mediated transfer of the CFTR-gene to lung of nonhuman primates: toxicity study. *Human Gene. Ther.* **4,** 771–780.
16. Nabel, E. G. (1995) Gene therapy for cardiovascular disease. *Circulation* **91,** 541–548.
17. Knowles, M. R., Hohneker, K. W., Zou, Z., Olsen, J. C., Noah, T. W., Hu, P.-C., et al. (1995) A controlled study of adenovirus-vector-mediated gene transfer in the nasal epithelium of patients with cystic fibrosis. *N. Engl. J. Med.* **333,** 823–831.
18. Hug, P. and Sleight, R. S. (1991) Liposomes for the transfection of eukaryotic cells. *Biochim. Biophys. Acta* **1097,** 1–17.
19. Schulick, A. H., Newman, K. D., Virmani, R., and Dichek, D. A. (1995) *In vivo* gene transfer into injured carotid arteries: Optimization and evaluation of acute toxicity. *Circulation* **91,** 2407–2414.
20. Morishita, R., Gibbons, G. H., Kaneda, Y., Ogihara, T., and Dzau, V. J. (1993) Novel and effective gene transfer technique for study of vascular renin angiotensin system. *J. Clin. Invest.* **91,** 2580–2585.
21. Felgner, P. L, Holm, M., and Chan, H. (1989) Cationic liposome mediated transfection. *Proc. West. Pharmacol. Soc.* **32,** 115–121.
22. Felgner, J. H., Kumar, R., Sridnar, C. N., Wheeler, C. J., Tsai, Y. J., Border, R., et al. (1994) Enhanced gene delivery and mechanism studies with a novel series of cationic lipid formulations. *J. Biol .Chem.* **269,** 2550–2261.
23. Duzgunes, N., Goldstein, J. A., Friend, D. S., and Felgner, P. L. (1989) Fusion of liposomes containing a novel cationic lipid, N-[2,3(dioleyloxy)propyl]-N,N,N-trimethylammonium: induction by multivalent anions and asymetric fusion with acidic phospholipid vesicles. *Biochemistry* **28,** 9179–9184.
24. Labroille, G., Bonnefille, S., and Belloc, F. (1996) Tfx™-50 reagent increases the uptake of oligonucleotides by leukaemic cells. *Promega Notes* **56,** 8–13.
25. Sambrook, J., Fritsch, E. F., and Maniatis, T. (1989) *Molecular Cloning. A Laboratory Manual.* 2nd ed., Cold Spring Harbor Press, Cold Spring, Harbor, NY.

32

Gene Delivery to Rabbit Arteries Using the Collar Model

Mikko O. Hiltunen, Mikko P. Turunen, and Seppo Ylä-Herttuala

1. Introduction

Emerging knowledge of molecular pathology of vascular diseases provides new targets for vascular gene therapy. Sufficient expression of a gene of interest in the vessel wall can be achieved using either extravascular or intravascular gene delivery approaches *(1)*. Plasmid DNA, transferred by an extravascular approach, gives transfection efficiency high enough to cause biological effects. Plasmids and adenoviruses can be used for both extravascular and intravascular gene therapy. The collar model allows one to use controlled gene transfer. In this chapter we describe two gene delivery methods used for extravascular and intravascular gene transfer experiments.

2. Materials
2.1. Rabbits, Collars, and Catheters

1. New Zealand White (NZW) male rabbits, weighting 2.5–3.5 kg.
2. Inert silastic collars (MediGene Oy, Kuopio, Finland): used to induce smooth muscle cell proliferation and to serve as gene transfer reservoir.
3. Introducer sheath and perfusion catheters: a 3.0 F channeled balloon local drug delivery catheter (Boston Scientific Corp., Maple Grove, MA) is introduced into the abdominal aorta via a 5^{Fr} percutaneous introducer sheath (Arrow International, Reading, PA) in the right carotid artery.
4. Fentanyl-fluanosine anaesthetic (Janssen Pharmaceutica, Belgium).
5. Midazolam muscle relaxant (Roche, Switzerland).
6. Lidocaine local anaesthetic (Medipolar, Finland).

From: *Methods in Molecular Medicine, Vascular Disease: Molecular Biology and Gene Therapy Protocols*
Edited by: A. H. Baker © Humana Press Inc., Totowa, NJ

2.2. Plasmids and Adenoviruses

2.2.1. Production of Plasmid DNA

1. LB medium (5X stock): Dissolve 2.5 g of tryptone, 12.5 g of yeast extract and 25 g of NaCl in 500 mL H_2O and adjust to pH 7.4.
2. Ampicillin: 50 mg/mL.
3. Bacterial inoculation: 100 mL 1X LB medium, 150 μL ampicillin (50 mg/mL).
4. Glycerol stock solution of plasmid.
5. Qiagen-tip 10,000 (Qiagen, Germany) plasmid purification kit.
6. Phenol-chloroform.
7. Chloroform.
8. Ethanol.
9. Tris-EDTA buffer: 10 mM Tris-HCl, 1 mM EDTA, pH 8.0.
10. 4% paraformaldehyde/phosphate buffered saline, pH 7.4.

2.1.2. Production of Adenoviruses

Replication-deficient E1-E3 deleted adenoviruses are produced in 293 cells and concentrated by ultracentrifugation as described in other chapters (*see* Chapters 22 and 25). Adenoviral preparations are analyzed for the absence of helper viruses or bacteriological contaminants (*see* also Chapter 22).

1. Adenovirus titer of 1.0×10^{10} pfu in volume of 2 mL of 0.9% NaCl is used for gene transfer.

2.3. Immunocytochemistry and General Histology

2.3.1. Antibodies

1. Avidin-biotin-horseradish peroxidase system (Vector Elite, Vector Laboratories, CA).
2. Smooth muscle cells: α-actin-specific monoclonal antibody (mAb) HHF-35, dilution 1:500 (Enzo Diagnostics, NY).
3. Endothelial cells: mAb CD31, dilution 1:50 (Dako A/S, Denmark).
4. Macrophages: mAb RAM-11, dilution 1: 1000 (Dako).
5. 4% paraformaldehyde/15% sucrose, pH 7.4.
6. 15% sucrose, pH 7.4.

2.3.2. β-Galactosidase Assay

1. 4% paraformaldehyde/0.15 M sodium-phosphate buffer, pH 7.2.
2. 0.15 M sodium-phosphate buffer, pH 7.2.
3. Optimum cutting temperature (OCT) compound (Miles, Elkhart, IN).
4. 5-Bromo-4-chloro-3-indolyl-β-D-galactoside (X-gal) reagent (100 mg/mL): dissolve 1 g of X-gal (MBI Fermentas, Lithuania) in 10 mL of dimethylformamide.
5. X-gal stain: dilute X-gal reagent drop-wise 1:100 with X-gal solution [5 mM $K_3Fe(CN)_6$, 5 mM $K_4Fe(CN)_6$, 2 mM $MgCl_2$] by slowly mixing to avoid precipitation.
6. Mayer's Carmalum.
7. Permount embedding reagent (Fischer Scientific, Pittsburg, PA).

3. Methods
3.1. Production of Plasmid DNA

1. Inoculate 100 μL of plasmid glycerol stock solution into 6 L of 1X LB-amp-medium (inoculation medium) overnight with continuous shaking at +37°C.
2. Purify plasmid DNA using the Qiagen-tip 10,000 plasmid purification kit.
3. Extract the plasmid DNA three times with phenol-chloroform, once with chloroform and precipitate overnight in the presence of ethanol at –20°C.
4. Wash precipitate with 70% ethanol and dilute with Tris-EDTA buffer (to 1 μg/μL).

3.2. Collar Installation and Extravascular Gene Transfer (see Fig. 1 and Notes 1–4).

1. Anesthetize rabbits with 0.7 mL subcutaneous injection of fentanyl-fluanosine (fentanyl 0.315 mg/mL and fluanosine 10 mg/mL) and 1.0 mL intramuscular injection of midazolam (5 mg/mL).
2. Shave the neck and achieve a local mid-line anesthesia with an intracutaneous injection of lidocaine.
3. Through a mid-line neck incision of 5 cm between the sternohyoid and sternocleidomastoid muscles expose the common carotid arteries.
4. Gently prepare the arteries from surrounding tissues and vagus nerve for a length of 2.5 cm.
5. Install collars (2 cm) to the prepared positions.
6. Gene transfer can be performed immediately after the collar installation or at varying time points depending on the function of the gene of interest. For a gene transfer at a later time, the collar is exposed and opened using the same approach as in the collar installation *(2,3)*.

3.3. Intravascular Gene Transfer to the Aorta (see Note 5)

The same anesthesia as in the collar operation is used except with intravenous administration of fentanyl-fluanosine due to longer operation.

1. Through a mid-line neck incision, expose the right common carotid artery and prepare from the surrounding tissues and vagus nerve for a length of 4 cm.
2. Ligate the carotid artery at the distal end.
3. Close the proximal end with a surgical clip or tape.
4. Position the introducer sheath inside the artery through incision near the distal closure.
5. Position the gene transfer catheter to the abdominal aorta through the introducer sheath under fluoroscopical control.
6. Inflate the channel balloon to 6 atm and infuse the gene transfer solution for 10 min.
7. Deflate the balloon.
8. Ligate the right common carotid artery at the proximal end after removal of the introducer sheath *(4)*.

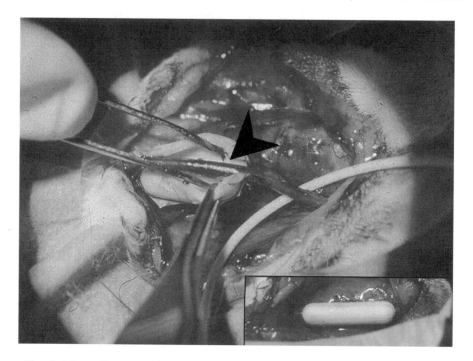

Fig. 1. The collar operation. The common carotid artery (arrowhead) is exposed and the collar is placed around the artery with the aid of surgical tape (white string). Inset: Closed collar around the artery.

3.4. Sacrificing and Sample Preparation (see Notes 6 and 7).

1. Achieve general anesthesia as described above (*see* **Subheading 3.2., step 1**) followed by a 0.4 mL intravenous dose of fentanyl-fluanosine.
2. Remove the collared carotid arteries, flush gently with saline and divide into three equal parts: immerse-fix the proximal third in 4% paraformaldehyde/15% sucrose, pH 7.4 for 4 h, rinse in 15% sucrose, pH 7.4 overnight and embed in paraffin. Directly embed the medial third in OCT compound or store at –70°C for later analyses. Aortic samples are treated in a similar way as carotid arteries.
3. Cut 10-μm sections and stain with hematoxylin-eosin for general histology and morphometry.
4. Cell counts are measured from hematoxylin-stained sections.

3.5. Measurement of Gene Transfer Efficiency

Gene transfer efficiency is calculated as a percentage of X-gal positive cells of all arterial cells *(5)* (*see* **Note 8**).

1. Fix arterial samples for the β-galactosidase assay in 4% paraformaldehyde/0.15 *M* sodium-phosphate buffer, pH 7.2, for 10 min and rinse with 0.15 *M* sodium-phosphate buffer, pH 7.2 for 30 min.

2. Embed arteries in OCT compound and cut 10-μm sections on a cryostat.
3. Add 100 μL of X-gal stain solution on to the frozen sections and incubate in the dark at +37°C for 8 h.
4. Rinse sections with 1X PBS.
5. Counter stain with Mayer's Carmalum, dehydrate with rising ethanol concentrations, and embed with Permount.

4. Notes

1. Preparation of both carotid arteries from surrounding tissues can damage the vagus nerve causing paralysis of vocal chords and severe breathing difficulties. This can be avoided easily by using surgical tape around arteries during the procedure.
2. For collar operations the initial anesthesia is usually enough for the whole operation, but in the gene transfer protocol to the aorta rabbits there is a requirement for additional anesthetics due to the longer operation. The most convenient way to keep rabbits anesthetized through the whole operation is to inject a 0.05 mL bolus of fentanyl-fluanosine through iv cannule placed in the ear vein. Intravenous injection of 0.05 mL naloxon (0.4 mg/mL) is then used for stopping the anesthesia after the operations.
3. During collar operations there is no danger of thrombus formation, but intraarterial manipulation during gene transfer to aorta may cause severe thrombus formation and neurological complications. Subcutaneous injections of heparin (200 U) before and after operation effectively abolish this problem.
4. To avoid inflammation, intramuscular administration of 125 mg of cefuroxim can be performed.
5. Positioning of the perfusion catheter in aorta. Papaverin (10 mg/mL) injections into the prepared carotid artery are used to dilate the artery before positioning the Introducer sheath. The side branch-free position of the aorta for the gene transfer is selected with fluoroscopical control. Leakage around the gene transfer catheter may decrease gene transfer efficiency. To prevent parasympathetic effects caused by the operation, 0.04 mg of glycopyrronbromide can be injected intramuscularly before the operation.
6. Various methods for tissue fixation have been reported. We have used 10 min fixation for arterial samples and 30 min fixation for the other tissues. Longer fixation, e.g., in the liver, abolishes the background from the low expression of endogenous β-galactosidase activity.
7. The number of cells positive for the transferred gene varies between sections. It is essential to count cells from at least 10 different sections and give the average count. Analysis of large number of samples can be automated using image analysis systems.
8. Using plasmid/liposome complexes the gene expression time in the vessel wall lasts up to 2–3 wk. Using adenoviruses the expression time is longer, lasting up to 4 wk. Endogenous expression of β-galactosidase has to be controlled. Too long incubation times in X-gal often result in background from endogenous β-galactosidase activity. The use of positive and negative controls in X-gal staining is essential.

References

1. Ylä-Herttuala, S. (1997) Vascular gene transfer. *Curr. Opin. Lipidol.* **8**, 72–76.
2. Laitinen, M., Pakkanen, T., Donetti, E., Baetta, R., Luoma, J., Lehtolainen, P., et al. (1997) Gene transfer into the carotid artery using an adventitial collar: comparison of the effectiveness of the plasmid-liposome complexes, retroviruses, pseudotyped retroviruses and adenoviruses. *Human Gene Ther.* **8**, 1645–1650.
3. Laitinen, M., Zachary, I., Breier, G., Pakkanen, T., Häkkinen, T., Luoma, J., et al. (1997) VEGF gene transfer reduces intimal thickening via increased production of nitric oxide in carotid arteries. *Human Gene Ther.* **8**, 1737–1744.
4. Hiltunen, M.O., Häkkinen, T.P., Laitinen, M., Turunen, M.P., Hartikainen J., Mäkinen, K., et al. DNA hypomethylation and methyltransferase expression in atherosclerotic lesions, *submitted for publication.*
5. Turunen, M.P., Hiltunen, M.O., Ruponen, M., Virkamäki, L., Szoka, F.C., Urtti, A., and Ylä-Herttuala, S. (1999) Efficient adventitial gene delivery to rabbit carotid artery with cationic polymer-plasmid complexes. *Gene Ther.* **6**, 6–11.

33

Delivery of Antisense Oligonucleotides to the Vascular Wall

Cathy M. Holt, Julian Gunn, Darren Lambert, David C. Cumberland, and David C. Crossman

1. Introduction

1.1. Antisense Oligonucleotides (AS-ODNs)

Antisense oligonucleotides are short segments of synthetic DNA designed to contain sequences of bases complementary to the DNA or RNA of a particular target gene of interest. By binding to the target, the antisense oligonucleotides can prevent translation of the gene into protein via different mechanisms including destruction of the AS-ODN-nucleic acid hybrid by RNAse H, steric hindrance of the ribosome causing interference of protein elongation, or blockage of the initiation of protein translation *(1)*. **Figure 1** shows the possible mechanisms of action of AS-ODNs.

1.2. AS-ODNs in the Treatment of Vascular Disease

Coronary artery disease remains the most widespread cause of mortality and serious morbidity in the developed countries and is increasing in prevalence in the third world. The main form of treatment is revascularization with either coronary artery bypass grafting (CABG) or percutaneous transluminal coronary angioplasty (PTCA) and, in a few cases, cardiac transplantation. PTCA currently exceeds one million per year world-wide and out numbers CABG. Since 1987, coronary stent implantation has supplemented PTCA and now occurs in up to 80% of PTCAs *(2)*. All of these treatments are characterized by the formation of myointimal hyperplasia, causing 30–50% of lesions which have undergone PTCAs to restenose by 6 mo, 50% of saphenous vein grafts to fail by 10 yr, and for chronic rejection of transplanted hearts to occur *(3–5)*.

From: *Methods in Molecular Medicine, Vascular Disease: Molecular Biology and Gene Therapy Protocols*
Edited by: A. H. Baker © Humana Press Inc., Totowa, NJ

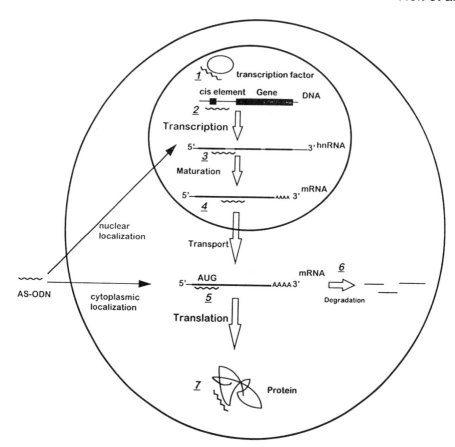

Fig. 1. Possible mechanisms of action of antisense oligonucleotides. 1, Aptameric or specific binding to transcription factors; 2, triplex formation via binding to double-stranded DNA resulting in steric inhibition of transcription of DNA into RNA; 3, specific binding to splice junctions or poly A signals inhibits mRNA maturation; 4, inhibition of transport from the nucleus; 5, specific binding to mRNA causing inhibition of translation via steric hindrance of ribosomal complexes; 6, duplex formation causing RNAse H mediated cleavage of mRNA; 7, aptameric binding to protein causing inhibition of protein function.

Myointimal hyperplasia involves the abnormal migration and proliferation of vascular smooth muscle cells (VSMC) and the deposition of extracellular matrix around the vessel lumen. Despite numerous, large, well conducted clinical trials of systemically administered agents, no acceptable therapies have convincingly been shown to be effective in large trials preventing restenosis in man *(6)*. Recently, there has been interest in the local application of AS-ODNs to prevent restenosis and vein graft failure.

1.3. AS-ODN Targets

The main targets studied to date for inhibition via AS-ODNs for the treatment of restenosis and graft failure are proliferation and cell-cycle related genes, especially genes that are expressed downstream from growth factors and their receptors. In particular, the proto-oncogenes *c-myb* and *c-myc* have been widely studied for their inhibitory effects on VSMC proliferation. *c-myb* and *c-myc* are both involved in the proliferation of VSMC, and they may also be involved in the regulation of apoptosis *(7)*. At least one clinical trial has just been completed to investigate the effects of *c-myc* AS-ODN on restenosis after coronary stenting *(8)*. Using "downstream" targets such as these surmounts, to some degree, the problem of redundancy that may be encountered if individual growth factors are targeted. Though myointimal proliferation is the major feature of restenosis, remodeling (shrinkage) of the artery can account for up to two thirds of the luminal encroachment in restenosis *(9)*. The targeting of proliferation-related genes, nevertheless, is attractive because proliferation is an early event after angioplasty and may be particularly appropriate following stenting, when geometric adaptation (recoil or remodeling) is minimal. The early occurrence of proliferation is confirmed by atherectomy specimens, which reveal a low level of proliferation in restenotic lesions late after PTCA *(10)*. Antiproliferative therapy could, logically, therefore be given locally immediately after PTCA. Whether the situation is similar in vein graft failure remains to be clarified.

1.4. Local Drug Delivery

One of the problems relating to the treatment and prevention of restenosis is the delivery of a therapeutic agent. Our group has a long-standing interest in local drug delivery (LDD) devices and, in particular, the delivery of AS-ODNs from such devices to the vessel wall *(11)*. The advantage of LDD is that an effective local concentration of an agent may be achieved in the precise area required, whereas systemic delivery may not attain the required local concentrations despite doses with potentially toxic side effects. The delivery issues in local vascular drug delivery are:

1. The drug must enter the wall of the artery.
2. It must enter the target cells.
3. It must remain there long enough to exert a useful effect, before being degraded or eluted.

Numerous devices with different modes of delivery are currently under trial. There are three major types:

1. Passive diffusion (double balloon).
2. Convection (infusion under pressure).
3. Mechanical delivery (direct injection).

Variants also exist, such as porous balloons capable of dilating a lesion and delivering a drug, gel-coated balloons, iontophoretic (charge-driven) devices, biodegradable implants, and, more recently, the delivery of drugs from coated stents. **Figure 2** shows the principles underlying the main LDD devices under investigation.

1.5. In Vivo Models

Despite the theoretical advantages identified in **Subheading 1.4.**, LDD remains clinically unproven. The devices can only be tested in animal models, and the porcine coronary artery model has been useful for testing device deployment, through delivery efficiency to efficacy in reducing myointimal hyperplasia. There are several advantages to this model, compared with small animal models. The porcine coronary circulation is anatomically similar to the human, as is its immune system, rheology, and genetic makeup *(12)*. Clinical devices can be investigated without the requirement for miniaturization. A lesion histologically similar to clinical restenosis may be produced by oversize balloon coronary angioplasty. We have also used human material to conduct experiments utilizing the explanted hearts of cardiac transplant recipients, with either atherosclerotic coronary heart disease or "normal" coronary arteries from patients with dilated cardiomyopathy. This model allows the pattern of delivery of antisense to diseased coronary arteries to be studied. Experiments using both the pig and the human model will be described.

2. Materials

2.1. Oligodeoxynucleotides

1. AS-ODNs are manufactured on a commercial DNA synthesizer. It is of the utmost important to ensure that the ODN is pure and intact. This can be achieved by HPLC analysis and capillary gel electrophoresis. This is essential to ensure that the effects observed are specific for the target under observation, rather than arising from fragments of oligonucleotide DNA binding nonspecifically to RNA or DNA other than the selected target. In any experiment using AS-ODN, a series of control oligonucleotides should also be investigated including scrambled, sense, and mismatch. The AS-ODN sequence that we have routinely used in our experiments is an unmodified phosphodiester ODN: 5' GTG CCG GGG TCT TCG GGC 3', directed against *c-myb* although the methods we describe can relate to any AS-ODN.
2. Labeling of ODNs is required in order that their delivery can be localized and quantified.
3. Fluorescent labels, e.g., FAM (a FITC analog): these can subsequently be observed in unstained, histological sections of vessel under UV illumination.
4. Digoxygenin: this is another useful marker that can be detected using antidigoxygenin antibodies. Because digoxigenin is nonmammalian, the problems encountered using naturally occurring endogenous compounds such as biotin are overcome.

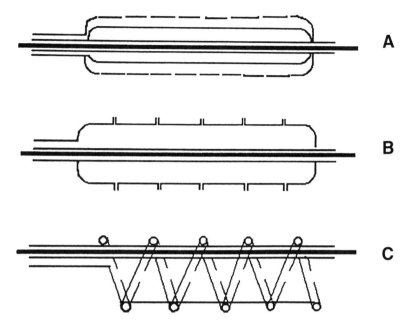

Fig. 2. Diagrammatic longitudinal sections of representative contemporary local drug delivery catheters from each of the main types. (**A**) A Transport balloon (Boston Scientific) is a pressure-driven, "convectional" device. A conventional inner dilatation balloon is surrounded by a second balloon containing 36–48 perforations 250 μm in diameter. The space between the two may be filled with the fluid to be delivered via a separate channel, so dilatation and delivery can be uncoupled. The inner balloon can be used to support the outer envelope against the artery wall to ensure intramural delivery. (**B**) An Infiltrator catheter (InterVentional Technology) is a direct injection-type device. It consists of a single balloon with three parallel rows of steel microports 250 μm in height. When the device is in position, the fluid to be delivered fills the balloon and is injected into the wall of the vessel via the microports. (**C**) The Dispatch catheter (Boston Scientific) relies on passive diffusion. When the device is in position, the fluid to be delivered enters a spiral channel around a cylindrical membrane. The arms of the spiral are perforated, so the fluid leaks into the space between the membrane and the vessel wall. Prolonged delivery may be safely accomplished because blood can perfuse the artery distal to the device through the central channel.

5. Radioactive labels (e.g., ^{32}P): may provide quantitative data regarding the efficiency of LDD devices.

2.2. Local Drug Delivery (LDD) Catheters

1. Transport® catheter: this device has concentric 20-mm long balloons near the tip. One lumen is used for inflation of the (inner) dilating and support balloon, the second supplies the (outer) infusion balloon and the third admits a 0.014-in.

coronary guidewire. The shaft is 2.9 F, tapering to 2.7 F distally. The undeployed profile of the Transport® is 0.032 for the 2.5-mm, 0.035 for the 3.5-mm, and 0.039 in. for the 4.5-mm balloon. The outer balloon possesses 36 (2.5-mm balloon) or 48 (3.0- to 4.5-mm balloons) pores of 250 μm in diameter within the central 10 mm. The balloons are made of polyethylene, reaching nominal diameter at 6 atmosphere (atm) and enlarging by 0.2 mm at 10 atm. For intramural delivery, the inner balloon may be inflated to support the outer envelope against the lesion or the artery wall (**Fig. 3**). This may be done at any pressure up to 6 atm. The rate of fluid infusion is proportional to infusion pressure for a given support pressure. As the support pressure increases, the infusion rate falls. Typical conditions used for intramural delivery in these studies are 1 atm support, 2 atm delivery, these are low pressures, to avoid arterial injury, producing an infusion rate of 2 mL/min.

2.3. Experimental Animals (see Note 2)

1. Cross-bred male or female Yorkshire White pigs (20–30 kg): in this model, balloon injury is inflicted on normal coronary arteries with the production of a neointima similar to that seen in clinical restenosis. Home Office licences (personal and project) are required for the procedure.
2. Azaperone (12 mg/kg, Janssen Animal Health, High Wycombe, UK) or ketamine (Willow Frances, Crawley, UK) for sedation.
3. Propofol (4 mg/kg, Zeneca Pharmaceuticals) for intravenous induction of anaesthesia.
4. Iso-or enflurane (4–7% in oxygen) by inhalation for maintenance of anaesthesia.
5. Sterile surgical instruments and sutures for exposure of the carotid artery and closure of the wound.
6. Catheters, guide wires, and inflation device (Boston Scientific, Nattick, MA).
7. Fluoroscopy for catheter guidance, positioning, and sizing.
8. Animal feed (normal diet).
9. Thiopentone (intravenous injection for humane killing of animals).
10. Normal saline: for washing of explanted coronary arteries at the end of the experiment.
11. Soluene 350 (Packard, Downes Grove, IL).
12. 30% hydrogen peroxide.
13. Hionic fluor (Packard).
14. LKB 1217 Rack Beta liquid scintillation counter (Hewlett Packard).
15. Colloidal carbon suspension (Indian ink, median particle size 74 nm).
16. Tissue-Tek® OCT compound (Miles Inc., Elkhart, IN).
17. Slowfade antifade (Molecular Probes Europe BV).
18. Olympus BH-2 light microscope with a Sony video camera XC-711P attachment.
19. Image analysis system (e.g., Seescan) and television monitor.

2.4. Human Vessels

1. Human vessels: obtained from the explanted hearts of cardiac transplant recipients with prior informed consent of the patient (*see* **Note 3**).

3. Methods

3.1. Porcine Coronary Artery Balloon Injury Model

1. For delivery studies, position a Transport® catheter in one segment of each suitable artery with a balloon/artery ratio 1.1:1, assessed by quantitative angiography, leading to formation of a neointima. (If injury is required, the balloon-to-artery ratio must be >1.25:1.)
2. Perform local drug delivery (*see* **Subheading 3.2.**).
3. After delivery, or at selected time intervals, kill the animals by intravenous overdose of thiopentone.
4. Perform thoracotomy and explant the heart.
5. Dissect out the coronary arteries and process for histological analysis (*see* **Note 4**).

3.2. Acute Delivery Experiments

3.2.1. Drug Concentration

1. To obtain an estimate of the correct concentration of drug for detection by fluorescence microscopy, deploy the Transport® catheter at 1 atm support, 2 atm delivery, to deliver 2 mL of saline containing 5, 50, or 500 µg FAM-AS-ODN-*c-myb* (or equivalent AS-ODN), one to each of three epicardial coronary artery segments in vivo.
2. Kill the animal immediately and prepare for UV microscopy.

3.2.2. Delivery Pressures

1. Determine the optimal delivery pressure using the ODN concentration established (*see* **Subheading 3.2.1.**).
2. Deliver FAM-AS-ODN-*c-myb* (or equivalent) at 2 atm (support), 3 atm (delivery) ("2/3 atm"); 3/4 atm; 4/5 atm; and 5/6 atm. The minimum effective ODN concentrations and balloon pressures thus established can then be used for all subsequent experiments. **Figure 3** shows the delivery of FAM labeled AS-ODN-*c-myb* to pig coronary artery via the Transport® balloon.

3.2.3. Prior Injury

1. To determine the effect of prior injury, inflate the inner balloon of the Transport® catheter to 8 atm for 30 s twice at a balloon/artery ratio of 1.25:1 to produce arterial injury in three coronary arteries of the pig.
2. Use the minimum effective delivery pressures and the best of the three concentrations of ODN established above for drug delivery at the three sites.
3. Harvest the arteries immediately after the last delivery.
4. Process as described (*see* **Subheading 3.3.**).

3.3. Delivery Efficacy

To determine the efficiency of delivery, use radiolabeled ODNs with quantification by scintillation spectroscopy.

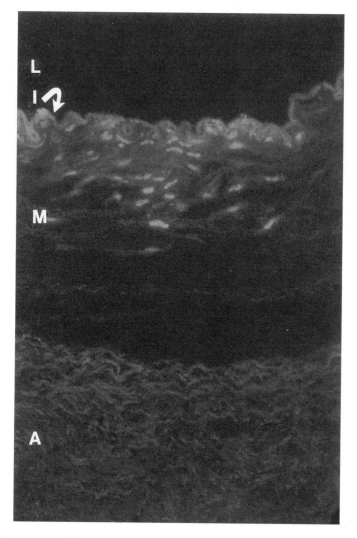

Fig. 3. Intra-mural drug delivery of FAM-AS-ODN-*c-myb* using the Transport®. Infusion of 2 mL saline containing 500 µg FAM-AS-ODN-*c-myb* at 1 atm (support) and 2 atm (delivery) into an uninjured porcine coronary artery. L, lumen; I, intima; M, media; A, adventitia. Uptake is seen in the inner media and adventitia, with concentration in the nuclei of the smooth muscle cells of the media.

1. Label AS-ODNs with ^{32}P using either 3' or 5' end-labeling techniques.
2. Combine 32 ng of ODN with 2 µL 10X kinase buffer, 2–3 µL ^{32}Pγ ATP, water, and 1 µL T4 polynucleotide kinase.
3. Incubate the reaction at 37°C for 15 min.
4. Stop the reaction by the addition of 2 µL 0.5 *M* EDTA.

5. Dilute the labeled ODN with 20 μL water and spin through a G50 column for 5 min at 1500–2000 rpm to remove any unincorporated nucleotides (*see* **Note 5**).

The optimal delivery pressures established are used (*see* **Subheading 3.2.2.**).

6. Dissolve each compound in 2 mL of saline.
7. Assess the baseline activity of each 2-mL aliquot using a scintillation counter prior to delivery.
8. After delivery, kill the animals immediately and explant the arteries with a wedge of surrounding myocardium about 5 mm deep.
9. Obtain samples of distant myocardium, aorta, other organs, blood, and urine.
10. Mince tissue samples and solubilize at 50°C in 20 mL scintillation vials containing 3 mL Soluene 350 overnight.
11. Bleach with with 750 μL 30% hydrogen peroxide for 18 h at 21°C.
12. Add 15 mL of Hionic fluor and mix.
13. Count on an LKB 1217 Rack Beta liquid scintillation counter.

The efficiency of delivery is the ratio of the activity of the tissue from the delivery site to the activity of the delivered aliquot, expressed as a percentage.

3.4. Persistence of AS-ODN

1. To determine the persistence of intramural delivery, repeat the above experiment (**Subheading 3.3.**).
2. Harvest the arteries at different time intervals following delivery.

3.5. Regionality of Delivery

To assess the extent of LDD, perform the following experiments.

1. Position a Transport® catheter in the left anterior descending coronary artery (LAD) of a pig.
2. Open the chest and pericardium, exposing the site of delivery.
3. Use video filming to record the spread of 2 mL colloidal carbon suspension (Indian ink, median particle size 74 nm) infused at 1/2 atm.
4. Kill the animal.
5. Explant the heart.
6. Section the myocardium and photograph.
7. Dissect the LAD, serially section and preserve for light microscopy.

3.6. Effect of Volume

1. To determine the effect of volume of infusate, deploy the Transport® catheter in the LAD and right coronary artery (RCA) of pigs.
2. Using the minimum delivery pressures established above, deliver increasing volumes of PBS, i.e., 4, 8, and 12 mL PBS using the minimum practical balloon/artery ratio of 1.1:1.
3. At 28 d, kill the pigs.
4. Section the arteries and prepare for light microscopy.

Calculate the number of sections containing a breach in the internal elastic lamina (IEL), the number with a distinct neointima, the maximal cross-sectional area of neointima, and total volume of neointima. Uninstrumented arteries serve as controls.

3.7. Chronic Efficacy Experiments

1. To determine the effect of AS-ODN *c-myb* on neointimal formation in the pig balloon injury model, perform LDD as described above (**Subheading 3.2.**) and deliver 500 µg of AS-ODN-*c-myb* in saline using the Transport® device.
2. Allow the pigs to recover and kill after 28 d (sufficient time for a neointima to develop).
3. Remove the hearts.
4. Dissect the coronary arteries and prepare histological sections.

Figure 4 shows the histological appearance of a control (uninjured) coronary artery and an artery 28 d after injury with and without delivery of AS-ODN-*c-myb*. There is a significant reduction in neointimal area following treatment with AS-ODN-*c-myb*.

3.8. Analysis of Tissue Specimens

1. Immerse-fix alternate tissue blocks in formalin, process, embed in paraffin wax, and stain with hematoxylin and eosin and Miller's elastic van Gieson for light microscopy, or freeze in Tissue-Tek® OCT compound in liquid nitrogen in preparation for sectioning and viewing under fluorescent light microscopy.
2. Mount sections using Slowfade antifade in order to prolong fluorescence.
3. Examine each section for the intensity and distribution of fluorescence for each concentration of ODN (*see* **Note 6**).
4. Perform quantitative histology on transverse sections using an Olympus BH-2 light microscope with a Sony video camera XC-711P attachment and output to a computerized image analysis system (e.g., Seescan) and television monitor.

A breach in the IEL is used as evidence of injury and only those sections with a breach are used for analysis of intima/medial cross sectional area. The injury score is also determined by recording the percent breach in the IEL.

3.9. Ex Vivo Human Experiments

1. Flush the coronary arteries and venous bypass grafts with saline.
2. Obtain angiograms to identify a segment of patent vessel suitable for drug delivery.
3. Flush the vessels again with saline.
4. Position a Transport® catheter at the selected sites.

Experiments may be performed either with or without prior injury as described above.

5. Infuse 2 mL of saline containing 500 µg FAM-AS-ODN-*c-myb* or 2 mL colloidal carbon into each site.

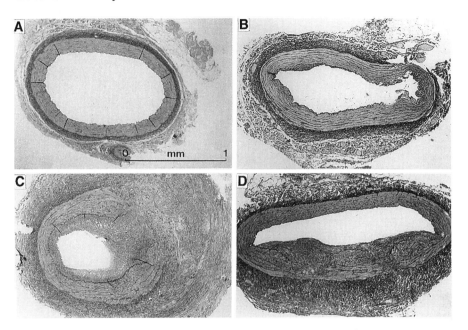

Fig. 4. Effect of oversized balloon angioplasty on pig coronary arteries: histological changes. (**A**) Normal coronary artery. (**B**) Artery harvested immediately after oversized-balloon PTCA, showing breached intima, IEL and media. (**C**) Artery harvested 28 d after oversized balloon PTCA showing extensive breach of IEL, a thick neointima, and a marked adventitial reaction. (**D**) Artery 28 d after oversized-balloon PTCA and local delivery of AS-ODN-*c-myb*. Despite two breaches of the IEL, neointima formation is modest.

6. Perform escalation of pressure to achieve delivery in diseased vessels.
7. Dissect free the vessels.
8. Serially section and prepared for light and fluorescence microscopy, as described above.

3.10. Limitations in the Use of AS-ODN

3.10.1. Specificity of Action of AS-ODNs

There has been much debate concerning the specificity of action of AS-ODNs. The following rules have recently been suggested by Stein *(13)* in performing AS-ODN experiments:

1. Decrease in target protein must be observed following AS-ODN treatment, and a control protein with a similar half life should remain at constant levels.
2. Several control ODNs should be tested: sense, scrambled, mismatched control, and mismatched target control (i.e., cells with a mutant or deleted gene).
3. Binding of the ODN to target RNA should be determined.

3.10.2. Degradation of ODNs: Assessment of Integrity

Detection of FAM or ^{32}P, etc., does not necessarily imply that delivery of ODN has occurred. The label could be detached from the ODN, which could be elsewhere and/or degraded. It may therefore be important to perform experiments to determine the integrity of ODN. This can be done by extracting AS-ODN from coronary artery and plasma samples at various time points following delivery and analyzing them for integrity using capillary gel electrophoresis (CGE) and HPLC mass spectrometry. CGE allows for analysis of the length of ODNs, i.e., the number of bases and also quantitation of ODNs isolated from biological samples. HPLC mass spectrometry allows further characterization and sequencing of metabolites.

3.10.3. Autofluorescence

Autofluoresence of vascular tissue may interfere with observation of fluorescent-labeled ODNs. This applies particularly to highly elastic arteries, for example, the aorta and carotid arteries. The problem of autofluorescence can be surmounted by using an anti-FITC antibody with subsequent detection using, for example, diaminobenzidene (DAB), which gives a brown end-product visible by light microscopy. We have found the use of Slofade antifade beneficial in delaying the loss of fluorescence. In addition, frozen sections should be stored in the dark at –20°C and exposure to UV illumination should be minimized to further prolong fluorescence.

3.10.4. Regionality of Local Delivery

Different LDD devices are capable of delivering drug to different regions of the vessel wall. The Transport® device used in our studies, for example, is capable of delivering drug to the innermost layers of the media as well as the *vasa vasorum* of the adventitia. Other devices, for instance, the Wolinsky balloon, will deliver drug deeper into the vessel wall but at the expense of vascular injury *(14)*. Equally, atraumatic delivery to superficial layers may be possible with, for example, the Dispatch® Catheter (Boston Scientific). Other devices are available that target the adventitia, e.g., the Needle injection catheter *(15)*. The choice of delivery catheter is dependent upon the localization of the target. It is always important, therefore, to know the distribution of the molecule that it is required to inhibit.

3.10.5. Timing of Delivery

With most LDD devices, for practical reasons and for similarity with what would be clinical practice, delivery occurs at the time of angioplasty, so the drug is present early in the restenotic process. This should be considered when targets for inhibition are being selected. In addition, when AS-ODNs are used, the longevity of ODNs in vivo needs to be taken into account and this may be modulated by any molecular modifications (e.g., phosphorothioation). In our in vivo studies, we used unmodified ODNs, because the efficacy of these is enhanced in vitro compared to phosphorothioated ODNs *(16)*. This parameter, however, should be considered for each individual target under investigation and considered together with the time course of expression of the molecule under target. If the target gene expression is late after PTCA, molecule protection might be worthwhile despite the problem of decreased uptake and efficacy.

3.10.6. Volume of Agent Delivered

The volume of fluid delivered via the Transport® catheter in increments from 2–12 mL causes a significant increase in the extent of neointimal thickening and injury to the internal elastic lamina *(11)*. The extent of injury is approximately proportional to the volume delivered. It is, therefore, important to minimize the volume of therapeutic agent but consideration needs to be given to the realistic handling volume for the device being used. Any therapeutic effect must also be compared with a control group in which delivery of an equivalent volume of vehicle has been performed.

3.11. Future Directions

In addition to LDD to the vascular wall from catheter-based devices such as described above, various other modalities are currently under analysis. These include the delivery of therapeutic agents from polymer coated endoluminal stents *(17,18)*. In order to determine the most efficacious device, detailed information regarding the location and timing of expression of the target under investigation within the vessel wall are important. In addition to the ideal delivery device, information regarding the mechanisms of action, including the specificity of AS-ODNs, and whether unmodified or modified (and which modification of) ODNs should be used, is still required before the use of LDD of AS-ODNs becomes a clinical reality.

4. Notes

1. It must be ensured that all label is attached to the ODN by performing (for example) HPLC analysis. For in vivo localization and efficiency studies, (FAM-) or ^{32}P labeled AS-ODN-*c-myb* can be used. To answer further specific questions, other methods may be necessary. Study of the immediate, macroscopic, intramuscular pattern of spread of an agent, FAM labeling together with view of the epicardial surface of the heart in a darkened room using UV illumination (and protective eye shielding) is possible. Alternatively, a simpler approach is to use colloidal carbon (Indian ink, median particle size 73 nm), it is retained in the

lumen and is readily visible both macro- and microscopically. The effect of fluid delivery alone must not be neglected, phosphate-buffered saline (PBS) or suitable vehicle alone should be used.

2. Criticism of the pig balloon injury model used in the previous studies and also a number of other models is that injury is induced in normal coronary arteries. In the clinical setting, PTCA and, hence, LDD are performed in diseased vessels. In order to partially overcome this problem, we have also performed LDD experiments on diseased human coronary arteries. These experiments can only be performed on coronary arteries in the absence of flow, thereby introducing an additional limitation. Furthermore, quantification of delivery to a diseased vessel is difficult because of the variability of the disease. An experimental model of LDD to diseased vessels in vivo may be a better option. We and others are currently working on developing a realistic model of atherosclerosis in the pig. This problem may be avoided by genetic manipulation, for example, in the development of a familial hypercholesterolemic animal.

3. Hearts are obtained within minutes of their removal and are transferred to the laboratory at room temperature. Hearts are either obtained from patients with coronary heart disease (severe atheroslerosis) or with dilated cardiomyopathy (minimal atherosclerosis). LDD is performed on coronary arteries *in situ* to observe LDD in disease states and to study drug distribution.

4. Histology: Usually requires cross sectioning at 2 mm intervals, prior to fixation in buffered formalin, processing, embedding in paraffin wax, sectioning, mounting, and staining. We have performed a comparison of the effects of perfusion and immersion fixation on quantitative histology. Perfusion was performed with 500 mL formalin in saline (4% v/v) via an aortic root cannula at 80 mmHg for 10 min, followed by 24-h immersion fixation. Comparison of morphometric analyses of total vessel cross sectional area, media, and lumen cross sectional area were not significantly different in perfusion fixed and immersion fixed vessels.

5. Typically, ^{32}P-AS-ODN-*c-myb* (37.5 ng, 4.14×10^6 counts per minute [cpm], the total dose is dictated by safety criteria) has been delivered to both LAD and RCA of pigs.

6. Use the concentration giving optimal assessment of intramural delivery for subsequent experiments.

Acknowledgments

We are grateful to Boston Scientific for providing the Transport® catheters, the British Heart Foundation and the Northern General Hospital Research Fund for financial support, and the Cardiac Transplant team and patients of the Northern General Hospital for access to human hearts.

References

1. Bennett, M. R. and Schwartz, S. M. (1995) Antisense therapy for angioplasty restenosis-some critical considerations. *Circulation* **92,** 1–13.
2. Foley, D. P. and Serruys, P. W. (1996) Clinical trials in stenting. Editorial; *Semin. Intervent. Cardiol.* **1,** 231,232.

3. Kent, K. M. (1988) Restenosis after percutaneous coronary angioplasty. *Am. J. Cardiol.* **61,** 67G–70G.

4. Loop, F. D., Lytle, B. W., Cosgrove, D. M., Stewart, R. W., Goormastic, M., Williams, G. W., et al. (1986) Influence of the internal-mammary artery graft on 10 year survival and other cardiac events. *N. Engl. J. Med.* **314,** 1–6.

5. Gordon, D. (1996) Transplant arteriosclerosis, in *Atherosclerosis and Coronary Artery Disease.* (Fuster, V., Ross, R., and Topol, E. J., eds.), Lippincott-Raven, Philadelphia.

6. Serruys, P. W., Hermans, W. R. M., Rensing, B. J., and deFeyter, P. J. (1993) In *Advances in Quantitative Coronary Arteriography.* (Reiber, J. H. C. and Serruys, P. W., eds.), Kluwer Academic Publishers, Netherlands, pp. 329–350.

7. Edelman, E. R., Simons, M., Sirois, M. G., and Rosenberg. (1995) *c-myc* in vasculoproliferative disorders. *Circ. Res.* **76,** 176–182.

8. Kutryk, M. J. B., Serruys, P. W., Bruining, N., Sabate, M., Ligthart, J., van den Brand, M., et al. (1998) Randomised trial of antisense oligonucleotide against c-myc for the prevention of restenosis after stenting: results of the Thoraxcenter "ITALICS" trial. *Eur. Heart. J.* **19,** A3264.

9. Post, M. J., de Smet, B. J., van der Helm, Y., Borst, C., and Kuntz, R. E. (1997) Arterial remodelling after balloon angioplasty or stenting in an atherosclerotic experimental model. *Circulation* **96,** 996–1003.

10. O'Brien, E. R., Alpers, C. E., Stewart, D. K., Ferguson, M., Tran, N., Gordon, D., et al. (1993) Proliferation in primary and restenotic coronary atherectomy tissue: implications for antiproliferative therapy. *Circ. Res.* **73,** 223–231.

11. Gunn, J., Chico, T., Malik, N., Yusof, N., Holt, C., Francis, S., et al. (1998) Transcatheter fluid delivery: volume directly influences vascular injury and neointima formation. *Eur. Heart. J.* **19,** P2816.

12. Wolinsky, H. (1996) Historical perspective: Local drug delivery. *Semin. Intervent. Cardiol.* **1,** 3–7.

13. Stein, C.A. (1998) How to design an antisense oligodeoxynucleotide experiment: A consensus approach. *Antisense Nucleic Acid Drug Dev.* **8,** 129–132.

14. Eccleston, D. S., Horrigan, M. C. G., and Ellis, S. G. (1996) Rationale for local drug delivery. *Semin. Intervent. Cardiol.* **1,** 8–17.

15. Hofling, B., Huehns, T. Y., and Gonschior, P. (1996) Needle injection catheter. *Semin. Intervent. Cardiol.* **1,** 44.

16. Gunn, J., Holt, C. M., Francis, S. E., Shepherd, L., Grohmann, M., Newman, C. M. H., et al. (1997) The effect of oligonucleotides to c-myb on vascular smooth muscle cell proliferation and neointima formation after porcine coronary angioplasty. *Circ. Res.* **80,** 520–531.

17. Armstrong, J., Holt, C. M., Stratford, P., and Cumberland, D. C. (1997) Phosphorylcholine stent coating as a method of local drug delivery: preliminary data from an ex vivo model. *Heart* **77,** P47.

18. Lambert, T. L., Dev, V., Rechavia, E., Forrester, J. S., Litvack, F., Eigler, N. L. (1994) Localized arterial wall drug delivery from a polymer-coated removable metallic stent. Kinetics, distribution and bioactivity of forskolin. *Circulation* **90,** 1003–1011.

34

Local Gene Delivery of Recombinant Adenoviruses to the Rat Carotid Artery In Vivo

Clare M. Dollery and Jean R. McEwan

1. Introduction

A number of animal models are available to investigators wishing to study the use of gene transfer to prevent neointimal formation after vascular injury. The majority are models of primary vascular injury rather than the human situation, where recurrence of a stenosis occurs in an abnormal blood vessel treated by angioplasty. The main animal models used to study vascular balloon injury or angioplasty are the rat carotid, the rabbit iliac, the pig coronary and carotid models, and, less frequently, the dog coronary and primate saphenous or iliac models. A healthy level of skepticism exists about many of these animal models following the success of angiotensin-converting enzyme inhibitors in preventing neointima formation in the rat model but their failure to prevent human restenosis (*1,2*). Each model, however, has a particular suitability to investigate different aspects of the balloon injury process and all are suitable for gene transfer studies.

1.1. Overview of the Rat Carotid Artery Injury Model

The rat model is perhaps the most commonly used and has the advantage of being extensively studied. The main advantages of the model are availability, low cost, and the ability to develop a rapid reproducible response to balloon injury. Proliferation reaches its peak approx 2 d after injury in the rat, and migration can be assessed at 4 d (*3,4*). The lesion in this model is likely to equally reflect proliferation and migration (*5*). Its disadvantages include the overestimation of the ability of pharmacological inhibitors to influence lesion development, which may be partially due the higher doses used in rodent studies (*1,2*). The model may overemphasize the role of proliferation and fails to reflect

From: *Methods in Molecular Medicine, Vascular Disease: Molecular Biology and Gene Therapy Protocols*
Edited by: A. H. Baker © Humana Press Inc., Totowa, NJ

the influences of lipids and vascular remodeling on vascular injury. Rat arteries are dissimilar to the human arteries in having no vasa vasorum, a smaller subintimal layer, and a low elastin content. The rat carotid has a concentric elastin layer rather than the internal and external lamina and intervening multilayered smooth muscle cells of the human coronary. It also differs from the human coronary in that injury does not result in an occlusive lesion. However, for many investigators the rat model is a starting point to prove the effects of potential therapies on migration and proliferation of smooth muscle cells and the formation of a neointima in vivo before moving to more complex models.

1.2. Recombinant Adenoviruses

Adenoviruses are the most widely used viral vector in vascular biology. Many of their advantages have already been discussed in chapters 22 and 29. Adenoviruses, made replication incompetent by removal of essential genes, can accommodate the insertion of relatively large genes (8.3 kb), and high titer viral stocks can readily be grown in the laboratory *(6)*. Adenoviruses are efficient at infecting numerous different cell types in many species. An important advantage over the retroviruses is their ability to infect quiescent nondividing cells. They are also highly efficient in transferring genes due to their cell surface receptor and endosomal disrupter. Their efficiency is superior to retroviruses and liposomes in normal, uninjured and atherosclerotic blood vessels *(7–9)*. Adenoviruses also have a safety advantage over retroviral vectors in that they do not insert their DNA into the host chromosomes, and although this reduces their duration of action, it also reduces the chances of insertional mutagenesis. Insertion of viral genes into the host genome has been reported, but is rare *(10)*. Use of live adenoviruses as vaccines over some years has not revealed an increased frequency of malignancy and is safe even in immunocompromised subjects *(11)*.

The principal problem with adenoviruses is their ability to provoke a humoural and cellular immune response, which may result in destruction of the infected cell. This limits expression of the transferred gene. In addition, they cause the production of circulating neutralizing antibodies, which prevent successful repeat administrations *(12)*. In rats that are specific-pathogen-free when delivered to the laboratory, preexisting adenoviral antibodies are very unlikely to be present and therefore should not effect gene transfer efficiency. A systemic response to viral infection will occur when these viral vectors are used in vivo. This can be reduced by local delivery techniques that minimize systemic leakage of virus. Although systemic administration of adenoviruses can successfully modify an animal's phenotype gene transfer to modify the response to vascular injury is best applied locally to target only the injured area of vessel *(13)*. This minimizes the systemic effects of the transgene as well as any unwanted effects of the gene delivery vector. Scrupulous purity of the viral stocks used is also essential for in vivo gene transfer. All virus should be screened for wild type/E1A contamination using polymerase-chain-reaction-(PCR) based techniques to identify low levels of E1A and this may be combined with a biological check on replication competence such as studying the virus's ability to form plaques on HeLa cells. In addition, cesium chloride centrifugation should remove as many empty capsids as possible, as these will increase the systemic immune response without augmenting in vivo gene transfer. The above techniques are described in detail in Chapter 22.

1.3. Analysis of Gene Transfer to the Vasculature

The initial step in establishing an animal model of gene transfer is to confirm the ability to transfer a marker gene. Marker genes should ideally encode a readily identifiable, biologically inert but functional native protein that will not provoke a host immune response. The commonest marker genes used are β-galactosidase *(7–9,14–28)*, luciferase *(22,23,29–32)*, and, more recently green fluorescent protein *(33,34)*. β-galactosidase has been most popular to date because it can be identified by a simple blue color change when exposed to X-gal reagent (*see* **Subheading 3.7.**) and so can be localized within the arterial wall but can also be analyzed by examining arterial extracts using an ELISA or a chemiluminescent assay *(16,19,21,25)*. The aim of marker gene studies is to optimize the gene transfer protocol prior to using an active construct. The most detailed studies of the relationship between viral titer and transgene expression have shown an optimal dose of 5×10^8 pfu per artery (1×10^{10} pfu/mL) with variable low levels of expression at 5×10^7 pfu *(16,21)*. It was also shown that the toxicity produced by adenoviral infection at 5×10^9 pfu per vessel (1×10^{11} pfu/mL) reduced transgene expression *(21)*. This is consistent with the authors' unpublished experience. Investigators should be aware that titration of adenoviruses by plaque assay is subject to variability and that repeat freeze/thaw will reduce viral titer. Each investigator will therefore need to confirm an optimum titer for their virus rather than simply extrapolating from published data. Pooling of virus and then performing titration assays of several types prior to aliquoting virus for storage is time well spent.

1.4. Targets for Gene Therapy

A number of different targets have been studied in trying to prevent the response to vascular injury. The commonest approach has been to reduce smooth muscle cell proliferation by cytotoxic (e.g. Herpes simplex virus thymidine kinase, HSV-tk *[35,36]*, cytosine deaminase) or cytostatic approaches (e.g. retinoblastoma protein *[37]*, p21 *[38,39]*, Gax *[40]*, H-ras DN *[41]*). Others have targeted thrombosis (Hirudin *[42]*, cyclo-oxygenase *[43]*), or aimed to restore or simulate normal endothelial function (VEGF *[44]*, eNOS *[45]*). Work in our own laboratory has shown that inhibition of migration of smooth muscle cells can also ameliorate neointimal hyperplasia *(46)*. When choosing a transgene, it should be remembered that, although more efficient than other vectors, adenoviruses may still only achieve transduction of 5–10% of medial smooth muscle cells. A transgene that encodes a secreted protein or whose product has a bystander effect is more likely to have a biological effect than one which can act only on a successfully infected cell. All these studies have shown between 30% and 89% reduction in intimal medial area ratio, and their relative merits has recently been reviewed *(47)*.

1.5. Additional Comments

For those intending to pursue the methods described in these and other chapters (chapters 30–33), it should be noted that all animal work undertaken in the United Kingdom is subject to the Animal Scientific Procedures Act 1986 (*see* **Note 1**). Similar regulations exist in other countries, which must be strictly adhered to. Those intending to carry out gene transfer experiments will also require health and safety executive approval (*see* **Note 2**).

2. Materials

2.1. Animals and Adenoviral Stocks

1. 300–350 g rats Male Wistar (*see* **Note 3**).
2. Dilute viral stocks in RPMI tissue culture medium (Gibco-BRL, Gaithersburg, MD) to give a final concentration of 5×10^9 pfu/100 µL.

2.2. Anesthetic Agents and Equipment

1. Fentanyl/fluanisone (Hypnorm, Janssen Pharmaceutica, Belgium): 0.03 mg per 100 g/1 mg per 100 g respectively, and midazolam (Hypnovel, Roche Welling, Garden City, UK) 0.3 mg/100 g, these agents are stored at room temperature until suppliers expiration date.
2. Two thermal barrier 37°C heating pads (Harvard Apparatus Ltd., Kent, UK).

2.3. Surgical Instruments

1. Surgical instruments: three $1^{1}/_{8}$th in. Dieffenbach curved serefines (Harvard).
2. Iris scissors (Aesculap and Downs Ltd., Sheffield, UK).
3. 9 mm Autoclips and Mikron autoclip applier (Becton Dickenson, Cowley, Oxford, UK).
4. Sterile surgical blade, size 20 (Swann Morton Ltd., Sheffield, UK).
5. Curved dissection forceps, two pairs, (Aesculap and Downs Ltd.).
6. Sprung forceps for cannulation of vessels (Aesculap and Downs Ltd.)
7. Toothed forceps.
8. Straight scissors (Aesculap and Downs Ltd.).
9. Mosquito Haemostat (Aesculap and Downs Ltd.).

2.4. Sterile Supplies

1. 3.0 silk (Davies and Geck, Gosport, Hants, UK): cut to individual 10 cm lengths and autoclaved.
2. Sterile operation drapes (Baxter Healthcare, Berkshire, UK): disposable plastic translucent drapes are used to allow observation of the animal throughout the surgery; sterile scissors are used to cut the drape to appropriate size with a window over the area of dissection.
3. Fogarty Balloon Embolectomy catheter, 2 French gage (Baxter Healthcare): Can be carefully reused for up to 10 balloon procedures or until there is evidence of any distortion of the balloon. Can be sterilized using ethylene oxide.
4. Portex cannula for viral delivery: 2 French gage (SLS, Nottingham, UK).
5. Anticoagulant: Heparin 100 IU/kg in 100 μL of normal saline, heparin is stored at 4°C and supplied with manufacturers expiry dates.

2.5. Harvesting Tissue and Fixatives

1. 1000 mL Bladder pressure perfusion bag (Baxter Healthcare).
2. 20G cannula (Vasculon 2 cannula, Ohmeda, Sweden).
3. 1% w/v paraformaldehyde and 2% w/v glutaraldehyde fixative solution for electron microscopy preparation. Can be stored at 4°C for up to 3 mo.
4. 2% formaldehyde, 0.2% glutaraldehyde in PBS: use as a fixative for light microscopy for morphometric measurements. Can be stored at 4°C for up to 3 mo.
5. 4% formaldehyde: for light microscopy using immunohistochemistry. Can be stored at 4°C for up to 3 mo.

2.6. Histological Reagents and Staining Chemicals

1. 5-Bromo-4-chloro-3-indoyl-β-D-galactopyranoside (X-Gal): dissolve to 150 mg/mL in dimethyl sulfoxide (DMSO).
2. X-gal buffer: dissolve 0.07 g of potassium ferrocyanide [$K_4Fe(CN)_6.3H_2O$], 0.05 g of potassium ferricyanide [$K_3Fe(CN)_6$], 1.852 mL of 4 M sodium chloride, 50 μL of 1 M magnesium chloride in 50 mL of PBS. Add 25 μL of 150 mg/mL X-gal per 1 mL of X-gal buffer.
3. Dewaxing chemicals for paraffin sections: xylene, 100% ethanol, 70% ethanol, 90% ethanol, DPX (BDH).
4. Counterstain: 0.1% nuclear fast red (Sigma, St. Louis, MO) in 5% aluminium sulfate.
5. Polylysine coated microscopy slides.
6. Aquapolymount (Polyscrenes Inc., Worrington, PA).
7. Morphometric analysis: a Labphot 2A microscope (Nikon Ltd., Surrey, UK), a JVC-TK 1281 video camera and a Lucia M color image processing system or equivalent.

3. Methods

3.1. Preparation of Sterile Area and Appropriate Equipment

These experiments should be carried out in a quiet area with a preparation/anesthetic area, operating area, and recovery area. A temperature-controlled area with overhead adjustable operating lights is ideal. Anglepoise lamps, however, can be used to illuminate the surgical field if necessary. Containers of bleach or Virkon should be available in the operating area and recovery area to soak instruments or swabs that come into contact with viral solutions or blood from infected animals. All potentially contaminated material is soaked in an appropriate solution for 10 min prior to disposal or preparation for reuse. A fume cupboard should be available in the area where aldehyde fixation is carried out to prevent inhalation.

1. Clean all surfaces with water and then spray with 70% ethanol.
2. Use aseptic techniques for all surgery and instruments, which should be autoclaved prior to use.

3.2. Surgical Exposure of the Rat Carotid (48) and Balloon Injury

1. Anesthetize male Wistar rats weighing 300–350 g with an intraperitoneal injection of fentanyl/fluanisone (0.025 mg per 100 g/0.8 mg per 100 g, respectively) and midazolam (0.42 mg/100 g) (*see* **Note 4**).
2. Place the anesthetized animal on its back on a piece of sterile drape and clean the ventral aspect of its neck with hibiscrub solution (or alternative antiseptic) and warm water.
3. Using a scalpel blade, shave the fur from the ventral neck.
4. Spray the neck with 70% ethanol and move the animal to the operating area and place it on its back on a heating pad with its head toward the surgeon.
5. Cut to size a piece of sterile translucent drape, making a cut through which the animal's head can be placed.
6. Make a 3–4 cm median or left paramedian incision with a scalpel blade. Sterile swabs and cotton buds should be available if hemorrhage obscures the view of the operating field.
7. Using curved scissors, expose the muscles by blunt dissection (*see* **Fig. 1**). The blunt dissection is most easily continued using a pair of curved forceps held in each hand and by gently inserting the tips into the triangle shown in **Fig. 1** and opening the forceps to expose the underlying bifurcation of the common carotid artery (shown as a dotted line in **Fig. 1**). The branches of the common carotid artery are illustrated in **Fig. 2A**. The carotid artery must be separated from the vagus nerve, which is also present in the neurovascular bundle of the common carotid.
8. Ligate the external carotid artery at the most distal extent of the dissection with a long 3-0 silk ligature.
9. Place the artery under slight tension by lightly weighting the ligature distally with a pair of artery forceps.
10. Place a loose 3-0 silk ligature proximally around the common carotid artery and secure a second loose ligature around the external carotid artery as close to the bifurcation as possible.
11. Place a third suture around the internal carotid. This will simplify the virus delivery technique.
12. A side branch, illustrated in **Fig. 2A**, is commonly present in the proximal portion of the external carotid, this should be identified. Place two tight ligatures

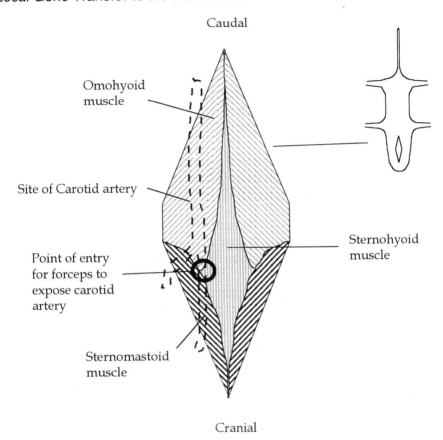

Caudal

Omohyoid
muscle

Site of Carotid artery

Sternohyoid
muscle

Point of entry
for forceps to
expose carotid
artery

Sternomastoid
muscle

Cranial

Fig. 1. Schematic diagram of the rat neck after initial incision demonstrating the site of dissection.

around it by passing a piece of 3-0 silk held in the tips of a pair of fine curved forceps behind the artery.

13. Cut the artery between the ligatures with small scissors. This minimizes bleeding during catheterization of the artery (*see* **Note 5**).

14. Place a Diffenbach arterial clip on the external carotid artery immediately distal to the bifurcation to occlude flow. This clip should be distal to the loose suture already positioned at the bifurcation.

15. Make a small arteriotomy in the external carotid artery using Iris scissors.

16. Introduce the closed blades of a pair of sprung curved forceps into the arteriotomy, open, and pass a Fogarty Balloon Embolectomy catheter between the blades of the forceps into the lumen (*see* **Fig. 2B**). The catheter then rests securely within the 2–5 mm of the artery distal to the Diffenbach arterial clip.

17. Gently remove the clip as the catheter is slowly advanced and passed down the common carotid artery.

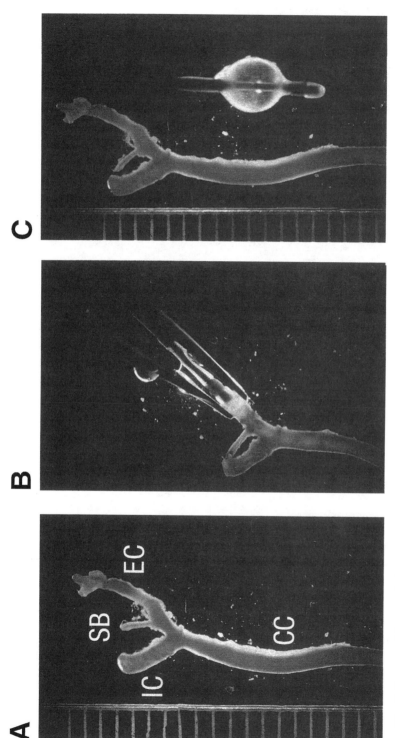

Fig. 2. Rat carotid artery balloon injury technique. The rat carotid artery excised from rat neck and photographed under dark ground microscopy to demonstrate the technique. (**A**) Branches of the rat carotid artery; IC, internal carotid; EC, external carotid; CC, common carotid; SB, side branch, which is commonly present and can cause hemorrhage (1 mm markers). (**B**) The balloon catheter is being inserted into the external carotid artery between the blades of sprung forceps. (**C**) Balloon catheter inflated with saline beside the artery to illustrate the balloon injury when the catheter is within the lumen.

18. Tighten the proximal external carotid suture around the artery and catheter to prevent hemorrhage at the arteriotomy site.
19. Pass the embolectomy balloon into the aorta and inflate with 30 µL of sterile saline (0.9% w/v).
20. Pull the balloon to the origin of the carotid artery, which is not visible but can be identified by resistance to movement of the catheter (*see* **Note 6**). Inflation of the catheter is shown outside the carotid artery in **Fig. 2C**.
21. Deflate the balloon momentarily and move 5 mm distally into the common carotid and reinflate.
22. Pull it up the common carotid artery with a small twisting motion, in order to denude the endothelium and stretch the media of the arterial wall and deflate before being passed back into the aorta. This procedure is repeated twice.
23. Slightly loosen the ligature securing the catheter in the external carotid artery to allow slow withdrawal of the catheter into the external carotid artery.
24. Reapply the Diffenbach clip to the external carotid artery before full withdrawal of the catheter tip.

3.3. Systemic Venous Anticoagulation (see Note 7)

1. After balloon injury of the artery, administer a systemic dose of anticoagulant to prevent thrombosis of the common carotid following 20 min of stasis for viral delivery.
2. Expose the right internal jugular vein by blunt dissection in the subcutaneous tissue ventral to the omohyoid muscle at the thoracic inlet.
3. Place a distal suture around the vein and tie off distally and place a loose suture proximally.
4. Make a small incision in the vein with iris scissors and insert one blade of a pair of curved dissecting forceps into the vein.
5. Lift the blade of the forceps to open the vein beneath it and insert a Portex cannula (2 French gage) connected to a 1-mL syringe.
6. Inject heparin (100 IU/kg in 100 µL) of normal saline and withdraw the cannula.
7. Ligate the vein proximally.

3.4. Viral Gene Delivery

1. Following administration of heparin, apply Diffenbach clips to the most proximal portion of the common carotid artery and to the internal carotid artery. This isolates a segment of artery 1.5 cm long (*see* **Fig. 3A**).
2. Now remove the external carotid clip. If necessary, incise the omohyoid muscle to expose a greater length of common carotid artery.
3. Insert a Portex cannula (2 French gage) into the external carotid artery between the blades of fine forceps using the same arteriotomy used to insert the balloon catheter (*see* **Fig. 3B**).
4. Gently flush the artery with saline to wash out any remaining blood.
5. Remove the cannula and connect to a syringe containing infection solution.
6. Reinsert the cannula and secure in the lumen of the isolated section of artery using the same loop of 3-0 suture previously used to secure the balloon catheter.

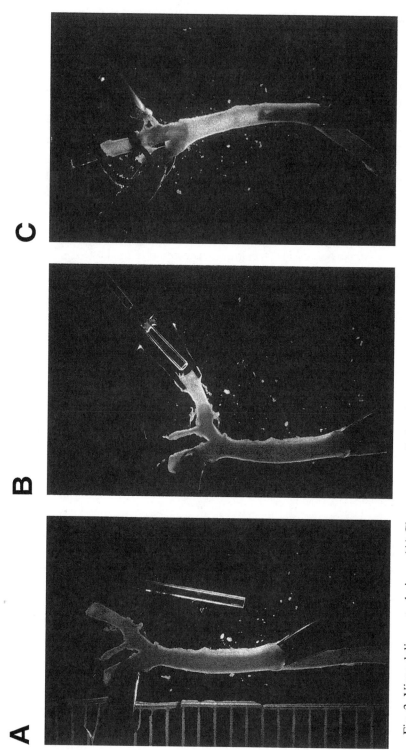

Fig. 3. Virus delivery technique. (**A**) Clamps are applied to the internal and common carotid arteries as shown to isolate a segment of lumen. (**B**) A cannula is inserted into the external carotid artery between the blades of sprung forceps. (**C**) The cannula is secured with a suture and any side branches are identified and occluded. The virus solution is instilled into the isolated segment of lumen and allowed to dwell for 20 min.

7. Advance the syringe barrel to distend the artery with 100 μL of solution.
8. Secure the syringe barrel in position and distend the artery with the infusate (viral solution) for 20 min (*see* **Fig. 3C**).
9. Aspirate the infection solution.
10. Withdraw the cannula and ligate the external carotid artery.
11. Remove the arterial clamp from the internal carotid and inspect the artery to ensure that it has become distended by back flow from the internal carotid.
12. Remove the proximal clip on the common carotid artery and restore the circulation through the common and internal carotid arteries. Pulsation should be clearly visible.
13. Close the wound with autoclaved metal auto-clips or a 2-0 prolene suture.

3.5. Recovery and Postoperative Care

1. Immediately after surgery place the animals on a second heating pad in the recovery area.
2. As they recover consciousness, put them into cages in which the sawdust has been covered by tissue paper. This paper can be removed the next morning.
3. Check the animals daily to ensure that they are healthy and not distressed.

3.6. Euthanasia and Harvesting of Tissues

1. Anesthetize the animal with an intraperitoneal injection of fentanyl/fluanisone (0.025 mg per 100 g/0.8 mg per 100 g, respectively) and midazolam (0.42 mg/ 100 g).
2. Place it on a heating pad in the operation area.
3. Make a midline abdominal incision penetrating the peritoneal cavity.
4. Expose the descending aorta by blunt dissection.
5. Place two sutures around the aorta either in the supra or infra renal region.
6. Tie off the distal suture and gently apply countertraction to the aorta while inserting a 20-G cannula retrogradely into the proximal aorta.
7. Secure it with the second silk ligature.
8. Exsanguinate the animal by aspiration of the aortic cannula with a 10-mL Luer lock syringe (5–10 mL of blood can be reserved for further analysis).
9. Infuse the appropriate fixative solution retrogradely, through the aortic cannula, at a constant pressure of 120 mmHg (using a pressure bag).
10. Continue fixation *in situ* for 10 min.
11. Reopen the original neck incision and excise the mid portion of the common carotid artery.
12. Dispose of animals exposed to adenoviruses according to health and safety regulations.

3.7. Histological Techniques to Demonstrate Transgene Expression (see Note 8)

The efficiency of marker gene transfer following virus infection is estimated by staining arteries with X-gal. This chromagen changes from a yellow to a blue color in the presence of β-galactosidase allowing localization of the transgene (*see* **Fig. 4**). All reagents used in making X-gal solution should be warmed to 37°C to ensure minimal precipitation of X-gal and X-gal solution needs to be filtered prior to use.

1. Fix arteries in situ in 2% formaldehyde, 0.2% glutaraldehyde in PBS for 10 min as described above (*see* **Subheading 3.6., steps 9** and **10**), and then wash in PBS solution for 10 min before transfer to X-gal.
2. Incubate the arteries in X-gal solution for 18 h at 32°C in an oven. Control samples not exposed to a β-galactosidase-encoding virus should always be used as controls in X-gal incubation.
3. Embed all tissue incubated in X-gal in paraffin using short cycles designed for biopsy tissues to minimize exposure to organic solvents, in particular xylene, which will wash out the blue pigment product of the X-gal reaction.
4. Cut 5-μm sections using a microtome and place on polylysine coated microscopy slides.
5. Rehygrate sections by immersion in xylene solutions for 20 s twice, and then place in the following alcohols for 20 s: 100% ethanol, 100% ethanol, 70% ethanol, and finally tap water.
6. Place sections in 0.1% nuclear fast red in 5% aluminium sulfate for 5 min.
7. Wash sections in dH$_2$O.
8. Mount slides in aquapolymount, an aqueous mountant in which the blue pigment product of the X-gal reaction is not soluble.
9. Photograph sections or store the images on a computer image analysis system shortly after staining.

3.8. Quantitation of Lesion Size in This Model

Lesion size is usually quantified in this model 14 d after balloon injury although longer time points may sometimes be relevant.

1. Paraffin embed the harvested carotid and cut 5-μm serial histological sections.
2. Stain with hematoxylin and eosin and Verhoeff's-van Gieson.
3. Analyze by digital morphometry. Trace the luminal area, area within the internal elastic lamina, and area within the external elastic lamina, and calculate the intimal and medial areas by subtraction.

4. Notes

1. Work must be undertaken only in a designated establishment, and the room used for surgery must be designated appropriate to both the species of animals used and the procedure undertaken. All work undertaken in an experimental program must be covered by a project license approved by the home office (and usually held by a group leader or head of department). The individual investigator must have obtained a personal license, which details all techniques used. This will require a certificate of satisfactory completion of modules 1–4 of an Institute of Biology training course for the type of recovery surgery described in this chapter.

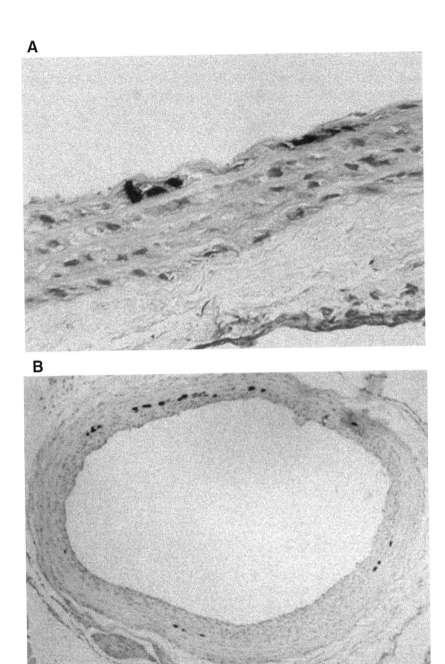

Fig. 4. Demonstration of gene transfer efficiency using β-galactosidase. The efficiency of marker gene transfer following virus infection is estimated by staining arteries with X-gal. The transgene is localized by the presence of a blue color. The arteries are embedded and sectioned and then viewed under a microscope. Gene transfer to smooth muscle cells of the arterial media (**A**) 2 d and (**B**) 14 d after balloon injury and gene delivery (magnification 20× and 40×, respectively).

In any institution the named Veterinary Surgeon will be able to advise on appropriate procedures that must be followed at all times.

2. Health and safety issues are governed by the genetically modified organisms (contained use) regulations 1992. Currently wild-type adenovirus, an ACDP (Advisory Committee on Dangerous Pathogens) hazard group 2 pathogen, must be handled at containment level 2 (as designated by the Advisory Committee on Genetic Modification). A virus that has been deleted in the E1A region and which cannot therefore replicate unless the mutation is complemented in *trans* is hazard group 1 with containment level 1. Risk assessments will need to be submitted to the Healh and Safety Executive (HSE) (UK) if the proposed vector is a group 2 pathogen or if it is the first use of a group 1 virus. Assessment of risk and assignment to group 1 or 2 must take account of the potential hazards of both the vector and the inserted sequences. The advice of the local Safety Committee should be sought.

3. Wistar or Sprague Dawley rats can be used. A single species, strain, and sex should be used for all groups in comparative studies and a single supplier of animals may also assist reproducibility. 300–350 g rats are commonly used in the authors' laboratory but others use 400 g animals; higher weights can make reliable anesthesia more difficult but do facilitate dissection.

4. The anesthetic regimen described provides a satisfactory level of anesthesia for 20–30 min and further doses may be given after that time with careful attention to avoid respiratory depression. Both agents are drawn up in the same 1-mL syringe for administration and immediately injected into the animal. Fresh syringes and needles must be used even if readministering these agents to the same animal because after initial mixing they rapidly form precipitates, and this is almost immediate in syringes previously contaminated with both agents. It may be complemented in longer procedures by inhalational anesthetics such as methoxyflurane, which can be administered with oxygen using an appropriate scavenging apparatus. An anesthetic chamber must be used to induce anesthesia with inhalational agents but a face mask can then be used for maintenance. Face cones/masks hamper the access to the rat neck for dissection and can compromise sterility during the initial dissection. They may be used to good effect during viral intraluminal dwell periods.

5. The side branch commonly present on the inferomedial aspect of the external carotid artery can also be occluded using diathermy, but this may cause spasm or damage to the external carotid artery preventing catheterization. Care should be taken in making the initial arteriotomy in the external carotid. If this is too large, the repeated cannulation required with this technique may cause the posterior arterial wall to tear and become detached from its distal portion. If this occurs and sufficient stump is present beyond the carotid bifurcation, a ligature may be tied around the remaining external carotid artery, and put under tension, and a more proximal arteriotomy made in the external carotid.

6. Inflation of embolectomy balloons in the rat aorta results in temporary and usually partial obstruction to left ventricular outflow. If the balloon is left inflated in this

position for a prolonged time, the animal will become hemodynamically compromised and may die. When pulling the embolectomy balloon into the carotid artery, deflation followed by reinflation within the common carotid prevents avulsion of the carotid origin from the aortic arch and also minimizes hemorrhage as the blood trapped distal to the balloon can be forced out of the external carotid arteriotomy.

7. The 20-min luminal dwell technique used has the disadvantage that it requires the administration of heparin. The use of heparin in clinical angioplasty, often given by both the intracoronary and intravenous routes, is standard, and other authors have incorporated use of a similar dose of heparin in this model *(21)*. Continuous infusion of heparin over 7–14 d is, however, known to reduce neointimal hyperplasia in the rat model *(4,49–52)*. Prevention of migration and proliferation of smooth muscle cells in the arterial wall is the likely mechanism of this change in lesion size *(4,52)*. The use of a single dose of heparin in this method is likely to have less effect on lesion size. Unpublished data from our own studies suggest a 30% reduction in intimal area or intimal medial ratio in animals receiving heparin and a delivery procedure (virus or control saline solutions) compared to those receiving balloon injury alone and no heparin. One group has demonstrated that dilution of adenoviral vectors in poloxamer 407 allowed reduction of luminal dwell times in the rat model from 20 min to 10 min *(25)*. This may remove the requirement for anticoagulation.

8. Immunohistochemical demonstration of β-galactosidase can also be used and appears to be a more sensitive test for presence of the transgene product *(53)*. It does not, however, demonstrate the successful production of functional protein by the transgene.

References

1. Powell, J. S., Clozel, J. P., Muller, R. K,. Kuhn, H., Hefti, F., Hosang, M., and Baumgartner, H. R. (1989) Inhibitors of angiotensin-converting enzyme prevent myointimal proliferation after vascular injury. *Science* **245**, 186–188.

2. (MERCATOR) Study Group. (1992) Does the new angiotensin converting enzyme inhibitor cilazapril prevent restenosis after percutaneous transluminal coronary angioplasty? Results of the MERCATOR study: a multicenter, randomized, double-blind placebo-controlled trial. Multicenter European Research Trial with Cilazapril after Angioplasty to Prevent Transluminal Coronary Obstruction and Restenosis. *Circulation* **86**, 100–110.

3. Clowes, A. W., Reidy, M. A., and Clowes, M. M. (1983) Kinetics of cellular proliferation after arterial injury. I. Smooth muscle growth in the absence of endothelium. *Lab. Invest.* **49**, 327–333.

4. Clowes, A. W. and Clowes, M. M. (1986) Kinetics of cellular proliferation after arterial injury. IV. Heparin inhibits rat smooth muscle mitogenesis and migration. *Circ. Res.* **58**, 839–845.

5. Clowes, A. W. and Schwartz, S. M. (1985) Significance of quiescent smooth muscle migration in the injured rat carotid artery. *Circ. Res.* **56**, 139–145.

6. Bett, A. J., Haddara, W., Prevec, L., and Graham, F. L. (1994) An efficient and flexible system for construction of adenovirus vectors with insertions or deletions in early regions 1 and 3. *Proc. Natl. Acad. Sci. USA* **91,** 8802–8806.

7. Lemarchand, P., Jones, M., Yamada, I., and Crystal, R. G. (1993) In vivo gene transfer and expression in normal uninjured blood vessels using replication-deficient recombinant adenovirus vectors. *Circ. Res.* **72,** 1132–1138.

8. Guzman, R. J., Lemarchand, P., Crystal, R. G., Epstein, S. E., and Finkel, T. (1993) Efficient and selective adenovirus-mediated gene transfer into vascular neointima. *Circulation* **88,** 2838–2848.

9. Feldman, L. J., Steg, P. G., Zheng, L. P., Chen, D., Kearney, M., McGarr, S. E., et al. (1995) Low-efficiency of percutaneous adenovirus-mediated arterial gene transfer in the atherosclerotic rabbit. *J. Clin. Invest.* **95,** 2662–2671.

10. Ali, M., Lemoine, N. R., and Ring, C. J. A. (1994) The use of DNA viruses as vectors for gene therapy. *Gene Ther.* **1,** 367–384.

11. Rhoads, J. L., Birx, D. L., Wright, D. C., Brundage, J. F., Brandt, B. L., Redfield, R. R., and Burke, D. S. (1991) Safety and immunogenicity of multiple conventional immunizations administered during early HIV infection. *J AIDS* **4,** 724–731.

12. Wilson, J. M. (1996) Adenoviruses as gene-delivery vehicles. *N. Engl. J. Med.* **334,** 1185–1187.

13. Kopfler, W. P., Willard, M., Betz, T., Willard, J. E., Gerard, R. D., and Meidell, R. S. (1994) Adenovirus-mediated transfer of a gene encoding human apolipoprotein A-I into normal mice increases circulating high-density lipoprotein cholesterol. *Circulation* **90,** 1319–1327.

14. Plautz, G., Nabel, E. G., and Nabel, G. J. (1991) Introduction of vascular smooth muscle cells expressing recombinant genes in vivo. *Circulation* **83,** 578–583.

15. March, K. L., Madison, J. E., and Trapnell, B C. (1995) Pharmacokinetics of adenoviral vector-mediated gene delivery to vascular smooth muscle cells: modulation by poloxamer 407 and implications for cardiovascular gene therapy. *Human Gene Ther.* **6,** 41-53.

16. Lee, S. W., Trapnell, B. C., Rade, J. J., Virmani, R., and Dichek, D. A. (1993) In vivo adenoviral vector-mediated gene transfer into balloon-injured rat carotid arteries. *Circ. Res.* **73,** 797–807.

17. Dichek, D. A., Neville, R. F., Zwiebel, J. A., Freeman, S. M., Leon, M. B., and Anderson, W. F. (1989) Seeding of intravascular stents with genetically engineered endothelial cells [see comments]. *Circulation* **80,** 1347–1353.

18. Newman, K. D., Dunn, P. F., Owens, J. W., Schulick, A. H., Virmani, R., Sukhova, G., et al. (1995) Adenovirus-mediated gene transfer into normal rabbit arteries results in prolonged vascular cell activation, inflammation, and neointimal hyperplasia. *J. Clin. Invest.* **96,** 2955–2965.

19. Li, J. J., Ueno, H., Tomita, H., Yamamoto, H., Kanegae, Y., Saito, I., and Takeshita, A. (1995) Adenovirus-mediated arterial gene transfer does not require prior injury for submaximal gene expression. *Gene Ther.* **2,** 351–354.

20. Schulick, A. H., Dong, G., Newman, K. D., Virmani, R., and Dichek, D. A. (1995) Endothelium-specific in vivo gene transfer. *Circ. Res.* **77,** 475–485.

21. Schulick, A. H., Newman, K. D., Virmani, R., and Dichek, D. A. (1995) In vivo gene transfer into injured carotid arteries. Optimization and evaluation of acute toxicity. *Circulation* **91,** 2407–2414.

22. French, B. A., Mazur, W., Ali, N. M., Geske, R. S., Finnigan, J. P., Rodgers, G. P., et al. (1994) Percutaneous transluminal in vivo gene transfer by recombinant adenovirus in normal porcine coronary arteries, atherosclerotic arteries, and two models of coronary restenosis. *Circulation* **90,** 2402–2413.

23. Willard, J. E., Landau, C., Glamann, D. B., Burns, D., Jessen, M. E., Pirwitz, M. J., et al. (1994) Genetic modification of the vessel wall. Comparison of surgical and catheter-based techniques for delivery of recombinant adenovirus. *Circulation* **89,** 2190–2197.

24. Flugelman, M. Y., Jaklitsch, M. T., Newman, K. D., Casscells, W., Bratthauer, G. L., and Dichek, D. A. (1992) Low level in vivo gene transfer into the arterial wall through a perforated balloon catheter [see comments]. *Circulation* **85,** 1110–1117.

25. Feldman, L. J., Pastore, C. J., Aubailly, N., Kearney, M., Chen, D., Perricaudet, M., et al. (1997) Improved efficiency of arterial gene transfer by use of poloxamer 407 as a vehicle for adenoviral vectors. *Gene Ther.* **4,** 189–198.

26. Tahlil, O., Brami, M., Feldman, L. J., Branellec, D., and Steg, P. G. (1997) The dispatch(tm) catheter as a delivery tool for arterial gene transfer. *Cardio. Res.* **33,** 181–187.

27. Laitinen, M., Pakkanen, T., Donetti, E., Baetta, R., Luoma, J., Lehtolainen, P., et al. (1997) Gene transfer into the carotid artery using an adventitial collar: comparison of the effectiveness of the plasmid-liposome complexes, retroviruses, pseudotyped retroviruses, and adenoviruses. *Human Gene Ther.* **8,** 1645–1650.

28. Ooboshi, H., Rios, C. D., Chu, Y., Christenson, S. D., Faraci, F. M., Davidson, B. L., and Heistad, D. D. (1997) Augmented adenovirus-mediated gene transfer to atherosclerotic vessels. *Arteriosclerosis Thrombosis Vasc. Biol.* **17,** 1786–1792.

29. Lim, C. S., Chapman, G. D., Gammon, R. S., Muhlestein, J. B., Bauman, R. P., Stack, R. S., and Swain, J. L. (1991) Direct in vivo gene transfer into the coronary and peripheral vasculatures of the intact dog. *Circulation* **83,** 2007–2011.

30. Chapman, G. D., Lim, C. S., Gammon, R. S., Culp, S. C., Desper, J. S., Bauman, R. P., et al. (1992) Gene transfer into coronary arteries of intact animals with a percutaneous balloon catheter. *Circ. Res.* **71,** 27–33.

31. Riessen, R., Rahimizadeh, H., Blessing, E., Takeshita, S., Barry, J. J., and Isner, J. M. (1993) Arterial gene-transfer using pure dna applied directly to a hydrogel-coated angioplasty balloon. *Human Gene Ther.* **4,** 749–758.

32. Takeshita, S., Gal, D., Leclerc, G., Pickering, J. G., Riessen, R., Weir, L., and Isner, J. M. (1994) Increased gene expression after liposome-mediated arterial gene transfer associated with intimal smooth muscle cell proliferation. In vitro and in vivo findings in a rabbit model of vascular injury. *J. Clin. Invest.* **93,** 652–661.

33. Kafri, T., Blomer, U., Peterson, D. A., Gage, F. H., and Verma, I. M. (1997) Sustained expression of genes delivered directly into liver and muscle by lentiviral vectors. *Nat. Genet.* **17,** 314–317.

34. Trouet, D., Nilius, B., Voets, T., Droogmans, G., and Eggermont, J. (1997) Use of a bicistronic gfp-expression vector to characterise ion channels after transfection in mammalian cells. *Pflugers Archiv.-Eur. J. Physiol.* **434,** 632–638.

35. Simari, R. D., San, H., Rekhter, M., Ohno, T., Gordon, D., Nabel, G. J., and Nabel, E. G. (1996) Regulation of cellular proliferation and intimal formation following balloon injury in atherosclerotic rabbit arteries. *J. Clin. Invest.* **98,** 225–235.

36. Guzman, R. J., Hirschowitz, E. A., Brody, S. L., Crystal, R. G., Epstein, S. E., and Finkel, T. (1994) In vivo suppression of injury-induced vascular smooth muscle cell accumulation using adenovirus-mediated transfer of the herpes simplex virus thymidine kinase gene. *Proc. Natl.Acad. Sci. USA* **91,** 10,732–10,736.

37. Chang, M. W., Barr, E., Seltzer, J., Jiang, Y. Q., Nabel, G. J., Nabel, E. G., et al. (1995) Cytostatic gene therapy for vascular proliferative disorders with a constitutively active form of the retinoblastoma gene product. *Science* **267,** 518–522.

38. Chang, M. W., Barr, E., Lu, M. M., Barton, K., and Leiden, J. M. (1995) Adenovirus-mediated over-expression of the cyclin/cyclin-dependent kinase inhibitor, p21 inhibits vascular smooth muscle cell proliferation and neointima formation in the rat carotid artery model of balloon angioplasty. *J. Clin. Invest.* **96,** 2260–2268.

39. Yang, Z. Y., Simari, R. D., Perkins, N. D., San, H,. Gordon, D., Nabel, G. J., and Nabel, E. G. (1996) Role of the p21 cyclin-dependent kinase inhibitor in limiting intimal cell proliferation in response to arterial injury. *Proc. Natl. Acad. Sci. USA* **93,** 7905–7910.

40. Smith, R. C., Branellec, D., Gorski, D. H., Guo, K., Perlman, H., Dedieu, J. F., et al. (1997) P21(cip1)-mediated inhibition of cell proliferation by overexpression of the gax homeodomain gene. *Genes Dev.* **11,** 1674–1689.

41. Ueno, H., Yamamoto, H., Ito, S. I., Li, J. J., and Takeshita, A. (1997) Adenovirus-mediated transfer of a dominant-negative H-ras suppresses neointimal formation in balloon-injured arteries in vivo. *Arteriosclerosis Thrombosis Vas. Biol.* **17,** 898–904.

42. Rade, J. J., Schulick, A. H., Virmani, R., and Dichek, D. A. (1996) Local adenoviral-mediated expression of recombinant hirudin reduces neointima formation after arterial injury. *Nat. Med.* **2,** 293–298.

43. Zoldhelyi, P., McNatt, J., Xu, X. M., Loose, Mitchell, D., Meidell, R. S., Cet al. (1996) Prevention of arterial thrombosis by adenovirus-mediated transfer of cyclooxygenase gene. *Circulation* **93,** 10–17.

44. Asahara, T., Chen, D. H., Tsurumi, Y., Kearney, M., Rossow, S., Passeri, J., Symes, J. F., and Isner, J. M. (1996) Accelerated restitution of endothelial integrity and endothelium-dependent function after phvegf(165) gene transfer. *Circulation* **94,** 3291–3302.

45. von der Leyden, H. E., Gibbons, G. H., Morishita, R., Lewis, N. P., Zhang, L., Nakajima, M., et al. (1995) Gene therapy inhibiting neointimal vascular lesion: in vivo transfer of endothelial cell nitric oxide synthase gene. *Proc. Natl. Acad. Sci. USA* **92,** 1137–1141.

46. Dollery, C. M., Mcclelland, A., Latchman, D. S., Henney, A. M., Humphries, S. E., and McEwan, J. R. (1997) Adenoviral gene transfer of human timp-1 inhibits

smooth muscle cell migration and neointima formation in injured rat carotid arteries. *Circulation* **96**, 2693.

47. Baek, S. and March, K. L. (1998) Gene therapy for restenosis - getting nearer the heart of the matter. *Circ. Res.* **82**, 295–305.

48. Waynforth, B. D. and Flecknell, P. A. (eds) (1992) *Experimental and Surgical Techniques in the Rat.* London, Academic Press.

49. Au, Y. P., Kenagy, R. D., Clowes, M. M., and Clowes, A. W. (1993) Mechanisms of inhibition by heparin of vascular smooth muscle cell proliferation and migration. *Haemostasis* **23 Suppl 1**, 177–182.

50. Clowes, A. W., Clowes, M. M., Kirkman, T. R., Jackson, C. L., Au, Y. P., and Kenagy, R. (1992) Heparin inhibits the expression of tissue-type plasminogen activator by smooth muscle cells in injured rat carotid artery. *Circ. Res.* **70**, 1128–1136.

51. Clowes, A. W., Clowes, M. M., Vergel, S., Muller, R. K., Powell, J. S., Hefti, F., and Baumgartner, H. R. (1991) Heparin and cilazapril together inhibit injury-induced intimal hyperplasia. *Hypertension* **18**, 1165–1169.

52. Clowes, A. W. and Clowes, M. M. (1985) Kinetics of cellular proliferation after arterial injury. II. Inhibition of smooth muscle growth by heparin. *Lab. Invest.* **52**, 611–616.

53. Couffinhal, T., Kearney, M., Sullivan, A., Silver, M., Tsurumi, Y., and Isner, J. M. (1997) Histochemical staining following Lac Z gene transfer underestimates transfection efficiency. *Human Gene Ther.* **8**, 929–934.

Index